PSYCHIATRIC NURSING

NURSES' AIDS SERIES

Anatomy and Physiology for Nurses
Cardiac Nursing
Gastroenterological Nursing
Geriatric Nursing
Mathematics in Nursing
Medical Nursing
Microbiology for Nurses
Multiple Choice Questions, Book 1
Multiple Choice Questions, Book 2
Multiple Choice Questions, Book 3
Multiple Choice Questions, Book 4
Obstetric and Gynaecological Nursing
Ophthalmic Nursing
Paediatric Nursing
Personal and Community Health
Pharmacology for Nurses
Practical Nursing
Practical Procedures for Nurses
Psychiatric Nursing
Psychology for Nurses
Sociology for Nurses
Surgical Nursing
Theatre Technique

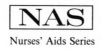

Nurses' Aids Series

PSYCHIATRIC NURSING

Sixth Edition

Annie Altschul
CBE, BA(Lond), MSc(Edin), SRN, RMN, RNT, FRCN
Emeritus Professor of Nursing Studies
University of Edinburgh

Margaret McGovern
BA(Lond), MSc(Edin), RGN, RMN, RCI, DipHV, RNT
Psychiatric Nurse Tutor,
Lothian College of Nursing
and Midwifery, Edinburgh,
and Examiner for the Scottish National Board

Baillière Tindall
London Philadelphia Toronto Sydney Tokyo

Baillière Tindall   24–28 Oval Road,
W. B. Saunders   London NW1 7DX

                         The Curtis Center
                         Independence Square West,
                         Philadelphia, PA 19106–3399, USA

                         55 Horner Avenue
                         Toronto, Ontario M8Z 4X6, Canada

                         Harcourt Brace Jovanovich Group (Australia) Pty Ltd,
                         30–52 Smidmore Street, Marrickville,
                         NSW 2204, Australia

                         Harcourt Brace Jovanovich Japan Inc.
                         Ichibancho Central Building, 22–1 Ichibancho
                         Chiyoda-ku, Tokyo 102, Japan

First published 1957
Sixth edition 1985
German translation, third edition, 1972 (Urban & Schwarzenberg,
Munich)
Spanish translation, fifth edition, 1977 (CECSA, Mexico)
Portuguese translation, fifth edition, 1977 (Publicações Europa-América,
Mem-Martins, Sintra)
Dutch translation, fifth edition, 1979 (Stafleu, Alphen)
Fifth ELBS edition 1979

Reprinted 1988, 1989 and 1991

Typeset by Scribe Design, Gillingham, Kent
Printed in England by Clays Ltd, St Ives plc

British Library Cataloguing in Publication Data

Altschul, A.
   Psychiatric nursing.—6th ed.—
   (Nurses' aids series)
   1. Psychiatric nursing
   I. Title   II. McGovern, Margaret   III. Series
   610.73′68   RC440
ISBN 0 7020 1060 X

Contents

Preface   vii

Part 1   General Introduction   **1**
1   Mental Health and Mental Illness   3
2   Classification and Description of Some Psychiatric
Disorders   10
3   The Psychiatrically Ill and Society   38
4   Nursing the Patient in the Community   46

Part 2   Nursing the Psychiatric Patient   **53**
5   The Therapeutic Environment   55
6   The Significance of Routine   66
7   The Nursing Process   70
8   Basic Activities of Everyday Living   87
9   The Significance of Food   94
10   The Significance of Sleep   103
11   The Long-stay Patient   109
12   Nursing Disturbed Children and Adolescents   115
13   The Mentally Ill Elderly Patient   135
14   Nursing Patients Who Feel Depressed   158
15   Care of Disturbed and Violent Patients   171
16   Nursing Epileptic Patients   182
17   The Patient Who is Dependent on Alcohol
or Drugs   197

Part 3   Special Forms of Treatment   **209**
Introduction to Part 3   211

vi   Contents

18	Drug Therapy	214
19	Electroconvulsive Therapy	235
20	Work, Recreational and Diversional Therapy	247
21	Psychotherapy	258
22	Behaviour Therapy	273
23	Nurse–Patient Relationships	284
24	Nurse–Patient Interactions	292
25	Social Therapy; The Therapeutic Community	304
	Appendix: Notes on the Mental Health Act 1983 and The Mental Health (Scotland) Act 1984	317
	Glossary	326
	Index	339

Preface

Just as preparation for the sixth edition was under way, Ruth Simpson died very suddenly. Her death results in a tremendous loss to psychiatric nursing in the United Kingdom. For me it has not only created a deep sense of personal grief but also a large void where once Ruth Simpson supplied ideas, stimulation and knowledge. For the publishers it has resulted in a long delay in the publication of the sixth edition. Fortunately Margaret McGovern has accepted the invitation to co-operate with me and has helped to re-examine critically every part of the book, which has now been on the market for nearly thirty years.

Many changes have occurred in these years, and even in the last eight years since the publication of the fifth edition, but these changes seem to concern the type of patient who seeks treatment, the form of treatment which is given and the location where it takes place more than the fundamental principles of nursing care, which were the substance of the book from the beginning. Physical treatments including certain drugs have come and gone, and psychotherapy, never very strong in the British psychiatric hospital setting, has lost further ground as patients' length of stay has become shorter. The concepts which generated the development of social treatment in hospital have found really fertile soil in the care of patients in their own community.

While it is acknowledged that the emphasis in psychiatric nursing has moved from the hospital to the patient's own home, the training of nurses for the Register of Mental Nurses still takes place predominantly in hospital. No satisfactory schemes have yet been designed to change this, even though many people would like to see change. Training of Community Psychiatric Nurses takes place at present in post-basic courses.

This book is written for students who are training for the Register, and for that reason the earlier format has been retained and the bulk of the book deals with care of patients in psychiatric hospitals.

It is hoped that students who read this book will become aware of the desirability to treat patients within their own community, whenever possible, and that they will become aware of the limitations imposed by hospital training on the role nurses fulfil in the community.

Because, within the hospital, the population of elderly patients with organic mental disorder has increased in recent years, the chapter dealing with the care of these patients has been considerably extended.

Of the forms of physical treatment, only electroconvulsive therapy and drug therapy are dealt with in this edition and the discussion of these forms of treatment has been extended.

There is now much talk of the 'nursing process'. Readers of earlier editions will be aware that the importance of assessment, planning and recording the care given has been stressed throughout. In this edition a chapter entitled 'The Nursing Process' has taken the place of the chapter on 'Observation and Reports'. The principles underlying the nursing process and the issues which need to be considered specifically in the care of psychiatric patients are made more explicit.

Many chapters have undergone extensive revision and some change in the sequence of the text has been made. The classification of mental disorders and the description of the manifestation of some of these are presented in greater detail.

The publisher's policy in the past was to give suggestions for further reading rather than document the text with references. We hope in the next edition to adopt the new policy of giving references in the text, but it was not possible to accomplish this for the present edition. The bibliography for all chapters has been brought up to date.

New Mental Health Acts passed in 1983 and 1984 have meant that the appendix dealing with legislation had to be completely revised. I should like to acknowledge the contribution of Sheamus Killen to the revised comments on the Act which pertains to England and Wales.

New readers are advised to read this book straight through to obtain an overview of the nature of mental disorder, of the problems which patients encounter and of the different ways in which nurses and others can assist the patients to cope. No one chapter is designed to be studied in isolation from the rest of the text. A certain amount of overlap, repetition and cross-referencing is intentional.

It is hoped that subsequently the use of the index will help readers to find the specific information they wish to return to and the particular topic they wish to study in depth. Students may find that they need to consult other textbooks for further study. They will find these more comprehensive textbooks easier to understand when they have used this book as an introduction.

I should like to acknowledge the help and inspiration which countless people have given me over the years and whose specific contribution to this book cannot be acknowledged. In particular I should like to thank all the students whose intelligent interest, perceptive comments and fervent enthusiasm have been responsible for sustaining my motivation to revise the book.

Annie Altschul

Part 1
General Introduction

1
Mental Health and Mental Illness

Psychiatric nursing is concerned with the promotion of mental health, the prevention of mental disorder and the nursing care of patients who suffer from mental disorder. Psychiatric nurses should know something about the disorders they are helping to prevent and cure, and about mental health which they are trying to restore.

Most textbooks of medicine and nursing begin with a description of the normal and proceed later to describe the abnormal conditions which arise in sickness. Originally, however, knowledge of what is normal and healthy in body and mind was nearly always gained by studying what was abnormal and diseased. Knowledge of the normal functioning of endocrine glands, for example, was discovered as a result of studying abnormalities associated with over- or under-production of hormones. Normal functioning of the brain becomes clearer as more and more is known about patients suffering from brain lesions.

Mental health, too, which has been defined by the World Health Organization, as 'the full and harmonious functioning of the whole personality', can best be studied by reference to mental disorder. If the nurse is seeking to promote the mental health of her patients, she needs to know what to regard as healthy and what signs to interpret as evidence of disease. As she becomes acquainted with abnormal behaviour she will develop a clear idea of the standards by which she can judge the behaviour of these patients, and of what to regard as normal.

THE DEFINITION OF NORMALITY

What is meant by normality? What does normal life entail?

It is often said that we are all 'a bit abnormal'. Is this true or is it obvious nonsense? Is it any easier if the word 'normal' is replaced by 'healthy', or is it normal to be a little unhealthy?

The difficulty which arises in answering these questions lies in the fact that the word 'normal' is used in more than one sense. It is sometimes employed for 'average' or 'most usual'. By 'normal height' is usually meant 'within certain limits around the average'. But the word 'normal' is not used in this sense when health is being discussed. For instance, it may be found that by a certain age most people have lost their teeth and are wearing dentures, but it is not therefore 'normal' to wear dentures by the age of, say, fifty.

It is often preferred to consider 'normal' as being 'ideal' or 'best possible'. An individual would be called 'normal' in respect of physical health if his organs were functioning in the ideal manner, and 'ill-health' or 'abnormality' are the terms that would be used if there were any serious deviation from the optimal function.

Any particular characteristic or clinical symptom may thus be abnormal when judged by absolute standards, but normal when judged by population standards, or vice versa. Outstandingly high intelligence, for example, may approach normality in the sense of 'optimal', but it represents considerable deviation from the 'norm' by population standards.

Deviation from the population norm is not always morbid, as the example of exceptionally high intelligence shows. In old age it may be that a person formerly of outstandingly high intelligence declines to a level approaching the norm for the population as a whole. He then suffers from a disorder characterized by deviation of intelligence from his personal norm.

How about mental health? Here it is difficult to define the ideal without reference to society. It could be said that a person is healthy if he manages to deal with the demands made upon him by society in a manner which is ideal both for society and for himself. He is ill to the degree that he has failed in his adjustment, to the detriment either of society or of himself. This definition is, however, not entirely satisfactory. There are those who regard society as sick, perceiving those who deviate from the norms of society as healthy. To equate mental health with adjustment to society also gives rise to the impression that psychiatrists and psychiatric nurses are committed to maintaining the status quo and preventing social change.

THE NORMAL ADULT

What is involved in the life of a normal adult must now be considered. First, it means the normal care of his body. An adult person attends to his personal hygiene in such a manner that he does not come into conflict with society. He washes regularly, attends to his hair, teeth and nails. He is clothed in a manner which conforms to the standards of the society in which he lives. His clothes are reasonably clean, in a reasonable state of repair. They are frequently changed and laundered. The fashions he wears approximate to the accepted styles. He does not walk in the nude, unless in private or in the presence of people who, he knows, do not object. He wears one style of clothes for funerals, another for weddings, and yet others for town or country.

It does not occur to the normal person that there is anything very difficult about this. He does not reflect how much learning was required for the simple achievement of washing and dressing appropriately. Yet there was a time in everybody's life when these actions were not habits. Every child learns by a slow and careful process to wash, and to do so without being reminded. Many people reach adolescence before they are encouraged to decide for themselves what clothes to wear and when to change them. They almost certainly reach adolescence before they buy their own clothes.

Personal hygiene involves skills not only in clothing and washing, but also in elimination. Western society demands that this should be done in private, and convention lays down the right place and time. Conversation about the subject is determined by convention and some people may be offended by a too open discussion of bodily functions in words other than those approved by society. This too has been learned during a long, painful apprenticeship, starting in infancy and completed some time during school years. Failure to maintain normal adult standards of personal hygiene is one of the characteristics of some mentally disordered persons.

Normal adults usually take a normal, healthy diet. They do so in spite of certain difficulties they may encounter. They consider meals as being social occasions, pleasurable because of the relief of hunger and the enjoyment of both food and company. They eat regularly, with moderation, and observe a vast number of rules or social conventions. Any mother knows how much effort on her part has gone into the education of her children in this respect. She is justifiably proud when one of her offspring has gone through a whole meal in the presence of visitors without disgracing her. It would be unreasonable to expect a small child to use a knife and fork, to eat tidily, or to refrain from putting his fingers into his mouth. It is often unreasonable to expect it from mentally ill patients.

THE ACTIVITIES OF NORMAL LIFE

Normal life, amongst other things, involves, broadly speaking, the following activities:
1   Adaptation to the work situation
2   Leisure-time activities
3   Management of social contacts
4   Adjustment to the opposite sex

Each of these headings includes a variety of highly complex activities.

Work

Working, for instance, consists partly of choosing the right kind of job, one which is within reach of the individual's ability, yet making some demands on him. It involves doing the job well and persevering in the face of difficulties. It involves attending the place of work at regular hours, in spite of possible disinclination to do so. At work, other people are encountered—those in authority, colleagues and subordinates. All kinds of complex skills are required in order to adapt to these in all situations.

Work represents the contribution which each person makes to the well-being of society as a whole. Many people find enjoyment in work which is interesting and well done, but many find discipline irksome. For the sake of the community as a whole, work must be carried out at a specified time, and some jobs must be undertaken though they may be intrinsically unattractive. For some people, problems related to work present the main difficulty.

Leisure

Many people use their leisure time for the pursuits they most enjoy and which make their life richer and more worthwhile. Leisure is often all too short for the variety of interests people may wish to pursue: art, music, drama, gardening or sports—to name but a few of the many possible and desirable leisure-time activities which may be carried on alone or in company with others. These are often felt to give real purpose to life when work fails to do so. In mental illness failure to find satisfaction in leisure activities is very common.

Social contacts

Making social contacts can be fraught with complications, a fact which becomes plain when consideration is given to the variety of possible relationships and the multitude of adaptations required. Thus, individuals behave in different ways towards their best friends, their neighbours, their clients, their green-grocers. It is difficult to learn the right kind of approach to each, and all embody many possibilities of failure.

Normal adults are continually making new social contacts and discarding others, but there are some friends who remain constant. Real friendship is a mutual relationship. It is easy to see why some patients appear friendless and lonely, and easy therefore to discern some of the ways in which they may be helped to take up their place in society again.

Sexual adjustment

Normal adults have learned to adjust to the opposite sex. Normal sexual development is fundamental to mental health. Love, companionship and sexual relationships in adult life depend on the social influences which are brought to bear on the sexual development of the child. Many people find sexual adjustment the most difficult task to master.

A brief reminder of what normal life entails should make it easier to understand 'mental illness' and to see clearly the task of the psychiatric nurse. Mental illness can be regarded as a failure to make a satisfactory adaptation to the demands of society.

THE PSYCHIATRIC HISTORY

By taking a detailed history the psychiatrist may be able to find out why a patient has failed to react in a normal manner. Heredity, early childhood influences, education, dramatic childhood experiences, e.g. loss of a parent, may all have contributed to the patient's difficulty. Recent stresses (so-called life events) may have caused him to break down at this particular time of his life. His previous personality structure may affect the particular areas of difficulty which he encounters in his adaptation to society.

What are called the symptoms of the disorder may be manifestations of faulty adaptation. Some patients have difficulties in managing the care of their bodies and maintenance of physical health. They require help with dressing, washing, eating and elimination. Others have difficulties in adapting to working conditions, or in finding interest in any leisure activity whatever. Some fail to make friends, and these find social intercourse a burden rather than a source of satisfaction. To many patients sexual adjustment is the greatest source of worry and anxiety. Whatever the patient's difficulties, they can be thought of as resulting at least partly from excessive demands made by the environment.

Psychiatric treatment involves, in the first instance, an understanding of the patient's problems; secondly, modifying the environmental demands so that the patient can successfully meet them. Often it is possible to do so without admission to hospital. When hospitalization has become necessary the nurse helps to create in the hospital ward a normal, flexible routine, adjusted to the patient's needs. Gradually he is helped to learn how to deal successfully with increasingly difficult situations. He is constantly encouraged to tackle more complex problems under the watchful eye of those who are ready to offer a helping hand should it be required. If he encounters failure, he is protected from its consequences and encouraged to try again.

Having achieved success in adaptation to hospital life, the patient is helped to meet the requirements of the world at large and to lead a full and satisfying existence.

Effective treatment not only consists of helping the patient, but concerns itself with the patient's family and with his total environment.

Further reading

Altschul, A.T. & Sinclair, H. (1984) *Psychology for Nurses*. London: Baillière Tindall.

Brown, G.W. & Harris, T. (1978) *Social Origins of Depression: a Study of Psychiatric Disorder in Women*. London: Tavistock.

Health Advisory Service (1982) *The Rising Tide: Developing Services for Mental Illness in Old Age*. Surrey: NHS Health Advisory Service.

2
Classification and Description of Some Psychiatric Disorders

The issue of classification of psychiatric disorders has bedevilled psychiatry for many years. It was during the period after the Second World War—a growth period for psychiatry—that it became evident that there was a need for a more internationally recognized classification of psychiatric disorders if studies on epidemiology, statistics and other aspects were to have any real value. The World Health Organization's International Classification of Diseases (now in its ninth revision) emerged and became the basis for a uniform classification. It is used worldwide as a tool of communication and is mandatory for psychiatrists' use; it is also extremely complex and comprehensive.

Individual countries, however, tend to have their own system of classification. The American Psychiatric Association, for example, dissatisfied with the International Classification, uses the Diagnostic and Statistical Manual (DSM III, third edition). Within the United Kingdom a range of different classifications is in use.

An outline of one possible, though not ideal, system of classification is given in this chapter, together with a brief description of some of the features of the disorders classified. A textbook of psychiatry should be consulted for details of various psychiatric disorders.

Psychiatric disorders may be classified initially into two very broad groupings. The distinction is made between those disorders in which the aetiology is known, for example the *organic* psychiatric disorders, having a demonstrable underlying physical cause (however obscure), and those disorders described as *functional*, whose aetiology is not yet proved and therefore cannot be primarily attributed to a physical cause.

10

ORGANIC PSYCHIATRIC DISORDERS

Acute organic psychiatric disorders

Synonyms: acute (toxic) confusional states, delirious states, acute organic reactions or psychoses or states, symptomatic or exogenous psychoses.

Physical causes of acute organic psychiatric disorders are numerous and some of these include infections, particularly chest and urinary infections in the elderly person; vascular disorders, for example cerebrovascular accidents; drug intoxication, either directly or by sudden withdrawal; anoxia, as associated with congestive cardiac failure; electrolyte imbalance, from self-induced vomiting and purging in anorexia nervosa, and hypo- and hyperglycaemia. Hypothermia in the elderly may cause delirium.

Once the underlying cause of the acute organic disorder has been found and treated, complete recovery can be expected in the majority of patients.

The most prominent symptoms are clouding of consciousness, disorientation for time and place, and disturbance of memory for recent events. The patient is unable to understand what is happening around him. His attention wanders; he misidentifies people and often fails to recognize familiar objects. His actions may appear strange because he may carry out correct movements but in the wrong circumstances, for example he may try to write with a cigarette, or eat soap, because he is unable to identify the objects he is using. He may have hallucinatory experiences. He may see terrifying visions, or behave as if he were responding to voices. In some conditions, especially in acute drug intoxication, he feels small animals crawling over his skin or describes minute moving visual hallucinatory experiences. Following some infections, the cardinal symptoms are tiredness, irritability and depression. Whenever the picture is one of acute confusional state it is important, by means of careful examination, to establish a diagnosis of the physical disorder and institute appropriate treatment (see also Chapter 13).

Chronic organic psychiatric disorders

Synonyms: chronic brain failure, chronic organic reactions, dementia, organic intellectual impairment.

A chronic organic psychiatric disorder tends to follow a prolonged and progressively downhill course, and is usually, though not invariably, irreversible. Necropsy findings of patients who had been diagnosed as having had senile dementia show evidence of brain shrinkage and of decreased cerebral weight. The sulci are widened and there is considerable dilatation of the ventricles.

Intellect, memory and personality of patients suffering from chronic organic psychiatric disorders become impaired without any disturbance in level of consciousness. It has been said of the patient with dementia that he lives in this world but he does so deficiently. At first the person affected may be aware of his deteriorating intellectual abilities, but eventually there is complete lack of insight until he finally ends up in a vacuous and semi-dreamlike world.

One of the most common types of chronic organic psychiatric disorder is senile dementia, also referred to as senile dementia of the Alzheimer type (SDAT) because post-mortem changes in senile dementia are virtually identical with those occurring in Alzheimer's disease (a form of presenile dementia). The cause is as yet unknown, though, according to some researchers in this field, findings suggestive of brain-enzyme abnormalities have yielded some encouraging results. One in five persons over 80 years of age is affected. Women are more likely to develop this disorder than men.

The term presenile dementia is used for dementias occurring before the arbitrary age of 65 years. Included in this category are Alzheimer's, Creutzfeldt–Jakob's and Pick's diseases and Huntington's chorea. The last-mentioned condition is hereditary, transmitted by a single dominant gene; modern techniques of molecular biology now make it possible to predict, in a proportion of cases, which individuals at risk are destined to develop the disease.

There are a variety of other chronic organic psychiatric disorders which may occur irrespective of age and which are due to specific, and sometimes treatable, causes. These include the following.

Dementia resulting from cerebrovascular disease

Post-mortem examination of the brain of hypertensive patients may reveal the widespread presence of small sac-like swellings of the walls of the arterioles which have often led to local bleeding and corresponding multiple small areas of brain infarction (multi-infarct dementia). Though these findings are commonly held to have been the basis of dementia during the lifetime of the patient, it remains nonetheless true in practice that the great majority of patients whose organic intellectual impairment is a result of cerebrovascular disease have suffered a major stroke with paralysis and often speech impairment, the pathological basis of which is atheroma of the cerebral arteries (cerebral atherosclerosis) and consequent sizeable infarction of brain tissue.

Vitamin deficiency

When associated with chronic alcoholism and due to thiamine (Vitamin B_1) deficiency, this vitamin deficit brings about damage to small localized areas of the midbrain. One dramatic clinical feature is failure of recent memory. The patient's memory up to the onset of dementia is reasonably good, but he may be unable to recall information, for example an address given within the last 5 minutes.

Cerebral anoxia

Possible causes include cardiac arrest and carbon monoxide poisoning.

Laceration of brain substance

This occurs as post-traumatic dementia after head injury.

Space-occupying lesions

These may be divided into: (a) subdural haematoma, which may be overlooked, especially in the elderly person liable to frequent falls whose blood vessels are more fragile and easily ruptured; (b) cerebral abscess, and (c) cerebral tumours.

Dementia may briefly be described as a failing of intellectual ability. The patient's performance in intelligence tests deteriorates, although his vocabulary initially remains good. He becomes unable to use symbols in thinking. Abstract thought becomes difficult, but the patient retains the ability to solve concrete problems, for example he may be unable to perform an addition using figures, but is able to do it if he has beads. He may be unable to say how he would share a sum of money among several people, but can actually do it correctly if given the money. He may be unable to experience emotional bonds with people not actually present. He may show tenderness to his wife when she is beside him, but appear to be unconcerned about her in her absence.

The patient becomes increasingly unable to vary his responses. He can see only one way of doing things and cannot modify his reactions. In psychological tests this is shown by the way in which he classifies objects, for example if he is given differently shaped objects of different colours, he may classify either according to colour or to shape. Once he has done this he finds it impossible to change the classification. Such disability in daily life might tend to make the patient irritable and apparently stubborn. His mood varies rapidly—tears and laughter are easily aroused. His understanding of other people's actions and particularly of other people's feelings declines, therefore he may appear self-centred and uninhibited. His relations may notice a decline in moral standards. Progressive dementia ultimately leads to complete helplessness and dependence (see also Chapter 13).

FUNCTIONAL PSYCHIATRIC DISORDERS

It is convenient to subdivide the functional psychiatric disorders into two broad categories:
1   The functional neuroses (psychoneuroses)
2   The functional psychoses

The functional neuroses

The neuroses, or neurotic reactions (reactions to stress), are those disorders in which anxiety is a predominant feature.

The patient's emotional experiences and behaviour are quantitatively rather than qualitatively different from normal. It is normal to feel anxious, for example before sitting an examination, but this anxiety is not normally excessive and subsides as the situation progresses. In the neuroses the patient's anxiety is multiplied thousandfold in a variety of situations, and may become so severe that it interferes with his daily life. It is unusual, however, for neurotic disorders to become so severe that continuation of life in the community becomes impossible. Many neurotic patients benefit more from treatment as out-patients and from the community psychiatric nurse's support than from in-patient care.

Neurotic disorder, however, may occur in a crippling form so that normal life becomes impossible. Neurosis should not, as so often happens, be lightly dismissed as a comparatively trivial form of mental illness.

Only the most severely disturbed neurotic patients, those who are unable to be cared for in the community, are likely to be accepted into a psychiatric hospital. There are, however, increasing numbers of day units for treatment of neurotic disorders where group psychotherapeutic and environmental influences are brought to bear on the patient.

In neurotic disorders constitutional factors appear to be partly responsible for rendering the patient particularly vulnerable to stress. It is usually possible, however, to demonstrate also that the illness is in some way related to traumatic experiences and to the parental attitude towards the patient in early childhood.

Psychodynamic interpretation relates the patient's symptoms, for example anxiety, to unconscious conflicts. Symptoms may solve difficulties, for example they may help the patient to avoid a difficult situation, but this does not help to deal with the problems which at an unconscious level caused the conflict to arise.

Anxiety states

This is a most distressing condition in which the patient experiences an intense feeling of 'anxiety' and presents in exaggerated form all the physical symptoms which normally accompany any feeling of fear or apprehension in preparation for action.

The patient complains of feeling worried and afraid, but does not know of what. He anticipates the worst, feels that some action is required, but does not know what such action should be. At times his feelings amount to 'panic attacks'. He is restless, his muscle tone is increased, sometimes tremors are present. His pulse is rapid and his systolic blood pressure raised. His mouth is dry, the palms of his hands often perspire, and beads of perspiration may appear on his forehead. He complains of headache, nausea and often also of frequency of micturition.

The patient's anxiety is not related to any adequate conscious cause, but often he becomes aware of the physiological changes which have taken place, and believes himself to be physically ill. He interprets his palpitations as evidence of heart disorder or his nausea as evidence of carcinoma of the stomach. He may then explain to himself and others that his anxiety is caused by his physical illness.

Anxiety results in increased output of energy. As the patient's fear of physical disease increases, his nausea, and possibly also diarrhoea, lead to a diminished intake of food and consequently his physical condition often suffers. He may lose weight and become seriously undernourished. Sleep is usually disturbed; he may have difficulty in going off to sleep or may wake repeatedly during the night. The patient may be intensely irritable and easily disturbed by noise. He may be acutely aware of his abnormal state of mind and be afraid of losing grip and of becoming insane.

The treatment depends on the existing circumstances and how far these can be modified, and on the extent to which the cause is rooted in the past. It is necessary to consider how far the patient's earlier childhood experiences have contributed to the development of his attitude, and how far back it is necessary to retrace steps in order to help him proceed along healthier lines.

A defence mechanism frequently used to disguise the cause of anxiety is rationalization: the development of an apparently reasonable and acceptable justification for an action or feeling. The nature of anxiety symptoms makes it easy for the patient to explain them on the basis of organic illness rather than emotional conflict, and the tenacity with which the patient persists in a well-established rationalization, despite reassurance, indicates the importance of concealing the conflict.

The patient's physical condition must be considered first of all. A few physical disorders, for example hyperthyroidism, may mimic an anxiety state and must first be excluded. Only after a very thorough physical examination can a patient be effectively persuaded that he is physically healthy. To some patients this is reassuring; others find it difficult to accept the fact that the symptoms could have psychogenic causes. Some explanation of the physiology of stress may then be helpful.

The short-term use of an anxiolytic drug and the practice of relaxation techniques may be helpful in producing relaxation, while psychotherapy may help the patient to a better understanding of his problems.

Nurses can contribute to the patient's recovery by remaining calm and emotionally unaffected by the patient's anxiety. They may be able to communicate to him a feeling of security, which is often lacking in his home background. Active listening may have the effect of helping such a patient to see his own problems in better perspective by the verbalizing of his fears and anxieties. The mere presence of a calm person whom he knows well may have a soothing effect on him.

Conversion reactions

Although rationalization of anxiety represents an effort to conceal its true source, it does not eliminate the patient's discomfort. Some patients can eliminate or at least reduce anxiety by the use of a defence mechanism called conversion which produces the neurotic picture of a conversion reaction. This mechanism is always unconscious but sometimes the purpose served is obvious to all but the patient, so that the impression may be given that he is malingering.

Conversion produces an apparently physical impairment of a part of the body which would normally be under the control of the will. The particular part or parts involved will depend on the patient's knowledge of physical disorder, but also on the particular stress from which he needs to escape. The anatomical placing of this reaction makes it impossible for the patient to act out the unconscious drive which causes anxiety, so that a hand which might strike is paralysed and an eye which might see too much is blinded.

Motor symptoms include paralysis of the limbs, twitchings, tics, fits and aphonia. Sensory symptoms include numbness, anaesthesia, pains, blindness or deafness. Careful neurological examination reveals discrepancies between the distribution of the symptoms and that which would occur if there were an organic basis. The symptoms complained of correspond rather to the patient's own idea of anatomical structure. Such symptoms are referred to as 'hysterical conversion symptoms'.

Although the symptoms may be exceedingly incapacitating and his description of them is often highly dramatic, the patient appears fairly complacent about his illness. This is possible because the symptom in fact represents the way in which he has solved an otherwise insoluble problem. He cannot give up the symptom without becoming overwhelmed by difficulties.

An example which might illustrate a conversion reaction occurred on an adolescent ward into which was admitted a young girl 'paralysed' from the waist down. She had been about to return to boarding school but found herself unable to walk on the morning she was due to leave home. Mary was an only child whose parents insisted she should follow a science course when she returned from the summer vacation, thereby totally disregarding Mary's natural abilities and desire to pursue her studies in modern languages and history. After lengthy discussions with the psychiatrist, the parents were helped to understand the patient's unconscious reaction to their plans for her future. Mary was able to 'give up' her symptom when her parents eventually agreed to the subjects of her choice.

Dissociation reactions
In this type of reaction to anxiety, the most commonly encountered symptom is amnesia, a combination of denial and repression which relieves rather than, as in conversion, diverts anxiety. Young women frequently show dissociative symptoms, in that they may be admitted to a psychiatric hospital having come to the attention of the police, unable to tell who they are or why they are in a strange city. The most spectacular form of dissociation occurs in the type of dual personality illustrated by Robert Louis Stevenson's *Dr Jekyll and Mr Hyde*, a condition which is very rare.

Treatment of conversion and dissociation reactions does not consist of removing the symptom, but of discovering the conflict situation which the symptom is designed to solve and then helping the patient to find a more satisfactory solution to the problem. The patient's illness demonstrates the need to attract interest and empathy. He must receive the attention, interest and understanding of the psychiatrist and the nursing staff. It may be possible to demonstrate to the patient that it is not necessary to maintain the symptom for this purpose and that the nurses accept and respect him.

Many nurses, however, find this a particularly difficult task and tend to treat the patient as if he were deliberately trying to deceive. It cannot be over-emphasized that the hysterical patient who is seeking attention and trying to be loved really needs all the love and attention he can get. He needs to feel successful and requires sufficient encouragement to surmount obstacles in a realistic way.

Obsessive–compulsive disorder

This is one of the most incapacitating of mental disorders. Patients who, prior to their illness, have often been known for their reliability, trustworthiness and meticulous neatness, during their illness show these traits in exaggerated form, so much so that they become aware of the absurd nature of their compulsive actions but are unable to desist without becoming severely anxious.

Sometimes a patient becomes preoccupied with some thought or phrase, occasionally of an obscene or blasphemous nature, considered totally alien to his character. Nevertheless the thought persistently intrudes into consciousness and no amount of will-power can rid him of it.

Some patients find, with increasing frequency, that they are in doubt whether an action just completed was correctly performed and feel obliged to repeat it. After checking, the patient still feels doubtful and so repeats the action again. He may be fully aware of the fact that his doubts are without foundation. Often such a compulsive action develops into a ritual which is carried out in precisely the same manner on each occasion and is then repeated, lest a mistake has occurred. Even the most minor interruption necessitates the ritual being started again from the beginning as the patient becomes intensely worried, feeling that something terrible may happen if the ritual is not correctly performed.

Some patients are terrified of going out, of crossing the street, of heights or bridges, or of being in an enclosed space. Some patients are afraid of knives or sharp instruments, always recognizing that these fears are irrational. These fears are known as phobias (focal anxiety or situation specific anxiety) and may sometimes be classified under the heading of phobic states.

The patient's symptoms may give an indication of the underlying conflict. Fear of heights may be associated with an unconscious desire on the part of the patient to throw himself down; fear of knives may be found in one who is afraid of hurting people and who may be protecting himself from his own unconscious impulses to do so. Compulsive acts such as hand-washing and the expressed wish to be scrupulously clean may represent the patient's attempt to rid himself of a feeling of being unclean. A feeling of guilt about some real or imagined wrongdoing, often of a sexual nature, may, without the patient's awareness of the connection, be expressed by an exaggerated concern about dirt.

Patients who develop obsessional neuroses are sometimes found to have been subjected to very rigorous and early toilet training. The parents may have been rigid, methodical and overconscientious people who may have made excessive demands for early socialization, and their own rigid moral standards may have been taken over by the patient. To what extent the parents' personalities are transmitted genetically, predisposing the patient to an obsessional illness, or to what extent the mode of training is responsible for producing the obsessional personality pattern is not always clear.

Only the most severely handicapped of these patients are likely to be admitted to hospital as in-patients. Many obsessional patients, in spite of the suffering they may undergo, succeed in remaining gainfully employed. The severity of the symptoms fluctuates with environmental circumstances.

During periods of stress the patient's rituals may become complicated and so extensive that he is quite incapable of keeping them under control. It may take him all his time to wash and dress, so that he never reaches his place of work, or at work he may feel compelled to go over each item so often that very little is done and he is unable to hold down his job. Sometimes, although the compulsive symptoms remain relatively mild, the anxiety associated with attempting to control them is so great that the patient's symptoms on admission to hospital are those of a severe anxiety state.

Treatment and nursing depend largely on the severity of the symptoms. In the calm and relatively well-ordered atmosphere of the hospital ward these are likely to become less intolerable. The fewer the demands made on the patient, the more likely he will be to become more relaxed. On the other hand, discussion of emotional conflicts may lead to a temporary exacerbation, but the patient may benefit ultimately from a better understanding of his problems.

It has been found that patients suffering from obsessional neurosis do not respond to individual psychotherapy. More consideration is therefore given to the rehabilitation of the patient, and treatment is aimed at reducing environmental stress and helping him to learn to live more successfully, in spite of his compulsive symptoms.

If the compulsive acts in themselves are relatively mild and not harmful, the patient may be helped to reduce his anxiety about them and to live a comparatively normal life. If the compulsive acts are seriously incapacitating, the aim must be to modify them. Sometimes less harmful preoccupations can be substituted for those that are more inconvenient. A patient who finds it difficult to stop washing his hands or to complete his morning toilet may perhaps be helped to work to a time schedule and to aim at completing a detailed routine within a given time.

It is necessary to discuss with the doctor whether it is more important to reduce anxiety and possibly to allow the patient unlimited time for his compulsive actions, or whether it is better to aim at a workable time schedule which would allow him to continue in gainful employment and to alleviate the resulting anxiety by sedation or other methods. If the latter is the case, a careful programme must be worked out and discussed in detail with the patient. He will derive some security from the knowledge that an attempt is being made to establish a workable routine and he will then be better able to tolerate his increased tension.

A carefully documented nursing care plan will ensure that all members of the nursing staff are consistent in their delivery of care. To be inconsistent, to drive the patient sometimes and at other times to let him take several hours to wash and dress, will increase anxiety and not help him in any way.

Behaviour therapy techniques may sometimes be used in the treatment of patients suffering from certain neurotic disorders (see Chapter 22).

Depressive reactions to stress
Synonyms: neurotic depression, reactive depression, atypical
depression, exogenous depression.

This diagnostic category is used by psychiatrists who hold the view that there are two forms of depression. One is found in patients with a neurotic disposition as a reaction to stress, and the other is associated with the functional psychoses; these two forms may overlap, however, and produce a mixed clinical state.

Almost all of us at some time in our lives admit to feeling 'depressed' in response to a stressful situation, but this experience is usually self-limiting and generally overcome without medical interference. In a minority of people, the depression persists and physical and psychological symptoms of anxiety may also be present. The sufferer cries easily, feels 'low in spirits', lacks energy and complains of a lack of interest. Overeating is not uncommon, and oversleeping with initial insomnia is sometimes present.

Reactivity to one's surrounding is retained, however, and if the person has to be admitted to hospital, she (more women than men are affected) may be observed to enjoy a comedy show on television, though afterwards to revert to a weepy and anxious state once she is alone.

A growing number of psychiatrists prefer to confine the use of the term 'depression' in psychiatric diagnoses to those patients with sustained depression of mood, lacking reactivity. They regard depressive disorders on a continuum, with patients showing symptoms of depression, but without psychotic features of delusions and hallucinations at one end of the spectrum, and those patients who do show these serious symptoms at the other end. This classification allows for a changing clinical picture. It is of more value to the psychiatric nurse, who, if told that a patient is depressed by the nurse in charge, is more concerned with the fact that this implies the patient might harm herself should her depression worsen, than with the adjectives used to assign the patient to a diagnostic category.

The functional psychoses

The functional psychoses may be described as psychiatric disorders which are characterized by their severity; they produce markedly disordered and disturbed behaviour, which is qualitatively rather than quantitatively different from normal, and cannot be understood (as in the neuroses) as an extension of ordinary everyday experience. Patients with a psychotic disorder generally lack insight into their illness and are often out of touch with reality.

The psychotic disorders may be further divided into the affective disorders and schizophrenia.

The affective disorders

The affective disorders, the commonest of all the disorders seen in psychiatric hospitals, include manic–depressive psychosis (bipolar illness) and endogenous (psychotic) depression (unipolar illness).

Manic–depressive psychosis or bipolar illness. The term bipolar indicates that the patient experiences sustained periods of disturbances of mood, i.e. excitement (mania) and depression at different times. Although mood (affect) is predominantly disturbed, other aspects of the patient's life may also be affected. Disturbances of thought may be reflected in delusions of grandeur (in mania), or of poverty (in depression). Activity may be excessive, as seen in mania, or almost non-existent, as in the retardation found in the depressed patient. The presence of hallucinations indicates disturbance of the patient's perceptual functioning. Visual hallucinations may be present in manic states and auditory hallucinations are not uncommon in psychotic depression.

In health, people predisposed to manic–depressive disorders are frequently warm, outgoing people, liable to be moody, but gay, cheerful and hearty when the mood is good. The friendliness and warmth of feeling are appreciated by many friends, and they are popular with their colleagues.

The first attack of mania or depression is often precipitated by a crisis in the patient's life; further attacks may occur at regular intervals or may only be triggered off by stressful life events.

In mania the patient is happy, elated and feels on top of the world. Everything is wonderful in his eyes; he is full of self-confidence, makes plans for great actions and indulges in feverish activity. His speech is so rapid that it is difficult to understand, his thoughts appear to follow each other too rapidly to be communicated in words. The patient's movements are large, often graceful. There is constant activity, but inability to concentrate on any particular task. The patient feels constrained and hemmed in, he is hypersensitive to noise, sometimes the feeling of his clothes irritates him sufficiently to cause him to tear them up. He is highly distractible. Any stimulus, a spoken word, a movement or some sound, will set off a new train of thought, words or deeds.

Speech does not follow the usual logic. The sound of words is often the cue to association of ideas. Rhyming and punning are common. For a while the patient's happiness is infectious. However, he easily becomes irritable and sometimes aggressive if he is in any way prevented from carrying out his intentions.

There is serious danger to the patient's health. Often it is difficult to persuade him to take adequate nourishment because he rarely takes the time for a substantial meal (see Chapter 9, The Significance of Food). His mouth becomes dry and furred as a result of constant talking. He may become seriously dehydrated; excessive energy output not balanced by adequate diet may lead to exhaustion. Injuries and intercurrent infections may occur if proper safeguards are not taken.

The use of drugs may be essential to calm the patient, but in view of his poor physical condition this may carry its own dangers.

Treatment consists of providing adequate rest and nourishment and protection from danger. The patient's distractibility can be utilized to avoid injury to any member of the staff or the other patients, should he become aggressive. But this distractability interferes with rest unless very skilled nursing is provided. The nurse's tone of voice, the deliberate, slow speech, slow movement, monotony of surroundings, subdued lights and absence of noise all help to calm the patient. Sedation and other forms of physical treatment are discussed elsewhere.

In acute mania the patient is too disturbed to be nursed with others.

Hypomania. A state of excitement and overactivity which is less severe but more prolonged sometimes occurs; this is called hypomania. All the symptoms of mania are present but in a less serious form. Most of the nursing problems are similar to those occurring in the nursing of manic patients, but since the hypomanic patient is able to be nursed in a ward with others, his effect on these must be taken into account. Often the other patients are at first amused by him. His drive and energy make him a suitable person to choose as a spokesman and to organize activities for the rest. Gradually the fact that he is not always able to carry out his ideas and that he interferes with the other patients makes the latter angry and irritable. Kind intentions are looked upon as interferences and he becomes a target of general hostility.

He requires protection from the less well-controlled patients; friction and quarrels should be prevented. The patient may overestimate his strength and some curtailment of his activities may be necessary.

Occasionally the hypomanic state becomes chronic and keeps the patient in hospital for years. Among the chronic psychiatric hospital patients, the hypomanic patient stands out because his drive and his interest in all that is happening are strangely in contrast with the apathy of many of the others. In dress the hypomanic patient is outstanding. He uses every scrap of colourful material to adorn himself. He is the one who comes forward to welcome visitors and to give all the information.

The depressive phase of manic–depressive psychosis, also known as bipolar or recurrent depression, is clinically indistinguishable from endogenous depression (see below) and until recently the terms were used interchangeably.

Endogenous (psychotic or unipolar) depression. The term endogenous ('arising from within') was traditionally used to distinguish this type of depression from reactive depression—a reaction to stressful situations—but it is considered unsatisfactory since recent social studies have found that the majority of all depressions are preceded by traumatic life events. The term psychotic depression is used to indicate the presence of psychotic features, such as hallucinations and delusions.

Unipolar depression contrasts with bipolar depression (i.e. episodes of mania alternating with episodes of depression) and the term is used for patients who have recurrent depressive episodes but have never so far suffered from an attack of mania. ('Unipolar mania' is used for episodes of mania without depression.)

The depressed patient often feels and looks sad. His movements and thoughts are slow, he stoops, or sits with his head bent low. He does not wish to converse and says as little as possible, slowly and in monosyllables. He is uninterested in his surroundings, unobservant of all but the most depressing events. His thoughts, if he reveals them, centre on unpleasant topics. Guilt and sin are commonly mentioned. The patient considers himself to be wicked, feels that he has committed unforgivable sins and that he deserves to be punished. He may hear voices which accuse him or comment on his unworthiness. His pessimistic concern with his wickedness or his poverty may be held with the force of a delusion.

Some patients suffering from depression do not look sad. Their apparently smiling expression may cause a profound underlying suffering to go unnoticed. In extreme forms of depression the patient does not feel depressed or sad. He may say that he lacks feeling altogether or feels empty. He may have feelings of unreality, the world may seem to have changed, or he himself may feel that he no longer exists or that parts of him have died away.

Loss of appetite, constipation and often nausea may give rise to delusions, in keeping with the depressive feeling, of having no intestines, of the intestines being eaten away, or of suffering from an incurable disease. He may sleep badly, particularly in the early hours of the morning. There is considerable danger of malnutrition occurring. Lack of interest in personal hygiene or personal appearance may lead to infection. Above all there is the danger of suicide.

Depressive illness of a different kind may occur in people of late middle age. In women the onset of the illness may roughly coincide with the menopause, and the term 'involutional melancholia' is used by those who believe it to be a discrete illness and not simply endogenous depression (with agitation) arising in later life in the involutional period. Involutional melancholia, however, is no longer included in the International Classification.

Involutional melancholia occurs in people who have never suffered from a depressive illness before, and have not been subject to fluctuating moods. On the contrary, there is often evidence of exceptionally stable temperament, and occasional irritability may have been the only emotional disturbance noticed by the patient or his relatives. The patient may have held the same job for many years, and may be conspicuous for his conscientiousness, reliability and perseverance.

The illness is possibly related to some physiological changes which take place in late middle age, and often an awareness of physiological disturbance is one of its cardinal features. There is very marked anxiety and preoccupation with bodily function. Worry is expressed about bowels, flatulence, indigestion, or about palpitations, flushing, giddiness and blood pressure. Some patients, in the depth of despair, attribute anxiety and depression to physical ill-health and contemplate suicide because of their intolerable fear of chronic disease. In some patients preoccupation with bodily function takes on a delusional character. Such a patient may be convinced that he smells, that his illness is contagious, that he is a danger to others or that his physical debility is the result of divine punishment, or caused by the wickedness of men. Sometimes the illness may be related to changes in the routine of life which had become indispensable for the patient's sense of security. Retirement or loss of a job after some unavoidable absence may precipitate the onset of the depression. Others react to the death of a close friend or relative by becoming depressed. Some women, when they realize that the childbearing period is approaching an end, that the children have grown up and are no longer dependent, feel overwhelmed with a sense of futility and loneliness.

Involutional depression differs from other depressive illnesses in that there is very marked agitation and anxiety but no retardation. The patient feels miserable, hopeless and desperate. The risk of suicide is very great, because the patient has the necessary energy and determination to put plans into action.

The patient's thought content is very similar to that of other depressed patients, but he speaks more, sometimes very rapidly, although he may only repeat incessantly some expression of despair, e.g. 'Dear, oh dear', or he may utter supplications to God for help.

Involutional depression responds particularly favourably to electroconvulsive therapy, as do other forms of depression with psychotic features, although even without this, most patients recover after some months.

In manic states and depression, drug treatment is often found to be effective (see Chapter 18, on drug therapy). During the illness constant vigilance is required to protect the patient from suicidal acts. He requires help to go through a period of intense suffering. The nurse's attitude of empathy, but unshakable hopefulness, her indication that the patient's life is important, her understanding of the conflict may provide the necessary support during the illness.

Schizophrenia

Schizophrenia is a term used to describe a variety of clinical reactions with certain characteristics in common but with considerable variations in other respects.

As with the affective disorders, all aspects of the patient's life are disturbed, but whereas in depression or mania his mood is primarily affected, in schizophrenia the patient's thought processes are predominantly disordered, as in thought blocking (see below) or in the expression of delusional ideas. Affect is also abnormal; the patient may show emotional coldness, often referred to as blunting of affect, or he may respond incongruously, laughing when given sad news and vice versa. Perception is often seriously disordered with hallucinations occurring frequently.

The patient's behaviour may be unpredictable, as for example when he acts in response to an auditory hallucination; he may also tend to withdraw completely from company if preoccupied with his 'voices', especially if he finds the environment too stimulating and socially demanding.

There is a great deal of evidence to support the claim for an interaction of genetic and environmental factors in the causation of schizophrenia. For example, there is a relatively high incidence of mental disorder among relatives of schizophrenic patients. The onset of observable symptoms may coincide with some period of emotional stress. The history of many patients reveals some traumatic incidents during earliest childhood. It may be found that the patient during his earliest years has failed to receive or show the amount of affection considered necessary for normal development, and that his parents appeared disinclined or unable to provide emotional warmth. It is not clear to what extent the patient's emotional detachment is an inherited characteristic and whether the lack of emotional responsiveness was caused by the mother's coldness or the child's own inability to show affection.

When the history of a schizophrenic patient is taken the onset of the illness is usually put down to a specific event in his life. Closer inquiry, however, reveals an insidious onset of the symptoms, and friends and relatives usually agree that over a long period they had observed increasingly strange behaviour on the part of the patient. He has probably very gradually become more aloof, less interested in other people or in events which interest others. He may have spent less and less time with people, and more by himself. His work may have deteriorated over a period of time.

Other symptoms, and the further course of events, vary greatly, but a number of patterns tend to recur.

The well-known traditional classification of schizophrenia into four subtypes is now less frequently used; the categories are not clear cut and often overlap, but a brief description will be given for historical reasons.

Simple schizophrenia. This term is used to describe a progressive course of gradual onset. The patient shows evidence of thought disorder, eccentricity, withdrawal from society and a lack of emotional response. Loss of drive and apathy cause these patients to drift from job to job, till eventually they become drop-outs and vagrants, living rough at a very low economic level.

Hebephrenic schizophrenia. These patients are commonly adolescents and young adults. This disorder has a poor prognosis. The patient shows a multitude of florid symptoms. Thought blocking may occur; the patient suddenly stops, appears to forget completely what he is saying and continues by discussing an apparently unrelated idea. Incoherent speech, bizarre delusions and hallucinations, especially auditory, are often present. The patient may complain he hears voices maligning him in the third person and giving a running commentary on his actions in unflattering terms, or the voices may accuse the patient of misdeeds, use obscene language, give orders, or pronounce prophecies. They may be so authoritative and clear that the patient unquestioningly obeys their commands and performs actions which he considers to be quite alien to his nature. He may attribute the voices to 'God' or to 'the Devil', or may endeavour to find the 'people' who are speaking to him.

Bizarrely, the patient may believe that his thoughts are being broadcast to others or that thoughts are being inserted into his mind. Other symptoms thought to be of special diagnostic significance include the patient's belief that his actions are being controlled or influenced by external forces, for example television or laser beams. These symptoms are known as passivity feelings.

Difficulties may arise because the voices command the patient to perform antisocial actions, for example attacks on others, or may suggest that people harbour evil intentions. The patient may refuse to eat and become completely incapable of continuing any normal activity as a result of his preoccupation with his hallucinatory experiences. Some patients become totally inaccessible, unable to follow ordinary conversation, uninterested in other people's ideas and preoccupied with bizarre thoughts of their own, which they may or may not be able to express. Some are able to give verbal accounts of their thoughts, ascribing significance to events which other people look upon in entirely different perspective. Thoughts do not follow each other in the normal manner and connections appear illogical and bizarre. Often new words are used in an endeavour to communicate highly complicated ideas (neologisms).

Catatonic schizophrenia. This is the least common form and is now rare in Britain. The extreme forms of catatonic behaviour are stupor and excitement. The patient exhibits wild and bizarre postures in the excited phase; this may alternate with periods when he lies motionless in bed, apparently unaware of what is going on around him. Prognosis is somewhat better than for simple or hebephrenic schizophrenia; the patient may only have a single attack lasting a short time and may never have another during his lifetime.

Paranoid schizophrenia. This type of schizophrenic disorder shows the most regular pattern of development. It begins with delusions of a fairly coherent nature. In paranoid schizophrenia it is usually conceivable that the delusional idea expressed by the patient might be true, unlike those of hebephrenic patients which are so bizarre that they could not possibly be true.

If it is assumed that the patient acts as if his delusional ideas were true, his actions become meaningful and it can be understood why he elaborates and enlarges on them and develops resentment against the people around him, whom he considers hostile because they disbelieve his ideas.

Many patients experience hallucinations which they try to explain and to integrate with the delusional ideas, so that one vast delusional system is developed which may persist for years and continue to grow. Some, however, become perplexed by their own feelings and thoughts which they may recognize as strange and, therefore, attribute to the influence of outside forces. Various delusional ideas, instead of becoming systematized, may be fleeting only, changing from day to day. The patient's emotional state depends largely on his delusions, varying from abject misery to states of overwhelming happiness and ecstasy, and on the extent to which he continues to be distressed by the presumed hostility of the world around him.

In chronic paranoid illness the patient may appear able to adapt himself to a situation in which he feels safe and protected from the evil influences of those he fears. He may appear to be quite normal so long as no major changes occur in his life. Alternatively, the patient may appear well in a new environment if he feels he has escaped from his persecutors. Gradually, however, his new environment is drawn into the delusional system and only another move will satisfy the patient. The prognosis is good in paranoid schizophrenia. This condition responds well to the major tranquillizer drugs.

Alternative classification of schizophrenia. An alternative classification of schizophrenia has been used in recent years. Symptoms are divided into two groups of syndromes, Type I and Type II. Type I includes such symptoms as thought disorder, delusions, anxiety, agitation, confusion, perplexity, hallucinations and a variety of odd behaviour patterns. These symptoms are also referred to as positive symptoms. Type II are negative symptoms and may be identified by a reduction in normal responses to environmental stimuli, such as poverty of speech (loss of range of ideas), flatness of affect (loss of emotional response), social withdrawal (loss of social interaction) and lack of self-care skills (loss of personal pride). The patient's behaviour may be stereotyped, indicating a lack of variation in behavioural responses, and also show a disturbance in communication, such as in the loss of range in his speech and lack of facial expressions. Some of these negative symptoms are said to be associated with the social understimulation of understaffed long-stay wards before active rehabilitation programmes were introduced.

Diagnostic imaging techniques have shown abnormalities such as dilatation of the ventricles of the brain in patients with a Type II syndrome. Generally, Type II syndrome follows Type I, but overlap is not uncommon. For example, a patient with negative symptoms may show some of the florid symptoms of Type I if he is overaroused. Overarousal can occur if the patient is introduced to an active rehabilitation programme without adequate preparation.

One of the nurse's most important functions is to establish and maintain emotional rapport with the patient and to prevent the emotional isolation which occurs in schizophrenic patients. Many nursing problems arise as a result of the patient's delusions. Refusal of food, episodic outbursts of violence and incontinence are some of the difficulties, and these are dealt with elsewhere in this book.

OTHER PSYCHIATRIC DISORDERS

Other psychiatric disorders may be classified under the following headings.
1 Personality disorders
2 Psychosomatic disorders
3 Anorexia nervosa

Personality disorders

The term 'psychopathic personality' is used to describe a form of personality disorder affecting the patient's emotional and social adjustment to other people. Patients who are called 'psychopaths' (or 'sociopaths') are not suffering from mental illness, yet their conduct is so abnormal that they must be considered as being psychiatrically disordered.

The disturbance dates from a very early age, and one of its characteristics is a failure to learn from experience. The psychopathic patient is immature in every aspect of his behaviour. He is impulsive, lacks foresight, is unable to persevere in his endeavours or to postpone gratification of his desires. He may have had frequent changes of jobs, given up some because of differences of opinion with other people, lost others because of his inability to conform to discipline.

In the most extreme form, the psychopathic individual expresses his demands and his aggression without inhibition or consideration of his environment. He is entirely self-centred, using relationships with others only to exploit them. Since he has either been denied affection or has been unable to accept and internalize the love given him, he has not learned to become involved in deep relationships or to give affection to others. With no altruistic feelings himself, he distrusts, or cannot understand, altruism in others, and will take advantage of what he sees as a weakness in any way which will be of benefit to himself. Patients of this type are lonely and pitiful figures, and fortunately the extreme form is not too common. A continuum from minor infringements of social and cultural expectations to the most violent forms of antisocial behaviour exists, and patients enter hospitals who could be placed on widely varying points of such a scale.

During a stay in hospital, some patients can be helped if they can feel that they are accepted and can form satisfying emotional relationships with other patients or with staff members. This can best be achieved in a ward or hospital where a 'therapeutic community' can be created (see Chapter 25). The patients assume responsibility with the staff for the functioning of the ward, and for the treatment of each member of the community. They develop interest in and understanding of each others' problems, become more interested, more tolerant of difficult behaviour. As they come to feel accepted by the others their behaviour improves and they learn to form closer personal bonds.

With advancing years most psychopathic patients settle down to a more satisfactory pattern of living.

Psychosomatic disorders

Psychosomatic disorders are conditions in which physical symptoms are noticeably related to emotional disturbances. The following examples are not uncommon.

Asthmatic attacks are frequently precipitated by periods of emotional stress and may cease when the patient feels relaxed and happy.

Vascular disorders, particularly congestion of the mucous membranes of the respiratory tract, are aggravated by anxiety. Fainting is associated with excitement and fear.

Hypertension and coronary occlusion appear to occur more frequently in people who are of a tense and worrying disposition. Hyperthyroidism, ulcerative colitis, peptic ulcers, urticaria and migraine are all conditions which tend to respond better to treatment when the patient's emotional adjustment is taken into account. The symptoms are not entirely due to psychological difficulties but improvement often coincides with improvement in the patient's mental state.

Anorexia nervosa

The term anorexia nervosa (nervous loss of appetite) was used in 1868 by William Gull to describe a condition of extreme emaciation in young women, associated with amenorrhoea, and in which there was no apparent physical cause to be found. Over 100 years later there is considerable concern over the steadily rising numbers of people affected by this eating disorder; young girls and women are ten times more likely to develop it than their male counterparts. Some of the increase is due not only to more public awareness and reporting, but also, it is thought, to an actual rise in the number of sufferers and in the incidence of the disorder. The fact that to be slim is 'in' may have contributed substantially to the present 'epidemic'. One recent survey of a schoolgirl population of 16–18 year olds found 1 girl in every 100 was affected.

An unrelenting search for thinness, morbid fears of becoming fat and gaining weight, and a distorted body image—the young girl strenuously refutes any suggestion that she is in fact desperately thin—all support a diagnosis of anorexia nervosa. Other classical symptoms are self-induced, severe, weight loss through rigid dieting, persistent amenorrhoea and a reluctance or refusal to seek medical advice.

To achieve her goal of losing weight, the anorectic (or anorexic) girl adopts a number of stratagems. Of these, a diet of non-fattening foods, such as lettuce and carrot, a rigorous exercise regimen, self-induced vomiting and the ingestion of massive doses of laxatives are most commonly adopted.

Paradoxically, the girl shows considerable interest in food, preparing (but not eating) elaborate meals for family and friends, and exchanging recipes with apparent enthusiasm. Occasionally she will have a secret binge followed quickly by feelings of guilt and self-induced vomiting with a return to renewed dieting.

Though several theories have been put forward, the cause of this potentially fatal disorder remains unknown. It may be triggered by a traumatic life event such as an examination failure or, alternatively, by a casual remark from a sibling about 'puppy-fat'. It has been suggested that the patient may have difficulty in accepting the 'fatness' which accompanies the secondary sex characteristics of adolescence, or have a fear of having to confront, at a later date, the potential and often inevitable conflicts and disharmony inherent in parent–teenager relationships. To avoid or postpone having to cope with a future fraught with problems, the girl may seek to retreat, through voluntary starvation, into an earlier and more secure stage of development.

The parents have been thought by some authorities to play a crucial part in the aetiology of this eating disorder. They have been variously described as controlling, overprotective and overbearing in their attitude towards their daughter. Many are said to be high achievers and to have similar expectations for their offspring.

An organic basis for anorexia nervosa has been postulated. The hormonal abnormalities, such as amenorrhoea, and the slower gastric emptying found in a recent study have been viewed as being indicative of possible hypothalamic malfunctioning (see also Chapter 12).

Bulimia nervosa

The term bulimia nervosa has only been in use since 1979, and this disorder has been described as a variant of anorexia nervosa. Russell, in a seminal paper, identified the syndrome and isolated certain criteria to be satisfied before the diagnosis is made. These include a profound loss of control over eating habits resulting in an overpowering urge to overeat, avoidance of 'fattening' food, self-induced vomiting and/or abuse of purgatives. As in anorexia nervosa, there is a morbid fear of obesity and usually females are affected. However, unlike anorectic patients, those with bulimia nervosa are of normal weight and shape, do not have amenorrhoea, tend to be rather older (20 years and over) and seek help of their own accord. They show an excessive concern about body shape. Again in comparison with girls with anorexia, who tend to be solitary, girls with bulimia nervosa are outgoing and socially competent.

Chaotic eating habits are a feature of bulimia nervosa. Sometimes the girl adheres to a strict reducing diet and at other times she indulges in binge-eating. The latter activity is carried out in secret and continues until all food supplies in the house are exhausted. This is immediately followed by self-induced vomiting.

Girls who suffer from bulimia nervosa are usually seen on an out-patient basis. Psychotherapy is the preferred form of treatment; antidepressant drugs are only of value to relieve depressive symptoms and, as with anorexia nervosa, they do not influence the outcome.

Further reading

Crisp, A.H. (1983) Anorexia nervosa: diagnosis and prognosis. *Psychiatry in Practice* 2(12), 13.

Curran, D., Partridge, M. & Storey, P. (1980) *Psychological Medicine*, 9th edn. Edinburgh: Churchill Livingstone.

Fairbairn, C. & Cooper, P. (1984) The clinical features of bulimia nervosa. *British Journal of Psychiatry 144*, 238.

Harper, P.S. (1983) A genetic marker for Huntington's chorea. *British Medical Journal 287*, 1567.

Kendall, R.E. & Zealley, A.K., eds. (1983) *Companion to Psychiatric Studies*, 3rd edn. Edinburgh: Churchill Livingstone.

Russell, G. (1979) Bulimia nervosa: an ominous varient of anorexia nervosa. *Psychological Medicine 9*, 429.

Stafford-Clark, D. & Smith, A. (1983) *Psychiatry for Students*, 6th edn. London: George Allen & Unwin.

3
The psychiatrically ill and society

Nearly half the hospital beds in Britain are occupied by mentally ill or mentally handicapped patients. Psychiatric nurses learn in hospital the art of caring for these patients and of contributing to their recovery and rehabilitation.

Later chapters will describe the way in which hospital treatment can be of value to the psychiatrically ill patient. But not all people who require psychiatric help are admitted to hospital; they are being cared for in the community by a rapidly expanding corps of psychiatric nurses specially trained for this role.

Although an understanding of the social problems of psychiatric disorder is more specifically the concern of community psychiatric nurses, something of this knowledge is also of interest to the nurse in hospital. Only the barest outline of this can be given in this chapter. Psychiatric nursing has only a short history. Traditionally, nurses look after the sick and helpless and the concept of mental disorder as sickness is a very recent one.

HISTORICAL ATTITUDES TO MENTAL DISORDERS

Until the end of the last century, with isolated exceptions, those who suffered from mental disorder were ignored or ridiculed unless they were obviously dangerous to the community. Those who were thought to be dangerous were, at various periods, executed, ill-treated or imprisoned. They were considered as being totally different from other human beings, chained and kept under physical restraint, physically and mentally tortured in order to render them manageable.

Pinel in France (1745–1826), and Tuke in York (1732–1822), proclaimed that the insane person was human, and would respond to kindness. Pinel, watched by a frightened and disbelieving audience, removed the chains and convinced his followers that the time was ripe for humane treatment of the insane. Education was required, both of those who were responsible for the care of the insane, and of society as a whole, before some of the fear of the insane person was lost and sufficient sympathy and interest acquired to abandon restraint. In 1889 the first course of instruction was given to attendants of the insane in Britain.

As public opinion changed, so people became less disposed to hide their affliction, and it became clear how large was the number of people who would benefit by humane care. Lunatic asylums were built where many thousands took refuge from an unsympathetic world too difficult for them to understand.

Not until the end of the nineteenth century was the public conscience sufficiently aroused in England to accept, by Act of Parliament, official responsibility for the care of the insane, to delegate this duty to local authorities, and at the same time to admit that the person of unsound mind required the protection of the law from those who might be sufficiently unscrupulous to take advantage of his afflictions.

The Lunacy Act of 1890 clearly laid down the circumstances in which society had the right to protect itself from those who might cause damage as a result of mental disorder. It defined the responsibility of the local authority to provide care and protection, free of charge, for those who were certified to be in need of them, and it laid down in detail the extent to which a person deprived of his liberty by virtue of certification was entitled to protection and to the safeguard of many of the rights of citizenship.

As time passed, many of the safeguards against wrongful certification, exploitation and ill-treatment appeared no longer to be necessary. Better staff were employed in mental hospitals, and public opinion had moved towards sympathy and understanding.

While wrongful certification became an unlikely occurrence, fear of mental illness and the stigma associated with it prevented maintenance of interest in the patient after certification. Feelings of fear, shame and guilt caused relatives to delay certification as long as possible but, once this had become necessary, quickly to forget the patient. The situation of many asylums made visiting difficult, and there was a tendency to think of admission to an asylum as final. Many asylums, with their large, beautiful grounds, became self-contained communities, a refuge for patients from the harsh world outside.

MODERN ATTITUDE TO PSYCHIATRIC DISORDERS

While public opinion gradually moved to an acceptance of responsibility for the humane care of the mentally disturbed, expert opinion approached the recognition of mental disorder as an illness requiring medical and nursing care. Medical interest was devoted to careful description of abnormal behaviour, in an attempt to classify and diagnose it, and to prescribe treatment. Psychiatric nurses were needed in place of attendants for the insane. The new function of the nurse consisted of accurate recordings of signs and symptoms, and in helping to detect early manifestations of psychiatric disorder with a view to treatment and prevention.

Fear of certification, however, militated against early treatment of psychiatric disorder, and a new method for the admission of patients became necessary. In 1930 the Mental Treatment Act made it possible to receive treatment in a mental hospital as a voluntary or temporary patient, without legal formalities, and yet retain the protection granted to certified patients. The Mental Treatment Act was preceded by a similar Act in Scotland, and in England by a special Act of Parliament granting the London County Council permission to treat voluntary patients at Maudsley Hospital.

To emphasize the recognition of psychiatric disorder as illness the name 'asylum' was changed to 'mental hospital', the word 'patient' substituted for 'lunatic', and 'nurse' for 'attendant'.

As the attitude of the public towards the mentally ill became increasingly sympathetic and understanding, many people became aware that the legislation relating to mental disorder was still unnecessarily complex and restrictive. In particular, concern was expressed about the fact that many people detained in institutions for the mentally defective did not appear to be discharged as readily as seemed to be desirable. A Royal Commission was set up in 1954 to enquire into the way the law was operating and to make recommendations for change. As a result of it, the Mental Health Act was passed in 1959 and the

Mental Health (Scotland) Act in 1960. They came into operation in 1961.

The essence of the Acts was reflected in the title. *Mental health* rather than disease was the subject of the Acts. All previous legislation relating to mental illness and to mental deficiency became obsolete and the aim of these Acts was to abolish all distinction between the way people suffering from physical and mental disorder were treated.

The Act abolished mental hospitals as specially designated hospitals. All patients had the opportunity of being admitted to any hospital able to offer them treatment. All hospitals could offer treatment to any patient they felt they could help and could refuse to admit patients whom they did not feel able to help. Clearly, many hospitals continued to specialize in certain types of treatment and many psychiatric patients required specialized care, but there was no legal restriction on other hospitals or patients.

Most patients suffering from mental disorders were admitted to hospital in precisely the same manner as if they were suffering from any other kind of illness. A few patients only required to be admitted or detained against their will. Patients who felt that they were wrongfully detained had, however, recourse to specially constituted Mental Health Review Tribunals or, in Scotland, to the Mental Welfare Commission.

The above Acts remained virtually unamended until 1983 (1984 in Scotland). The new Mental Health Acts seek to give the patient greater protection whenever compulsion is involved. Protection of patients has been a matter of deep concern to MIND (National Organization for Mental Health)—a voluntary organization which can be justly proud of the fact that many of the new Acts' provisions are based on its proposals. A brief description of the sections of the Acts of particular relevance to psychiatric nurses is given later in the book (see Appendix).

Investigations into the causes and treatment of psychiatric disorders developed along divergent lines. On the one hand, the chance discovery of malarial therapy for the treatment of general paralysis of the insane led to a search for organic causes and physical treatment. On the other hand, the findings of Freud and his followers led to increased understanding of personality development and the factors causing faulty adjustment. Investigation of psychological and social causes of mental disorder and treatment by psychotherapy and social influences made rapid strides.

The general interest in the prevention of illness which has yielded such marked results in other fields of medicine has spread to psychiatry. There is a widening interest in child care and in the social and educational responsibility for developing healthy mental attitudes. Preconception classes for prospective parents and health education programmes in schools are but two examples of this.

COMMUNITY CARE

Since the ambit of mental disorder has widened to include neuroses and social maladjustment, hospital care is no longer considered to be the best form of treatment for all. At present there is a growing awareness of the responsibility of the community as a whole for the rehabilitation of those who have suffered, and increased involvement in their treatment. Many people believe that hospitalization should be resorted to only if no other method of treatment is possible. Removal of the patient from his own environment makes it unnecessarily difficult for him to return to it when he has improved. Treatment of the patient in his own setting is considered to be preferable whenever this is possible, and general practitioners aspiring to a principalship must nowadays undergo a 3-year period of vocational training which will include in almost every case a period in a psychiatric hospital.

However, close contact between the patient's own doctor and the psychiatric specialists is still desirable, and this is being achieved in many health centres where the expertise of community psychiatric nurses, clinical psychologists and visiting consultant psychiatrists is available under one roof.

If more intensive therapy is required, day hospitals provide all the therapeutic resources of in-patient treatment, without the disruptive effect of removal from home and admission to hospital. Day hospital treatment avoids the complete removal of responsibility from the patient and spares him the effort of readjusting to his environment on discharge.

If community care of psychiatric patients becomes the method of choice for most patients, more help will have to be available to relatives. More community psychiatric nurses and social workers will be required to give help and support to the patient's family, and to understand their problems and difficulties. Education of the general public towards greater tolerance of the mentally ill is still necessary.

Many psychiatric patients are able to carry on only in a relatively sheltered atmosphere. More group homes and hostels will be required where those who do not need hospital care can nevertheless receive some measure of shelter and protection before graduating to independent housing accommodation. Many psychiatric patients are able to work well and efficiently provided they do not have to work in competition with normal people. More sheltered employment will be required (such as is provided by the industrial therapy organization movement) where, in spite of their disablement, mentally ill people can earn an independent living and benefit from the increased self-respect which is supplied by gainful employment.

TRENDS IN PSYCHIATRIC CARE

The present trends of psychiatric care are summarized below.

There is an increased awareness of the responsibility of the community to the mentally ill. On the whole, there is a tendency to keep patients out of psychiatric hospitals, or to return them to the community as quickly as possible. Within the community greater understanding of the needs of the mentally ill is being developed, and also a greater awareness of the social causes of psychiatric disorders.

Within the hospital there are three main trends of thought, which are as follows.

1 There is a growing amount of information available about neurophysiological disturbance in psychiatric patients, accompanied by an increasing use of drugs.

2 There is an interest in the psychological causation of faulty attitudes, an exploration of unconscious goals and motives. Psychotherapeutic techniques of individual, group and family therapy are developing along various lines.

3 The significance of social factors in the causation and treatment of mental illness is recognized. The interaction of patient groups is being studied, interpersonal problems are

being discussed, the effect of staff on patients and *vice versa* is better understood, and the hospital ward in many instances is developing into a therapeutic community. This is often referred to as sociotherapeutic treatment.

General principles of care are the same whether the patient receives treatment in hospital or in the community. Whatever the causes or manifestation of the patient's illness, some failure in adjustment to the demands of society always occurs. Therefore, in order to help the patient, some attempt must be made to adjust society to the patient in the first instance. Wherever possible, this should happen within the patient's own community. His friends, relatives, employer, might, with the help of the psychiatric team and as a result of changed attitudes, adapt to the patient. Where this is not possible, the patient needs treatment in the special environment of a psychiatric ward, be it in a day hospital, in a district general hospital or in a psychiatric hospital.

The aim of treatment is, however, to help the patient to learn new methods of adjustment. The phase during which the environment adapts to the patient should not be unnecessarily prolonged, nor should the demands made on the patient be excessively reduced. Everything that is healthy should be preserved; wherever the patient is capable of acting in a normal, healthy, independent manner he should have an opportunity to do so.

The patient may need help to improve his physical condition or, on the other hand, he may be physically fit and well and need only the opportunity to maintain his usual state of nutrition, exercise and physical care. He may have a reduced capacity to work, earn his living and assume responsibility for his dependants, and treatment may have to include help in this respect. On the other hand, the patient may be quite competent in all that is involved in working and should not, during treatment, be allowed to lose his skill or his sense of responsibility.

If the patient does not require active assistance in making friends or in using his leisure time, he should not, during illness, be allowed to lose his social skills, his interests or his circle of friends. If he does have difficulty, the hospital should offer the patient the opportunity to learn how to form new and more satisfying interpersonal relationships.

Community care offers the best opportunity for retaining all that is best in the patient's adjustment. Hospital care in what is described as a therapeutic community may be necessary where the patient needs to learn or relearn social living.

In this chapter the current approach to problems of mental illness has been discussed chiefly with reference to the United Kingdom. Cultural differences play a part in the emphasis given to specific treatment methods in different countries. Until recently it was believed that the incidence of mental illness was lower in developing countries than in the more industrialized parts of the world, but investigations carried out by the World Health Organization have shown that developing countries have a high incidence of mental disorder. It is hoped to develop community care programmes in the first instance and to avoid creating large mental hospitals.

Further reading

Brown, G.W. & Harris, T. (1978) *Social Origins of Depression: a Study of Psychiatric Disorder in Women*. London: Tavistock.

Gostin, L. (1983) *A Practical Guide to Mental Health Law*. London: MIND.

McIntosh, I. (1982) The clinical psychologist in practice. *Psychiatry in Practice 1* (9), 38.

Report of the Richmond Fellowship Enquiry (1983) *Mental Health and the Community*. London: Richmond Fellowship Press.

WHO (1975) *Organization of Mental Health Services in Developing Countries*. (Technical Report Series, 565). Geneva: WHO.

Wing, J.K. & Morris, B. eds. (1981) *Handbook of Psychiatric Rehabilitation Practice*. Oxford: Oxford University Press.

4
Nursing the Patient in the Community

Since integration of the Health Services took place in April 1974, the hospital, local authority and general medical services which had previously been administered as separate entities were united under the management of an executive group, the basic unit being the district. The aim of the services provided in the district for the mentally disturbed was to help them live as normally as possible, allowing for the nature and extent of their disorder.

In the previous chapter it was pointed out that treatment in the community is now often considered the treatment of choice because of the advantages to the person who suffers from psychiatric disorder. Firstly institutionalization is avoided. Secondly the danger of increasing dependency on the hospital may be diminished. It may be of considerable benefit to be spared the stigma of admission to hospital and of having officially a label of a psychiatric diagnosis attached. To many people it is important not to be classified as a 'patient' and to have to assume the appropriate role. To many psychiatrists as well as to many sufferers the term 'client' seems more acceptable. It may be a more appropriate concept of the help they are able to give and to accept. They see the client and the professional helpers co-operating in the solution of the client's problems. The role of 'patient' implies to them that the professional staff know best what is good for the patient, offer help and expect the patient, passively, to accept it, whereas a client is free to avail himself of help or to reject it if he sees fit.

It may be of benefit to see a family's problems in the home setting in that a more accurate evaluation of the relationships and dynamics of the family group is likely to be made. To this end, visits can be planned for varying times of the day or evening so that communication within the family can be observed, how tensions build up, where the family authority lies and how aggression is handled. The individual who has been referred for psychiatric help would, if treated in isolation in a hospital, have to return to an unchanged situation at home, with possibly the added disadvantage of being openly known as the 'sick' one of the family.

Problems may also arise when someone who is discharged after a lengthy period in hospital suffering from a schizophrenic disorder finds himself the subject of considerable criticism from his family if his behaviour does not come up to their expectations. It has been found that unless the family can receive considerable help and support from the community psychiatric nurse and the patient can perhaps be offered a day hospital place (thus reducing the number of 'contact hours' with his family), relapse and re-admission are a possible outcome for the patient.

ACUTELY DISTURBED PATIENTS

If, however, acutely disturbed people are to remain in the community, highly skilled community psychiatric nurses are needed. Any nurse who has cared for an acutely ill patient in hospital will readily understand how much strain and anxiety such a patient may cause to his relatives and how difficult it must be for relatives to look after the patient unaided. It is much easier for nurses in hospital. There they have the opportunity of relieving their anxiety about the patient by obtaining help from colleagues, by sharing responsibility with others, by delegating responsibility and tasks to others. They can call the doctor to their help at a moment's notice, they can refer to people in more senior positions problems with which they are unable to deal. They can obtain some rest and diversion by devoting their attention to other patients. They can go off duty after a predetermined period of work to obtain rest and support from others. However stressful the care of a patient may be to a nurse, she knows that she is performing a paid job to the best of her ability, but if she fails to bring about improvement in the patient, she is in no way penalized.

Relatives who take on the responsibility of caring for the patient have none of these benefits. Their personal stress is increased by the emotional tie with the patient, by the guilt feeling they may have about the patient's illness and by the fact that they know how serious consequences of his failure to recover may be for them. The general practitioner is often less readily accessible to the relative than the hospital doctor is to the nurse, and the help he can give when he does come may not be effective.

Relatives who are willing to undertake the care of a disturbed family member can do so only with adequate support from professional staff. It is becoming increasingly recognized that community psychiatric nurses play a valued part in providing this support, because of their professional experience in the management of psychiatric disorder and their specialized training.

In addition, the community psychiatric nurses' understanding of the symptomatology and causes of psychiatric illness is brought to bear on the observation and the management of the patient and the explanations and help given to relatives. The fact that their expertise is available may give the general practitioner without psychiatric experience confidence that he can cope with the patient.

The same expertise is used to make the decision to admit the patient should the therapeutic intervention within the community fail.

Community psychiatric nurses give practical help when it is required. Nurses appear to be the only professional group who actually give practical help at once, and they also have ready access to other agencies whose resources can be tapped when needed. Nurses carry out such work from a hospital base, or they might be employed wholly to work in the community as members of the primary health care team.

FAMILY THERAPY

In addition to the advantages to the patient of having a community psychiatric nurse involved in the care which he receives at home, the family in the crisis situation of facing a new and difficult experience is likely to benefit from the skill in group work which the nurse has acquired during specialist training. It may emerge on investigation of family dynamics that the person originally designated as the patient is not the central problem, but that the family structure and relationships have decided the symptoms to be presented. The concept of family therapy is a comparatively recent development and it should be stressed that a sound knowledge of the principles involved is essential for the nurse who participates in this form of treatment.

LONG-TERM CARE

Community care is not only concerned with the treatment of patients during an acute phase of illness, but also with the follow-up of patients discharged from hospital and with the long-term care of the chronically disabled who do not require active medical treatment. Many community nurses are more frequently engaged in this work than in work with any other single group.

Community psychiatric nurses are employed in an attempt to prevent relapse into schizophrenic disorder of those who, on discharge from hospital, have been advised to continue taking the drugs which have helped to control the illness. A person who feels well may find it difficult to accept that his recovery is dependent on continued drug therapy and may be inclined to stop taking drugs. A nurse who visits the patient regularly can not only use persuasion to ensure that drug therapy is not discontinued, she can also spot very early symptoms recurring and alert the doctor. With the advent of the long-acting drugs, the nurse is advantageously placed in that she may administer these at regular intervals. If, as may happen, another member of the primary health care team gives the injection, or the patient receives his medication at a depot injection clinic, the community psychiatric nurse is still in a unique position to monitor possible side-effects of these antipsychotic drugs. She can be particularly vigilant if she has known the patient during his stay in hospital.

It has been suggested that previous acquaintance with the patient is the greatest asset the nurse can bring to the situation. It enables her to assess the patient's behaviour reliably, it allows her to use the same skills in her dealings with the patient which she has used in hospital. The patient and his family who are familiar with her may trust the nurse and consequently be able to accept her help more easily.

SOCIAL CARE

There are situations where a community psychiatric nurse may be required to establish contacts with a variety of agencies to help the patient. Lodgings may have to be found by giving explanations and help to landladies. Employers may need to be contacted. The patient may need help to obtain money or other material assistance. Though social workers may be best qualified to mobilize help for the patient, the nurse's relationship with the patient may make her more sensitive to his needs and more acceptable to him.

Patients without families or close friends may be helped to overcome their social isolation by attending a club established initially by the community psychiatric nurse.

To maintain a patient in the community appears a highly desirable objective. However, it should not be forgotten that any success community care may have is also due to the willingness of many relatives to sacrifice their energy, their freedom of movement and, in many cases, much of their income to the care of the patient. The continuous obligation to be available day and night can put an intolerable strain on relatives. It is extremely tiring and often unbearably aggravating to be continuously exposed to a psychogeriatric patient who incessantly asks the same question, never remembers where he put his belongings, who constantly fumbles with his possessions, who is unable to keep tidy. Wandering off, leaving doors open, leaving gas taps turned on and saucepans boiling dry are among hazards which demand incessant vigilance. If one adds to that disturbed nights and the possibility of incontinence, one can see how very difficult life can become for the relatives.

It often happens that relatives find the strength to continue after a visit from the community psychiatric nurse, who nowadays may be a specialist in the community care of the elderly mentally ill. It helps when they realize that their difficulties are understood and appreciated.

The community psychiatric nurse may arrange for the elderly person to attend a day hospital, or for temporary hospital admission to an intermittent care bed to give the relatives the strength to resume care later. Additionally, the nurse may suggest membership of the Alzheimer's Society at whose meetings members can give one another considerable support.

However, the value of community care should be seriously questioned when there is danger to the health of the relatives. The community psychiatric nurse can perform a valuable service if she offers support to relatives and if she helps them to hand over to the hospital the care of the patient, without guilt feelings and with a sense of trust in the hospital staff.

In the past few years the community psychiatric nurse's functions have expanded greatly. Originally her work was predominantly with the newly discharged psychotic patient. More recently, however, the community psychiatric nurse has been shown to be particularly effective in the use of communication skills on a one-to-one basis when following up patients in the community suffering from neurotic disorders. Behaviour therapy techniques, such as those employed to help the person with agoraphobia for example, are also included in the community psychiatric nurse's repertoire of specialist skills. The community psychiatric nurse's expertise is now widely recognized within the community and she may be called upon to give advice to other professionals.

Further reading

Carr, P.J., Butterworth, C.A. & Hodges, B.E. (1980) *Community Psychiatric Nursing*. Edinburgh: Churchill Livingstone.

Leff, J. & Vaughn, C. (1980) The interaction of life events and relatives' expressed emotions in schizophrenia and depressive neurosis. *British Journal of Psychiatry 136*, 146.

Paykell, E.S. & Griffith, J.H. (1983) *Community Psychiatric Nursing for Neurotic Patients*. London: Royal College of Nursing.

Pollock, L. (1982) Caring for themselves. *Nursing Times, Community Outlook 78* (6), 43.

Part 2
Nursing the Psychiatric Patient

5
The Therapeutic Environment

For those who require in-patient treatment, the psychiatric hospital provides not only nursing and medical care but, temporarily, also a home and security. The patient's treatment begins from the moment of admission into the therapeutic surroundings of the hospital.

Most patients, before admission, have lived through a period of tension and strain. The patient may have realized his increasing inability to adjust to the demands made by society, and after desperate attempts to cope may have broken down suddenly under the stress, or may gradually have understood the need for treatment.

The patient's family may also have been exposed to considerable strain. Often, as a patient's symptoms develop, he is subjected to comment, criticism and reproach. Gradually, as it becomes clear that he is ill and unable to control his behaviour, the relatives become worried and anxious. They watch suspiciously for further proof of insanity and consequently the patient becomes more irritable and tense. Eventually, as the need for the patient's admission to hospital becomes obvious, the relatives feel guilty and partially responsible for his breakdown, ashamed and emotionally disturbed.

The patient's arrival in hospital may mark the climax of an intensely disturbed home situation. The feeling of guilt, added to misconceptions about psychiatric hospitals, may have led the family to delay as long as possible the patient's admission. The actual removal to hospital is sometimes an unpleasant procedure; force may have to be used, or considerable effort expended in persuading the patient to enter hospital. In almost every case, admission to a psychiatric hospital represents a crisis in the patient's life and that of his family. In any crisis people are more able and willing to accept help if it is offered than they would at any other time. The way patients and their relatives are received into hospital is therefore a significant aspect of treatment.

The hospital must provide the environment suitable for the patient's needs. His illness makes it impossible for him to adapt himself to his environment, therefore in hospital the environment is adapted to the patient. Outside, he has reacted to specific stress by becoming ill; in hospital, stress can be removed or controlled so that the patient can learn to deal with it.

The psychiatric hospital must be able to adapt to all kinds of patients—the most helpless and those who have almost recovered, the most antisocial or withdrawn and the most excited and active. Each patient from the moment of admission should feel that the hospital can provide security and the kind of atmosphere in which recovery is possible.

Several factors combine to create the therapeutic atmosphere of the hospital. Among these are:
1   The structure and arrangement of the ward
2   The attitude of the staff
3   The morale of the ward community as a whole

THE STRUCTURE AND ARRANGEMENT OF THE WARDS

Most patients are pleasantly surprised to find that wards look more like home than hospital. In all wards the aim should be to create an atmosphere of warmth, comfort and relaxation. Colour, tastefully decorated rooms, attention to the arrangement of furniture, pictures and flowers help to give the ward a home-like atmosphere. Cleanliness and order are necessary, but should not deprive the patients of comfort.

In some hospitals it is the practice to arrange each ward differently, each suitable for one group of patients only, graded as to the amount of difficulty presented to the patient who moves from ward to ward as he improves or as his symptoms become worse.

This is not, however, the only way in which accommodation in hospital can be utilized. Some believe that it is beneficial for the patient to remain in one ward throughout his stay. This allows time for him to get to know the staff really well, and to form sound, enduring relationships with nurses and with other patients. It helps him to feel secure, because he knows that, whatever his behaviour, he will not be transferred and that the people looking after him are capable of helping. As he improves he can take an increasingly active part in caring for others and assuming responsibility for himself.

Where the opinion prevails that it is in the best interest of the patient to remain in one ward throughout his stay, the patient's age rather than the mental disorder may determine to which ward he is admitted. Where the hospital is very small or where there is a single psychiatric ward in a general hospital, it is inevitable that patients remain in one ward throughout their stay.

There are some advantages, however, in thinking of the hospital as a total community able to accommodate patients in different wards according to their need for protection or their ability, or otherwise, to act more independently. The patients readily see that the move to a more unrestricted environment represents progress and improvement.

Careful preparation is necessary to ensure that transfer from one ward to another proves to be therapeutic. The patient needs to prepare himself for the move, plan how to collect his belongings, inform his visitors and take leave from the patients with whom he shared a ward. A little party or other celebration may be a suitable way to mark the occasion. He may wish to become acquainted with the staff and patients of his new ward before the move is actually made and he may wish to retain some contact with the staff and patients of the ward he is leaving by promising frequent return visits.

Unfortunately, while it is beneficial to the patient to feel he is progressing when he moves to a ward offering more scope and responsibility, it is distressing for him to be aware of a relapse when a move in the reverse direction is necessary. It requires considerable skill to convey to the patient that different wards are neither better nor worse, but just more suitable to help patients at specific stages of illness.

Great care must be taken never to give the impression that transfer to another ward might be used as a form of punishment, or to allow any stigma to become associated with a ward for disturbed patients. Patients who have improved after a very disturbed phase of illness often live in dread of a relapse, afraid of losing control once again. The added fear of being moved to a ward reputed to be unpleasant cannot be helpful to the patient.

Size of wards

The size of wards is of significance in the treatment of the patient.

While he is very ill, helpless or disturbed, he may benefit from a small ward where he is exposed to only a few people and where it is easy to comprehend the physical layout. The patient may derive a considerable feeling of security from the knowledge that he is physically safe and always accompanied by a dependable person whom he knows well.

As the patient improves, the space he occupies can be enlarged. Bedroom, dayroom, dining-room, kitchen and bathrooms become accessible to him. Within the precincts of the ward and ward garden the patient may be free to explore. He may be able to make his own decisions as to where he spends his time. Contact with more patients and an opportunity of trying to establish friendships, assuming leadership or making other social relationships may lead towards independence.

Before the patient's discharge is considered, he requires yet more complex surroundings. As part of a rehabilitation programme, the patient may move to a ward almost independent of any supervision by nursing staff; a ward where he and his fellow patients cook and carry out all domestic skills with the minimum of help. Far from being shut in, the patient should have full opportunity to move freely within the hospital and in the neighbourhood. He should use his own discretion about going into the nearby village or town and to visit his friends and family.

In order to cater for all patients the psychiatric hospital should be large enough to have all the facilities required in a community, but not so large that the patient feels out of touch with part of his environment. Hospitals of 100 to 300 beds have been found to be of greatest benefit. Such hospitals are large enough to have suitable wards for patients of all kinds. Ground floor wards might be provided for the old and infirm who need direct access from ward to garden. Small, sheltered, enclosed gardens should be available for those who are disturbed. Sports facilities should exist for those who can benefit from exercise. There should be workshops catering for diverse needs, work available from the simplest to the most complex types, with working conditions as near normal as possible for those about to be discharged, but able also to give the most sheltered employment to those who need it.

A community centre may be of advantage, a large entertainment hall for special occasions, smaller rooms for more informal social occasions, rooms for organized gatherings and rooms where men and women can mix in an informal manner. Library, reading-rooms, shop and canteen can be most valuable additions to hospital amenities.

Before discharge from hospital the patient's environment should be widened to include the local community, traffic and contact with people outside. The patient can then lead a full life organized by himself. He meets plenty of people and relies on his own initiative in associating with them. Facilities for hobbies and entertainments are provided, but it is left to the patient to decide how they are used. He should feel responsible for the care of the ward and be invited to interest himself in the welfare of others and to make suggestions for the running of the hospital. In short, the hospital is a training ground, albeit a safer one than the outside world, for life in the community.

ATTITUDE OF STAFF

In order to make the best possible use of the facilities of the hospital the nurses need to understand fully the aim of treatment and the reasons why the hospital is used in the way it is. The patients' attitude to treatment may well depend on the attitude conveyed by nurses.

In a few hospitals the ward for the most disturbed patients is kept locked. This is distressing to many patients though a few feel more secure and protected in a closed ward. The patient's relatives may find it difficult to accept the need for locked doors and it may increase their feelings of guilt and distress to think of the patient as 'locked away'.

The hospital's responsibility towards the community and for the safety of helpless and potentially dangerous patients must be recognized. Many psychiatrists and nurses believe that they can fulfil their responsibilities without resorting to the locking of doors. Increased skill in observation, a greater degree of patient participation in the management of the ward, and a programme of active occupational therapy help them to give adequate attention to those patients who are known to be in danger of wandering away or who might behave dangerously if they were permitted to leave.

Others believe, however, that the security of locked doors permits the nursing staff to give all their attention to active treatment rather than to custodial care.

In order to enable the majority of patients to benefit from an 'open door policy' a few secure units have been set up in various parts of the country. Within such units it is hoped to provide the patient with maximum freedom compatible with the fact that access to other parts of the hospital or to the outside needs to be restricted.

In a locked ward patients may become extremely disturbed. Excitement, anger and possibly violence may result from the frustrating experience of being locked in; and patients who might otherwise be quite willing to accept treatment become determined to leave the ward. Patients may develop resentment towards the nurse who holds the key and even the most unobtrusive handling of keys and the greatest care in preventing noise of locking and unlocking may result in casting the nurse in the role of custodial authority. The nurse's positive attitude is of cardinal importance if the closed ward is to be used therapeutically.

The newly admitted patient

The nurses' attitudes are also of great importance to new patients. Many patients feel extremely apprehensive about entering hospital. Some have heard rumours of ill-treatment, some are afraid that, once in the hospital, they will be there for ever, some simply fear the stigma of the psychiatric hospital and are convinced that their friends and relatives will despise them for having been admitted. Many patients, despite explanations from their doctor, are certain that mental health is simply a matter of willpower, and they despise themselves for having 'given in' instead of 'pulling themselves together'. If the nurses can succeed in creating a happy, warm, hopeful atmosphere, confident, relaxed, yet purposive, patients can soon be convinced that their decision to enter hospital was the right one.

Some patients, on arrival in hospital, are worried by the sight of patients more disturbed than they are themselves. However, the opportunity to observe the kind way in which another patient is being helped by a nurse is often most reassuring. It is important to learn that the nurses can remain calmly in control when other patients become disturbed. It may help the patient to feel sufficient confidence in the staff to risk letting go of his self-control for a while, and this may be a necessary preliminary to successful treatment.

Patients sometimes complain that very little is being done for them in hospital. This is because they fail to understand how the experience of living in a ward which has just the right kind of atmosphere for recovery can be part of 'treatment'. Explanations do little to convince the patient. Even so, it is necessary that the nurses themselves should be clear about the effect of atmosphere and should understand how they themselves are responsible for engendering therapeutic rather than anti-therapeutic attitudes.

Some nurses find it easy to understand patients who are very ill. They can readily maintain a calm and accepting attitude in the face of even the most disturbed behaviour. But when patients begin to improve nurses sometimes become irritable and intolerant. (More will be said about patient–nurse interaction later in the book.)

When a patient is very ill the constraints of firm rules and regular routine may be helpful, but they become irksome as the patient improves. It is essential that the patient should be enabled to experiment with freedom and responsibility as he gains independence and self-confidence. These experiments are not always entirely successful and some attempt may have to be made to exert control. But if nurses enforce discipline in an authoritarian manner, the patient's recovery can be very much delayed.

A new patient can feel very bewildered by the many new experiences of admission to the psychiatric hospital. Though he may need to ask many questions, he may feel unable to give voice to any of them, because he feels embarrassed, insecure and unable to know which of the many people he meets could be asked. In some cases the remedy may lie in admitting the patient to a small ward unit where he will find only very few people to whom he can easily be introduced. If the patient goes to bed when he first arrives, he is spared the embarrassment of moving around and introducing himself. Instead, staff and patients approach the patient one by one. If each person who speaks to the patient introduces himself, the patient can very quickly be helped to feel that he belongs.

It is, however, emphasizing the patient's dependence and illness if he is asked to go to bed soon after arrival in hospital. In many instances it seems more desirable to emphasize the normal healthy aspects of ward life. This can be done more easily if a fellow patient, rather than a nurse, takes on the role of host and is responsible for introductions, explanations and orientation.

Whatever admission procedure is adopted it must be recognized that every new patient has many unspoken fears and anxieties. The nurses' attitude will either assist the patient to ask, or it will stop all questioning.

Nothing the patient wants to know is too trivial for discussion, but the patient cannot always formulate his problems clearly. At the early stage of a patient's stay in hospital, answers to his questions may not in fact be known, but that should not prevent the patient from asking.

What is appreciated by patients is a nurse who has time to listen and whose attitude suggests that she would like to know more clearly what is worrying the patient.

Whenever an answer is possible it should be frank and clear. But hasty answers, before questions are fully expressed, merely serve to convince the patient of the futility of asking.

Some patients may have heard rumours of ill-treatment. They cannot put into words the question they would like to ask. For example: 'How are these people going to treat me? Are they as kind as they look? Can they be trusted? Are they competent? What will they think of me when they realize how bad I am?' Instead of asking these questions patients may put the nurses to the test, becoming, for example, either mute or hostile and aggressive.

The best way of convincing the patient of his nurse's interest in him is by her being interested. He must be convinced that his abnormal behaviour, which is the reason for his admission to hospital, is considered neither shameful nor wicked. The patient must never be condemned or ridiculed. The non-critical attitude of the staff may help him to relax and so recovery may be hastened. However inappropriate or disturbed the patient's behaviour, he must feel that he is accepted and wanted in the ward.

The nurse should convey to the patient that she considers all the information she obtains from or about him as being strictly confidential. It may be a great relief to patients and relatives that nothing about his illness will be known to anyone, except those concerned with treatment.

Many of the patient's actions during the worst phases of his illness are capable of leading later to considerable embarrassment. Some of the information which psychiatrists, and sometimes nurses, receive about the patient's private life is divulged with the greatest misgivings. The patient must be able to rely on the integrity of every member of the staff as to the observance of the necessary confidentiality.

MORALE OF THE WARD COMMUNITY AS A WHOLE

It is impossible to over-emphasize the importance of harmony amongst all members of the staff. There is no simple way of telling nurses how to get on with each other. A harmonious ward is the result of every individual working to the best of his ability with the interest of the patients at heart. Harmony results from a confidence that all are capable of coping with difficult situations, and that the efforts of one are appreciated by the others. It is the result of mutual confidence and trust. When the staff work in harmony with each other, the patients' behaviour usually presents very few problems, and those nursing problems that do arise are easily settled.

In every working community friction occasionally arises and usually results from personality clashes. In psychiatric nursing it arises more commonly from differences of opinion about the correct method of nursing the patient, and the latter becomes anxious because it affects him so intimately. Careful observation of the incidence of excitement in disturbed wards has shown very clearly the relationship between patients' anxieties and disagreement among staff.

Whenever difficulties arise in the ward it is worthwhile to examine the attitude of staff members to each other, and to have a free discussion about the way each feels. Exchange of opinion about the correct manner of handling a situation is possible only if each nurse feels secure in her relationships with the others. Inevitably mistakes are sometimes made; often there is an awareness of the wrong thing having been said to a patient. These mistakes can be discussed and their repetition avoided only if no nurse feels personally insulted or criticized. Sometimes the feeling of envy at another nurse's success, or of frustration at individual inability to make contact with a patient, may lead to staff tensions.

Some patients create ill-feeling among nurses by playing them off against each other, criticizing one nurse in the presence of another, making each feel that the other gives more attention. Free and open discussion among staff, and if possible between the patient and the staff, can bring this to light and can help to increase the patient's confidence in the treatment team.

For many patients the continuous support of the nurse represents the first sign of friendship in what appears to be a hostile world. Admission to the hospital may mark the end of a period of loneliness and the beginning of social participation in which the other patients as well as the staff have a vital part to play.

In the opening chapters it has been shown that some mental illness can be regarded as a failure in adjustment to social change. Difficulties in work, leisure activities and social contacts with friends and relations represent the main problems with which the psychiatrically ill person has to deal.

Irrespective of the specific diagnosis of a patient, the aim of treatment may often be to restore or to enhance the patient's ability to cope with changing circumstances of his life.

The psychiatric hospital provides the training ground within which the patient can learn to form healthier relationships with people and to modify his behaviour where appropriate.

In-patient therapy, even when it is intended to be of physical or psychotherapeutic nature, takes place in the social environment of the ward and the hospital. When that environment is therapeutic the patient's progress is often quite dramatic. When a therapeutic environment is not created patients fail to progress.

The greatest contribution the psychiatric nurse has to offer lies in the ability to create the social climate in which the patient can get well. In the chapters which follow it will be shown how this might be achieved.

Further reading

Goffman, E. (1970) *Asylums*. Harmondsworth, Middlesex: Penguin.
Towell, D. & Harries, C. (1979) *Innovations in Patient Care*. London: Croom Helm.

6
The Significance of Routine

Routine is an important stabilizing factor in life. It is well known that children become unhappy when their familiar routine is disturbed.

Nurses derive great security from knowing the routine of the ward in which they work and feel disturbed each time they move to another ward, until the new routine is mastered.

Ward routine is important to patients too, and if it is adjusted to the special needs of the patients, it plays an important part in therapy.

In order to understand the value of the established routine to any particular patient, the nurse should know something about the life led by patients in their own homes. Some will have led a very well-regulated life prior to admission. They may have been slaves to routine, and punctuality may have been the keynote of their lives. Some obsessional patients, for instance, have spent much time and energy arranging time-tables and organizing themselves and others. Difficulties of adhering to the schedules may have been major factors in the development of the illness. While some patients may have always worried about routine, others may never have adhered to any form of time-table. Some patients have never been sufficiently independent to organize their own lives, others have never been sufficiently concerned with the rules of society to consider other people.

Ward routine must therefore be planned according to the patient's individual problems.

Should the routine be inflexible or is it advisable to allow some variation?

For some patients it is essential that routine be firmly established, for example for the elderly person whose intellectual functions are deteriorating. Many have become insecure and anxious because they have failed to keep up with changes in their home circumstances. Some have succeeded in disrupting the home by their illness. The fact that hospital routine is stable and not dependent on the patient's behaviour may do much to aid recovery. To know that the immediate environment is predictable, that it is independent of the patient's own actions, may be most reassuring in the early stages of his illness.

It is essential, however, that variation in routine should occur sometimes to avoid boredom.

People have not only a daily but also a weekly routine. If all the days of the week resemble each other, time becomes difficult to measure. It is important that Sundays should be different from weekdays and preferable that each day of the week should be marked by some special event. The weekly menu, or the favourite TV programme, or the evening entertainment can help to differentiate between days. Shopping days or a ward outing can mark the highlight of the week.

To what extent should the routine be arranged for the patient, and to what extent should the patients be responsible for their own arrangements?
In some wards, a number of arrangements must be made by the staff. Patients, however, need to know what these are.

A clock and a calendar are of course essential items of ward equipment. Time-tables are made out and posted on the wall. Everybody sees at a glance what they should do at different times of the day. Work is distributed, a rota made out, nothing left to chance. This may be very helpful initially for an anxious or obsessional patient, and it may be of help to some withdrawn schizophrenic patients who would otherwise be inactive, hiding where nobody would pay attention to them. But it would not be a good preparation for resuming responsibilities outside hospital.

So, in other wards, only the bare skeleton of the ward routine is rigid. Meal-times are the usual landmarks, but everything else is left to the patients to arrange. Time-tables may be made out by the patients at ward meetings, or some patients may be entrusted with a particular section of routine, e.g. the arrangements for ward cleaning, or the organization for serving meals or for entertainments.

In some wards, no formal arrangements are made, division of labour evolves as a natural process and by mutual agreement among patients.

The nurse's role varies considerably in these different types of routine. She may become an elected leader, or she may become a member of the group, indistinguishable in function, as far as ward routine is concerned, from the patients themselves. She should know what is expected of her in the ward in which she is working, and she should be able to sustain this part and cope with the anxieties she encounters in those patients who have difficulties in adapting themselves.

Patients who move from ward to ward sometimes react very strongly the first time they are expected to make their own decisions. They may look to the nurse for guidance and become hostile or disturbed when they do not receive it. This can be anticipated and dealt with by adequate preparation of the patient and by the nurse who properly understands her function in this type of ward. A nurse who does not thoroughly understand this either becomes upset by the patients' criticism, or, as a result of her own insecurity, critical of the nurse in charge. Only frequent discussion of the problems at issue at staff meetings can help the nurse to maintain her proper position.

How important is it that patients should adhere to routine? How much initiative on the part of the patient should be encouraged?

Every now and then patients who break hospital rules are encountered. They come in late from pass, or they go out without letting anyone know. They are late for meals, or stay in bed longer than others. They decide to stay away from occupations or disapprove of the entertainment organized for them. In short, they rebel. Nurses often become disturbed by this type of behaviour. Their problem is how to persuade the patient to conform, but often they omit to ask whether it is essential for him to do so. Might it not be a good thing if the patient shows a little independence?

It should never be forgotten that the aim and purpose of treatment is not to create docile hospital residents, but to help patients to deal adequately with an infinite variety of difficulties in life outside the hospital walls. A little experimentation is essential if the patient is to succeed. This does not mean that hospital routine should be discarded, or that persistent breaking of hospital rules should be condoned. The nurse, however, is better equipped to deal with the problem if it is seen as a welcome sign of growing independence. Often the first attempt of a patient to break a rule is merely tentative. He may be afraid of the consequences. It would be all too easy to prevent any further show of a growing sense of self-confidence if the first attempt were dealt with tactlessly. All that is required is a willingness to find out why the patient behaved as he did and, instead of showing indignation, to try to get the patient to understand why the rule is necessary and why it must be kept.

Among other difficulties, the patient must learn to cope with the displeasure of the staff, e.g. the nurse in charge. It is perfectly all right to show disapproval of an action, provided the patient knows that the nurse is as interested as ever in him and his welfare, that he is accepted and valued, in spite of the fact that an individual act could not be permitted. A great deal, however, depends on the way in which the patient is censured, and on its timing. It is essential for nurses to plan what are to be their reactions to the breaking of rules. No two patients require the same approach. Spontaneous anger or indignation is rarely helpful and criticism should be resorted to only when it is known that the patient is well enough to tolerate it. Otherwise a different ward, with different routines, may be necessary for a patient who persistently violates the conventions of the one he is in.

7
The Nursing Process

Nursing care for patients in psychiatric wards follows the stages often referred to as the 'nursing process': assessment, planning of care, delivery of care, evaluation.

This chapter is concerned mainly with the first stage, that of assessment. Later chapters will deal with the various ways in which care is delivered, not only by nurses but by all the other people who are involved, for example doctors, occupational therapists, social workers, the patient's relatives, employers, employees, friends, visitors and fellow patients.

Assessment is a method of collecting information about a patient, evaluating and interpreting this information.

It is necessary to reflect on the issues involved in this part of the process of care. Information is always collected for a purpose—without a purpose, information gathering is not only wasteful of time, it is also an intrusion into a person's privacy. To gather information for a purpose means that one is selective, collecting only that information which is relevant to the purpose for which it is to be used.

There are serious difficulties, however, in making the choice of what information is relevant. A large number of factors enter into such selection.

The first factors which one may have to consider are the questions of who else is collecting information, to what extent other people's purpose in collecting information is the same or different, and whether some of the information may be able to be used for more than one purpose.

The psychiatrist always collects information by taking a detailed history from the patient. This is likely to take many hours, frequently spread over several sessions. In the course of history taking, the patient often becomes aware of the significance of life events which he had never thought of as significant. Neither the psychiatrist nor the patient can know in advance which aspect of the history will turn out to be important. In psychotherapy the process of reviewing the patient's history is part of the therapeutic intervention itself, as the development of insight is the essential basis for change.

The history which the psychiatrist takes is preceded by the collection of some information by the patient's own general practitioner or any other doctor who has referred the patient. Some of this information will be in the referral letter or in case notes which accompany the patient.

The issue which the nurse must address before she embarks on the assessment stage of the nursing process is whether or not she should, on the one hand, repeat the activity of interviewing the patient to obtain some of his history, or, on the other hand, consult the patient's records and ask the psychiatrist to share with her some of the information he has obtained.

It should be remembered that, at the time of admission, it is unlikely that the patient would be aware of the significance or relevance of many of the questions to which he is asked to reply. Resentment is likely to arise if he is asked repeatedly to reply to questions which may seem needlessly intrusive. On the other hand, patients are entitled to regard information given to a doctor as confidential. Some patients will divulge information to a doctor which until then had been jealously guarded as private and secret. It would never have been entrusted to the doctor if the patient had thought that it might be accessible to others.

In psychiatric care, teamwork between staff of different disciplines is important. Its value will not, however, be evident to the patient at the time of admission. Sharing of information should not, therefore, occur without the full knowledge and permission of the patient.

Another issue which must be considered is the fact that it is difficult, if not impossible, to be neutral while one collects information about the patient. An observer always has an effect on the person observed. The patient may hide some things and exaggerate others. It is impossible for an interviewer to pursue every opening offered to him, and he therefore selects certain points for further enquiry and omits others. How much a patient reveals depends on the empathy he perceives. Much of the information which needs to be obtained could be deeply disturbing to the nurse. Whether she can cope with such information depends on the extent to which she has learnt to develop self-awareness and to cope with disturbing aspects of her own personality. The patient is certain to observe the nurse for her reaction to what is revealed. If the patient notices that the nurse feels hurt, upset, disgusted, disapproving, there will be an immediate censorship in what is being revealed. Often nurses who begin to be disturbed by the information the patient provides change the subject or cut the patient off, thus distorting the assessment of the patient.

Doctors who practise psychoanalytic psychotherapy are required to have undergone a personal analysis themselves in order to ensure that they have dealt with their own emotional problems before they are exposed to those of their patients. To require that all doctors and nurses should have undergone such preparation is unrealistic and unnecessary. However, it is important for nurses to develop adequate self-awareness in order to be able to monitor their own reactions to patients' problems and to keep them under control.

The extent to which a patient is able to open up and permit the nurse to assess his problems depends in many disorders on whether he perceives the nurse to be genuinely interested and concerned. Empathy with a patient and liking for a patient arise spontaneously on first contact and determine to some extent how the assessment progresses. The feeling nurse and patient have for each other may later be modified, but at the beginning whether people take to each other depends on such factors as age, physical appearance, sex, social class and previous experience. Patients may like nurses of their own age, sex and social class but they may confide more easily in those who differ from them.

In research one attempts to eliminate all those factors which might result in biased data collection. In the assessment of a patient early in the process of nursing this is not possible, but awareness of the sources of bias is essential.

Another issue to be taken into account is that the collection of information during assessment is to some extent regulated by the theoretical framework in which one is operating. Theoretical knowledge helps one to organize one's observations and to ask questions, the answers to which will help to complete the picture.

While assessing the patient's physical fitness, for example, the theoretical knowledge the nurse has of the physiology of respiration helps her to notice the patient's breathlessness while talking or moving, guides her to enquire about the patient's usual tolerance of exertion, and prompts her to restrict conversation in order not to exhaust the patient.

In psychiatric nursing it is not always clear what theoretical framework is relevant as an organizing principle during assessment. To some extent, information about the patient's early life may be of importance, but how much so cannot be known at the beginning. To some extent a consideration of biological causation or social causation of psychiatric disorder is relevant, but such relevance cannot be evaluated in advance. There is no reason for accepting any of the current so-called theories of nursing as particularly useful in psychiatric nursing. Peplau distinguished between interpersonal and intrapersonal theories to guide understanding of patients' emotional problems, but which of these is applicable to a particular patient cannot be known in advance of the assessment stage.

It may be that a systems approach to the collection of information and to the delivery of nursing care is best suited for psychiatric nursing.

A system is thought of as a collection of items, for example people, events, objects or ideas which are examined for the relationship they have with each other and the way they affect each other. A system does not have an existence of its own, it is created by the person who wishes to analyse a particular situation. A 'boundary' is drawn around the system and everything not included in the system for the moment is referred to as the environment. A system is thought of as having an 'output'.

In psychiatric patients, disordered 'output' is the reason for seeking help. The observer attempts to assess what 'inputs' from the environment of the system affect the way the system works and which specific inputs affect output adversely.

In psychiatric nursing it is possible at one period, perhaps on admission of the patient, to concern oneself with the patient, his symptoms, his feelings and his behaviour only, putting the boundary within the patient and placing all staff, including oneself, all other patients and all the patient's usual social contacts, into the environment. At a later stage it may seem relevant to include the ward staff and fellow patients in the system, at a later stage still to include the patient's family.

A systems approach does not imply or exclude any theory about the nature of mental disorder, it is a way of trying to organize thinking about the very complex situation which has to be assessed.

Assessment serves the purpose of making appropriate plans for nursing care, designed to help the patient overcome the difficulties he is encountering. Assessment, planning, delivery of care and evaluation of the outcome are closely related. If the outcome is unfavourable, one must retrace one's step and find out whether care was properly carried out according to plan, whether the plan itself was faulty, or whether assessment had been inaccurate.

In principle this is very simple. In practice the nursing process in psychiatric nursing is not at all simple. Reasons for this can be found at every stage of the process. It may be useful to look at the last stage first.

Outcome

Patients may recover spontaneously, without any treatment at all. Recovery after treatment can therefore not necessarily be attributed to treatment. There is some danger that forms of treatment or care are perpetuated without any conclusive evidence of beneficial effect. The use of psychotherapy, for example, has been criticized on these grounds by some psychologists. Some physical treatments, for example insulin coma therapy, which in the past had been thought to be beneficial, were later shown to be ineffective.

Intervention stage

It is very difficult to isolate the effect of any one part of what happens to patients while they are in hospital from the others. To evaluate nursing care one would need to know not only what nurses had been doing but what, at the same time, the patient himself had been doing, for example what he had been reading; what other professional staff, for example the psychiatrist or the occupational therapist, had been doing. One would need to know what the influence of other patients or of the patient's relatives and friends had been.

Psychiatric illness is always of long duration, at least in comparison with many physical disorders. It develops over a long period, has multiple causation, manifests itself over a period of time in variable intensity and with shifting symptomatology. Nursing and other intervention may be needed for a relatively long period. The cumulative effect of the effort of several people over a long period may result in improvement, while the effect of any short-term intervention by any one person may appear to be insignificant. It is sometimes easy to spot immediately the negative effect of some ill-conceived intervention, while the success of beneficial effective intervention may not be so easily evaluated.

To some nurses, work with psychiatrically ill patients seems unrewarding, because they cannot obtain an immediate feedback about the effectiveness of their care.

PLANNING CARE

One must be realistic in the care which is planned for a patient. Resources for what one intends to provide must be at least potentially available. It is no use planning to give each patient several hours of undivided attention unless the necessary staff can be found to do this. It is pointless to plan to give some drug which has not yet been invented. On the other hand, resources may be available if only one knew how to mobilize them. There are, for example, many patients unnecessarily immobilized because suitable walking aids, wheelchairs or hoists are not used. These aids for the disabled do exist and can be obtained providing the staff who care for the patient know about their existence and how to obtain them.

To know what resources exist and how to mobilize them for any particular patient is one of the responsibilities of the nurse. It means that nurses must accept responsibility for keeping themselves up to date and must make determined efforts to continue their education.

In previous chapters it was shown that some of the resources which need to be considered are concerned with everyday living, with the physical, emotional and social environment of the patient. How the patient spends his time and what opportunities can be offered to the patient for choosing the way he spends his time are other considerations.

It would be a useful exercise for the reader to make a list of all the things he does in the course of a day and then compare them with what a particular patient does with his day. If there are large differences, the nurse should ask herself whether this is to the patient's advantage or disadvantage. In preparing a nursing care plan it is necessary to ask how different the patient's life in hospital needs to be compared with what is for him a normal day. For many psychiatrically ill patients, it is difficult to establish when their days were last normal. Their lifestyle may have changed slowly and insidiously, and a return to what was once a normal way of living may no longer be appropriate.

It has been suggested that the treatment of a psychiatrically ill patient within hospital rather than within his own community can only be justified if the daily living experience in the ward is used therapeutically.

Opportunities for using life in the ward therapeutically arise in relation to:

the patient's activities surrounding his personal hygiene;
the patient's consumption of food and drink;
elimination;
the patient's concern for personal appearance, hair, make-up, clothing;
the patient's ability to maintain his environment in a clean and tidy state;
the patient's cycle of work, rest, relaxation and sleep;
his pursuit of interests and hobbies;
the patient's educational pursuits;
his relationships with people in different situations, for example with male and female fellow patients of the same age as he is or older or younger;
the patient's relationship with staff of different disciplines and different degrees of closeness to the patient;
the extent to which the patient can retain or establish contacts with family and friends and can retain or establish responsibility for others;
the way in which he can try to cope with stressful or unpleasant situations.

Life in hospital can, of course, offer opportunities for therapeutic intervention for any physical complaint the patient may suffer from. Individual or group treatment with psychologists, nurses or others as the main therapist are available.

No patient needs every kind of therapeutic intervention which may be available. The purpose of the nursing plan is to identify what problems exist for the patient, what help he would like to have, and what help it may be appropriate to offer.

In summary, one can only plan nursing care if one knows, on the one hand, what the total range of intervention is from which a selection can be made, and on the other hand, what are the problems for which the patient seeks help or is willing to accept help. To identify the latter is what assessment is about.

ASSESSMENT

Assessment in psychiatric nursing cannot be carried out in one session on admission. Much of the information the nurse is seeking cannot be available until the patient has had the opportunity to participate in the daily life of the ward, to respond and to react to the people around him.

It is impossible in psychiatric nursing to delay giving care until a full assessment has been made. The care plan and intervention may have to be based initially on inadequate information. How the patient responds and reacts to the intervention then becomes part of the assessment.

For example, it may not be possible to know that the patient has difficulty in rising from a chair until he has been observed attempting to do so in response to the invitation to go to the dining room for lunch. It may not be possible to know that the patient feels angry about the way he has been treated by his children until a topic related to family dynamics has cropped up in a group meeting. It may be impossible to avoid talking about a subject which may cause the patient to be upset. Only after one has broached the subject can one know that it upsets him. For example, if the patient has attempted to hit a nurse or a fellow patient, one knows what was liable to anger him. Without having taken the risk of upsetting the patient, one would not have known.

In the next part of this chapter, methods of obtaining information about the patient during his stay in hospital will be discussed in more detail.

OBSERVATION

Because all observation is selective, it is important to be aware of the way one's expectations, attention, preoccupation and knowledge affect what is observed. It may be useful to compare observations of different nurses, paying particular attention to observations borne out by others, and to investigate reasons for conflicting observations.

Normal development and cultural differences in normal behaviour

A knowledge of normal behaviour patterns in different cultural groups is essential. What is accepted as normal behaviour differs with social class, with different educational background, and with nationality. It is important to observe to what extent the patient's behaviour deviates from that accepted by his own group. Without a background knowledge of sociology there is danger that the nurse's own social class and educational background may bias her observations. Where nurses and patients come from different countries, particularly if they do not share a language, special care is needed to make observation valid.

Psychopathology and symptomatology of psychiatric disorder

The nurse should be acquainted with the patterns of abnormal behaviour and their incidence in various psychiatric disorders. A knowledge of psychology and of psychiatric illness may help to detect the earliest manifestations of disorder, when these may well be atypical and different in each patient. Many disturbances can be avoided if nurses become sensitive to the earliest signs of anxiety in the patients.

It is important, however, to be aware of the effect of 'labelling' a patient. Once a patient has a diagnostic label attached, for example schizophrenia or psychopathic personality disorder, the nurse may believe that she observes symptoms which in reality are not there, or, on the other hand, the patient may display symptoms which he considers to be in keeping with his diagnosis—behaving in a disturbed way because it is expected of him.

Participant observation and observer effect

The nurse should be with the patient for sufficient time to be able to report on the total picture he presents. Only if she knows him intimately can she observe minor variations in behaviour.

The nurse should not disturb the patient by her presence. This means that she must be in the ward so much that her presence is taken for granted and that she is sufficiently unobtrusive for patients to behave as if she were not there at all. It is easiest to observe the patient's behaviour if one joins in all the activities. If the nurse supervises passively, doing nothing while the patient is expected to take part in some ward activity, her presence may be resented and the impression she gains then becomes distorted. If she comes and goes, she disturbs the patient's activities and cannot really observe.

Objectivity

Objectivity is impossible to achieve. However, in order to attain a certain degree of objectivity, it is important that the nurse does not allow herself to become disturbed or frightened by the patient's behaviour, or shocked or angry. Her interest in his recovery should not make her emotionally biased. She should not feel flattered at, or proud of, his improvement, since this might lead her to see improvements where there are none. One of the reasons why relatives are sometimes unreliable informants is their inability to remain emotionally detached. Close emotional contact with the patient, though often desirable, interferes with objective observation.

Bias and selectivity

The nurse should remember to observe not only the patient, but the situation in which the patient finds himself. To do this is relatively easy when the nurse's observation concerns the interaction between several patients, or that between the patient and another nurse. It is much more difficult if the nurse is observing an incident in which she herself has participated. The patient's behaviour which she observes may then be a reaction to her own words, actions or gestures. It may require considerable mental effort to report such behaviour not as it appeared to her, but as she imagines it might have appeared to a third person. Her own part in the interaction needs to be reported as well as the patient's.

Reporting

Recording observed facts and interpretation of facts

Although it is impossible to observe the patient's behaviour without to some extent interpreting or making guesses about underlying motives and forming judgements about his personality, it is essential that observed facts should be reported, and not merely opinions; or at least that, when opinions are given, these should provide some indication of the facts on which they are based. It is important for the nurse to remember that both ward reports and individual case notes might have to be produced in court at some time in the future, therefore accuracy in reporting facts is essential.

Good reporting

Clichés should, as far as possible, be avoided. Such words as 'pleasant and co-operative' mean nothing unless it is stated who finds the patient pleasant and for what reason, and what were the tasks in which the patient was expected to co-operate. 'Unco-operative', again, describes the relationship between the patient and someone else. It is important to know with whom he refused to co-operate, and what attempts were made to persuade him to do so.

Some expressions, such as 'bizarre behaviour' or 'incoherent speech', are meaningful to a certain extent, because they are used by most people to apply to the same kinds of phenomena. Nevertheless, definite examples are better than the mere statement that the nurse failed to understand the patient.

There should be some plan for carrying out and recording observations, in order to ensure significant aspects of the patient's behaviour are not missed and that the total picture becomes available rather than one distorted by the highlighting of episodes. There are many useful ways of arranging observations in categories under a variety of headings. One possible method is to consider all the various situations covered in a 24-hour period, and to list the activities in which observations can be made.

OPPORTUNITIES FOR OBSERVATION

At night

Sleeping with a number of other people in a ward is a comparatively infrequent experience for many patients, and entirely new to others. The patient's attitude to this and to being under observation, as well as how deeply and how long he sleeps, should be recorded.

In the morning

Observation should be made of the grooming habits of the patient and of his reaction to the still fairly public facilities afforded for this in many hospitals.

At meals

Much can be learned of the patient's social and cultural standards by observation at table, and discussion of the food served can provide a great deal of information about the attitudes and expectations of the patient.

Work

Work in the hospital setting can take many forms, ranging from the simplest domestic ward tasks to structured attendance at an industrial therapy unit. The attitude displayed by the patient in this context can provide information on his standards, perseverance, ability to work alone, and leadership qualities.

Leisure

A range of recreational activities is provided in almost all psychiatric hospitals and it can be most informative to observe the interest or lack of it taken by the patient in these: which, if any, of the entertainments provided appeal to the patient, as also his choice of reading material from the hospital library can form a natural basis for conversation.

Visiting

The anticipation with which visiting times are regarded and the reactions of the patient and his visitors while they are together can be revealing to the observant nurse. It is probable that more can be learned about the state of family and interpersonal relationships in the time just before and just after relatives and friends have visited than by attempting to probe these at any other time of the day.

Unusual events

The patient's behaviour on being admitted to hospital, his attitude to staff and other patients, to hospital life and hospital rules are points of significance. Later his approach to newly admitted patients, to unusual incidents in the ward, to a change of nursing staff, to transfer to another ward, are all matters of interest. Christmas festivities, sports day, a coach outing, may provide opportunities for observing hitherto unknown facts.

Observation of physical symptoms

Some incidence of physical illness is present at all times in any large psychiatric hospital, and the nurse must be alert to the dangers of dismissing any physical complaint by the patient as having its origin in the mental disturbance which brought him into hospital. Many mentally ill patients complain incessantly of their physical ailments so that it is only too easy, after several investigations, to dismiss the complaints as a function of the mental illness. It may then be found, perhaps too late, that a report of a physical symptom had been based on physical illness. Others may be organically ill without making any complaint, and only acute observation and vigilance on the part of the nurse will elicit the information which has, consciously or otherwise, been withheld.

Although it is rare for the recording of TPR to be carried out as a routine measure in mental hospitals, other precautionary procedures may be carried out regularly. These include weighing the patient, where any marked variation from the previous recording should be reported, and regular urine testing, which is particularly important in connection with certain drug therapies.

Many patients are capable of bathing alone and should be encouraged to do so, but an opportunity for observation of the physical condition can be achieved by offering help with this, when any variation from the last-recorded state can be noted and reported.

It has already been mentioned that appetite and elimination should be observed in relation to the patient's attitudes towards these functions, but any abnormality, such as discomfort on swallowing, vomiting after meals, or alternating diarrhoea and constipation, may be indications of physical disease and should be investigated without delay.

Amenorrhoea may be entirely without significance, since it is a fairly common feature of psychotic illness, but a record of menstruation may be useful, if only for the early detection of pregnancy. The presence of any vaginal discharge, particularly in elderly patients, may be symptomatic of uterine disease or vaginal infection which should be treated without delay. It is important for the psychiatric nurse to be thoroughly familiar with the signs and symptoms which may result from the administration of psychotropic drugs. Nausea and vomiting may arise as a side-effect of the prescribed drug and should be reported to the medical staff. It should be borne in mind that an apparently trivial sore throat may be the preliminary stage of agranulocytosis (see Chapter 18 on drug therapy).

Any deviation from the normal physical state of the patient merits some degree of investigation, and it may be helpful for a full description of the appearance and physical characteristics to be included in the observations on admission. This can be used later as a baseline from which any deviation can be accurately assessed.

OBTAINING INFORMATION BY TALKING TO THE PATIENT

The nurse obtains information about the patient, not only by asking questions, but also in an indirect way. She establishes rapport with him by showing that she is interested and a willing listener. She must be interested in anything he chooses to tell her and in everything he does. The first approach may be a trivial one. The patient wants to know which nurse, if any, he can talk to and may approach all nurses with some little story or some unimportant remark. Only when he becomes convinced that the nurse feels interested in him and that she does not laugh at or criticize him, does he continue to single her out and give her an opportunity of learning more about him. Every conversation she has with the patient, no matter what the topic, gives some indication as to his life, general upbringing and past experiences. Every time the nurse converses with the patient, alone or in a group, she acquires more information about his personality. Her task of convincing him of her real interest in him is the easier, the more topics of common interest she can find. In order to sustain conversations the nurse should have as wide a knowledge and as many interests as possible. She can increase her knowledge considerably by listening to patients who talk about their jobs, their hobbies or their opinions.

It is never the nurse's function to argue with the patient, or to expound her own opinions on controversial matters such as politics or religion. To show interest in the patient's point of view is valuable, not to convert the patient to one's own.

OBTAINING INFORMATION ABOUT THE PATIENT FROM OTHER PEOPLE

Obtaining information about the patient from records, from discussion with other staff in case conferences, and sometimes by interviewing the patient's next-of-kin or other informant is very important in psychiatric care, but this should not precede the nurse's effort to get to know the patient personally.

Patients should be able to make a personal choice about the information they entrust to particular staff members. It does not help, as a rule, to feel that one is being talked about, or that one's reputation has preceded one. There will of course be occasions when the patient's permission needs to be sought to pass information on to the doctor or to other nurses. As treatment progresses, patients come to realize that shared knowledge among members of the team can be more helpfully used than knowledge given to one staff member in confidence.

However, in the assessment stage of care planning, the nurse can only use information which the patient has offered to her personally or which she has obtained from records with the full consent of the patient.

WRITING CARE PLANS

The purpose of assessment is to devise for each patient a plan showing how ward and hospital life is to be geared to have a therapeutic effect on the patient.

To write a detailed plan for each patient, setting short- and long-term goals, documenting at frequent intervals the care which has been given and evaluating it regularly should be aimed at; but this may not be a realistic goal unless care plans are kept short. If too much writing takes place, nurses find they do not have time to read all the plans often enough and that they are unable to remember all details in their interaction with patients in everyday work. Several points should, however, be made.

It is impossible to learn how to plan nursing care without practising writing of detailed plans. Process recordings, for example, of conversation with patients should be carried out, noting in as much detail as possible what the patient said and what the nurse said during a specific encounter. Nurses should gain practice in identifying problems and writing problem-orientated plans. With adequate practice in writing detailed plans, it becomes easier to focus quickly on specific problems and to formulate clearly the objectives of specific nursing intervention. When patients have been in hospital for a long time it may become possible to follow individually prepared nursing care plans with more verbal and less written communication. Another point is that each patient should know which nurse is responsible for developing a plan, updating it, collecting information about the patient's progress, and discussing with the patient his progress and objectives, modifications in the plan and methods of evaluation. Patients should be actively involved in the preparation of the plan as they cannot otherwise be expected to understand what the purpose of the various activities in the ward is meant to be.

Patients should know what is being written about them. It is not possible to use information obtained about a patient from others if the patient is not aware that it has been passed on.

One reason for keeping a fairly detailed written record of the care plan and the nursing care which has been given, is that detailed records can later be used for research. It may be difficult, as has been said before, to be sure that one's actions have had the desired effect on an individual patient, but to collect in retrospect evidence of what has been done on a number of occasions by different nurses and with many patients is an important step in developing nursing practice.

Well-prepared nursing care plans and accurate progress reports help immeasurably in co-ordinating teamwork. It is of interest to compare the perspective brought to bear on any patient's treatment by members of different professions. It is of course important that the patient is aware of the fact that notes about him are discussed by the team.

A final reason for detailed individualized care plans and progress reports lies in the nature of psychiatric care. Much of what goes on in a ward affects all, or at least many, patients simultaneously. A ward meeting, for example, may concern itself with a problem common to several patients; an accident to one patient on the ward affects all, so does the admission of new patients, a patient's death or an episode of disturbed behaviour. How specifically an event affects a particular patient needs to be recorded by the nurse responsible for individual care planning, who also has to adapt the subsequent care plan in the light of the way the patient was able to cope.

Further reading

Altschul, A.T. (1978) A systems approach to the nursing process. *Journal of Advanced Nursing 3*, 333.

Smith, L. (1980) *A Nursing History and Data Sheet. Psychiatry under Review*, pp. 18–23. London: Macmillan.

8
Basic Activities of Everyday Living

In Chapter 1 it was shown that a mentally healthy person is able to function adequately in relation to some basic activities of normal life. Attention to self-care was among the activities listed. In this and the next few chapters we shall see how, in mental illness, the patient may need help with these activities.

Most people spend a considerable amount of time, energy and thought on the care of their own persons. They try to buy clothes which fit well, look nice and are made of good and lasting material. They dress as well as their financial situation permits and devote great care to their clothes. Much time is spent washing and ironing; clothes are hung or folded carefully in order not to crease them and to keep them in good condition.

Some people are much interested in the washing, ironing and cleaning of clothes. Others find this is a drudgery which they would gladly delegate if they could.

Personal hygiene, bathing, washing, care of hair and nails and elimination present few problems to normal healthy people. Few reflect on how much effort it has cost their parents to teach them the value of cleanliness, the habit of washing and shaving, the right time and place for defaecation. This highly organized aspect of behaviour has become habit and is carried out almost automatically. In sickness the individual becomes aware of the complexity of these details of daily occurrence.

Nurses who care for those who are physically ill devote a great deal of their time and skill to the personal hygiene of their patients. They learn early in their training how to wash and bathe patients in bed and in the bathroom, how and why to care for the mouths of helpless patients, how to give urinals and bedpans.

The psychiatric nurse needs to learn all these things and, in addition, she must learn why some of her patients do not appear to care for cleanliness, why others want to wash all day long; why some patients do not bother to make themselves attractive and others take so long over dressing that they would never reach the breakfast table if they were not helped. She must learn how to persuade the patient to wash or to stop washing, and she must try to understand why one nurse is sometimes successful in persuading a patient to undress, while another may dismally fail to do so.

Attention to the patient's personal care calls for skill and understanding and offers unique opportunity for establishing rapport with him, for obtaining valuable information and for helping him in a personal way.

Most patients are quite capable of looking after their own bodies and their own clothing. All that is required is adequate washing facilities, sufficient time, sufficient privacy and enough cupboard space for clothes. Most patients have regular baths, cut their nails if a pair of scissors is available, wash their hair, go to the lavatory, change their underwear quite regularly without prompting. In order to be sure that the patient is not neglecting any aspect of personal hygiene, it is the routine in some hospitals that a nurse is present in the bathroom at least on some occasions. (She is, of course, always present if there is any possibility that the patient may be suicidal.) The nurse uses this opportunity for observing the patient, noticing any scars, bruises, rashes or other abnormalities. Tact is required to help the patient overcome the embarrassment of having a nurse present.

Bathing is a pleasant activity; it should not be hurried. The patient should have a chance to relax and enjoy the pleasant sensation of hot water. Most people like to lie in the bath for a while. Many people sing or whistle in the bath. Patients often begin to talk. The intimacy of this situation can be most valuable. At times, the bathroom is the only place where the patient feels sufficiently relaxed to speak, and he may then sometimes confide to the nurse problems he would not have braced himself to mention in any other situation. It is most important that the pleasure and the intimacy of the bathing situation should not be ruined by hurry or by having several patients in the bathroom at once.

Shaving is usually supervised if razor blades are used. In the hands of suicidal patients they can be very dangerous indeed. In some wards razors are given out by nurses and collected again after use. Some patients may have to be shaved by the nurse.

Some hospitals have hairdressing shops, but, failing this, a keen and enthusiastic nursing staff can work wonders with the patients' hair. Patients may be enabled to try out new styles on each other and keen interest in hairdressing may then develop. The use of make-up may be encouraged and a complimentary remark from a nurse, doctor or another patient may give back to the patient some of the self-respect that may have been lost.

Clothes

It should almost always be possible for patients to wear their own clothes. These fit well and patients have good reason to look after them. Dress sense can be encouraged by the nurse if patients are helped to dress suitably for various occasions, differently for work, for dancing or for going out shopping. Mirrors must of course be freely available. A full-length mirror is necessary in order to ensure that patients feel well dressed.

Clothes assume considerable significance in most people's lives. Tastes differ and the way people dress is often characteristic of their personality. When looking at clothes in a shop window or admiring another person's dress, one tends to imagine the clothes on oneself. 'This dress would suit me', or 'This colour is not for me', are expressions which indicate that people's ideas of themselves often include their clothes. Their concept of their own identity is closely connected with the clothes they wear. Some people feel as acutely upset if their clothes suffer damage as if their own body were involved.

Because clothes are so intimately bound up with body image and feeling of identity, it is important that patients should have the opportunity of dressing as well and as distinctively as possible. Adequate time for good grooming is essential and patients benefit if they can choose their own clothes, go out personally to buy clothes or, sometimes, make their own at occupational therapy. Washing, ironing, mending and altering clothes may take up a fair amount of the patients' time and a good deal of their interest.

When patients have been in hospital for a long time it may be difficult for them to know how much clothes cost, and they may need help in planning how to save money and how to budget in order to buy a specific item of clothing. Some patients suffering from schizophrenia have particularly marked difficulty in assessing their own identity. They often have problems with their body image. For these patients, it is particularly important that they should possess their own clothing and that they should dress in their own distinctive manner.

For physically disabled patients, specially designed clothes now exist which look attractive, but are easy to put on and take off and which spare the patient pain and discomfort. Nurses and patients should inform themselves of available sources of supply

Some progress has been made in recent years in finding materials which are attractive yet durable and which retain colour and shape in spite of frequent laundering.

Elimination

Most patients go to the lavatory regularly, but the nurse should know if the patient passes urine normally and has his bowels open regularly. She should observe any abnormality, e.g. frequent visits to the lavatory, and show enough interest to encourage the patient to report any abnormality he himself notices.

Some patients need assistance in their personal hygiene at the time of the menstrual period. Behaviour changes often accompany menstruation, and these should be noted and reported to the doctor.

DIFFICULT PATIENTS

So far, consideration has been given to patients who require no more from the nurse than interest, encouragement and adequate bathroom facilities. There are, however, many others who need a great deal more than this. At one extreme there are patients who, left to themselves, are incontinent of urine and faeces, who defaecate and urinate wherever they stand. There are patients who would remain in the nude if they were allowed to do so. There are patients whose hair becomes matted, who would never wash unaided, never change their clothes of their own accord. Some of these are patients in a state of extreme excitement. For example, manic patients are so restless, preoccupied and excited that they have no time to wash or dress. The tongue and lips become dry and cracked, the skin sore. Clothes irritate them, they prefer to be naked. Some depressed patients simply have not the energy to wash or change their clothes. They are unable to make the effort to go to the lavatory. Some schizophrenic patients gradually lose interest in their appearance. They spend more and more time alone in their rooms and finally neglect themselves. Patients suffering from organic psychiatric disorders often neglect their own health and appearance. They sometimes use articles for purposes for which they are not intended. They may use the toothbrush for shoe cleaning, eat soap or drink the bathwater. They often soil their clothing, and if not watched may hide dirty underwear in quite unexpected places.

All these patients require very careful and skilled nursing if their health is not to suffer. They render themselves liable to infection and they also increase many times the danger of spreading infection should this occur.

Some patients refuse to dress. Some may hear voices telling them to undress, or may feel unworthy of the clothes they are wearing. Others believe that they are poor, that nothing, not even their clothing, belongs to them. Some patients think that their clothes are germ infested or that they smell. A patient may refuse to be dressed by a particular nurse because he thinks she is his enemy. He may fear that if he dresses he will be led away by the police. No amount of coaxing or persuasion can be successful unless the specific reason for refusal to dress is known and the patient can be convinced of the nurse's understanding. It may, however, be necessary to wait until the patient's mood has changed, or until a nurse trusted by him is available.

INCONTINENT PATIENTS

Incontinence as well as neglect of personal appearance sometimes occur in the withdrawn patient and should be recognized as an indication of the degree of the patient's illness. His behaviour should not arouse displays of emotional reaction in the nurse, and he should be protected also from the expressed disapproval of the group of fellow patients who may feel disgust at, or intolerance of, his disregard of social standards.

On the other hand, it may be equally wrong to accept incontinence as inevitable and to become resigned to its occurrence. Incontinence is sometimes a significant activity, a manner of communicating on a non-verbal level, something which is meaningful to the patient, but difficult to understand. The patient's incontinence may follow a regular pattern, it may occur only if he is alone, or always when a certain nurse is on duty. It may be a means of gaining attention or a manner of protesting against an action the patient may not wish to perform. One patient's incontinence may occur only in the ward, never in the garden, another patient may void urine each time the doctor passes through the ward without speaking to him.

It may be very rewarding to discover if there is any recognizable meaning in the patient's incontinence and to prevent its occurrence by giving him personal interest.

It is extremely embarrassing for the patient to be incontinent. Everything possible should be done to save him this embarrassment. In many instances incontinence diminishes once the patient is up and dressed. Physically ill patients who are confined to bed have great difficulties attracting the attention of a nurse in time to obtain a bedpan or a commode.

Some patients are incontinent simply because the lavatory is so far away that it is difficult for them to reach it in time, and confused patients may have difficulty in finding their way there.

Attention to the patient's toilet is the most personal service a nurse can give him. By giving it willingly, if possible anticipating his need, she can do more than she can by any other method to convince him of her interest.

It may be very difficult to find a way in which the patient who has been incontinent can be helped to wash and change clothes without causing loss of dignity and self-respect. It may be possible, if the nurse discusses the problem with those in a position to help, to obtain clothing specially designed to facilitate changing after incontinence, to use fabric in upholstery which reduces the danger of an unpleasant smell lingering in the ward and to make suitable adaptation to the toilet and bathroom area for easier access and greater comfort during the process of attending to the patient's toilet.

Behaviour therapy techniques such as token economy or restitution have sometimes been effective in reducing · a patient's incontinence.

OBSESSIONAL PATIENTS

One of the most difficult problems with which the nurse may have to deal is that of managing patients who insist on washing over and over again. Obsessional patients may wash many times a day, or may take so long over their morning toilet that they find it difficult to arrive at breakfast (see Chapter 2). In the evening, hours are spent in folding shirts. Every time the patient goes to the lavatory or touches a door handle he again washes his hands.

If these patients are stopped, they become intensely unhappy and anxious. If allowed to carry on, they occupy the bathroom all day, prevent others from using it and are quite incapacitated for other activities. When dealing with patients of this type, personal hygiene may become a matter of secondary importance. With the doctor's help, a plan of action must be drawn up, to say whether the patient is to be allowed to carry on his compulsive actions or whether the risk is to be taken of making him more anxious by interference, or the nurse, behaviour therapist or psychologist may be asked for help with a behaviour therapy programme.

It is important to try to understand what an obsession may mean to the patient. Water may have a symbolic significance, handwashing may perhaps be symbolic for the washing away of guilt. The doctor may be able to discover the reason for the patient's guilt feeling. If the latter's behaviour has some special meaning for him, he cannot give it up unless he can solve his unconscious conflicts. Once the nurse's curiosity is aroused and she is interested in why the patient behaves in the way he does, she ceases to be anxious about routine and has thus taken the first step in helping the patient, to whom her interest and willingness to understand are of great value.

Further reading

Roper, N., Logan, W. & Tierney, A. (1980) *Elements of Nursing.* Edinburgh: Churchill Livingstone.

9
The Significance of Food

FOOD AND SOCIETY

In order to appreciate the problems psychiatric nurses may encounter in relation to food, consideration must first be given to the importance of food in the lives of most people. Fortunately, extreme hunger is rare in Western civilization and it is difficult to realize how powerful a motive the hunger drive can be. In concentration camps, or in countries in which part of the population is literally starving, the importance of food and drink in human life can be only too tragically observed. Normal human beings, given the material means, provide themselves with an adequate, well-balanced diet. Their behaviour, their social and ethical standards and their cultural achievements are determined by factors other than the hunger drive. Because hunger is so rare in Western society, the actions of other drives, e.g. that of sex, can be observed in a more uninhibited way, and this may be the reason why some writers have attributed to it a disproportionate importance.

But even in a society which is rarely hungry, food plays an extremely important part. Political issues are decided on such problems as food prices and food production. Revolutions have begun over the price of bread or the dumping of tea into the sea. International treaties are formed and broken according to the nutritional needs of nations, and wars are won or lost by the maintenance or otherwise of a food supply line.

FOOD IN THE HOME

Individual lives centre around food. Housewives may spend a large proportion of their time planning meals, buying, preparing and cooking food. Marital relationships may be influenced by the quality of the cooking. Meals form central pivots for people's activity. Meal-times are relatively fixed landmarks in the day, and people tend to make them the central points of their lives. Friends are entertained to dinner, restaurants are visited when others are casually encountered. Evening outings begin or end with a meal. Business deals are closed over luncheons; successes are celebrated with food and drink. It is necessary only to observe the engagements of such a person as the mayor of a city in order to see how important is food in public life. Food, apart from its social significance, has great psychological importance.

FOOD AND THE CHILD

Sucking is one of the baby's first activities, and if, as is commonly practised nowadays, the baby is put to his mother's breast very soon after he is born, this is his first physical contact with the mother. Milk is the baby's first source of satisfaction. If infant feeding is properly managed, the mother who provides milk soon becomes the object of the child's love. The mother first holds and cuddles her child during feeding and she derives her greatest happiness from this contact.

When the mother withdraws the breast the baby is for the first time deprived of something he needs. Very early the baby loves and hates his mother, according to the satisfaction or frustration experienced in the feeding situation. The first conflict in the baby's life arises. If breast-feeding is difficult, both mother and child become anxious and derive little satisfaction. Many feeding problems may arise early in life. Parents worry about and discuss with friends and professionals the relative value of breast-feeding versus bottle feeding. They cope with weaning problems, they have to battle with food fads, with refusal of food or with excessive eating in their children. Table manners are taught and the child gradually learns to acquire the tastes of his elders.

If the child grows up in a warm, secure family setting, if he is loved and gains approval for his achievements, he succeeds in learning the complex skills related to adult enjoyment of food. If, however, the child is hampered in his development, some of his difficulties are expressed at meal-times.

Refusal of food is a very powerful weapon, arousing intense emotion in the parents. The mother may become excessively concerned about the child's health and, because of this, give him more attention. She may become angry about his obstinate refusal of food. In the scenes that follow the child asserts his strength, but everybody becomes unhappy and disturbed. Meals, instead of being pleasurable occasions, are dreaded by all because of the uncomfortable atmosphere created by the child. The unhappy child loses his appetite and feeding problems are intensified.

Later in life individual attitudes to food largely depend on early experiences and associations. Some people, when they are worried and unhappy, feel sick and lose appetite. Others find in food their only solace. Food may always remain symbolic for love. The offer of a meal by one person to another may be an indication of the relationship between them.

Preoccupation with health foods, with special diets, with slimming or with trying to put on weight are characteristic of many people of all ages.

FOOD AND THE PATIENT

In hospital the patient is dependent on others for the satisfaction of all his bodily needs. Nurses are very much aware of the fact that they establish emotional contact with the patient when they offer him food or have to feed him. They realize that the patient's praise of food represents an appreciation of the general care he receives. A great deal of thought is given to the serving and preparation of meals. Nurses do their best to whet the appetite of those who have no inclination to eat, but on the whole they expect the patient's co-operation, if not gratitude, for supplying him with food.

This is by no means the case in the psychiatric hospital, where a variety of problems may occur. There are patients who do not eat, or do not eat enough, or not the right kinds of food. Some patients eat too much, or too fast. Some eat each other's food, or bolt food without chewing it. There are those who no longer attach any social value to food, whose table manners are objectionable, or who perform rituals in such a way that food no longer serves as a social stimulus.

FOOD AND THE NURSE

The nurse can do a great deal in the treatment of her patients by giving meals the important place they deserve. Patients should be aware of meal-times and punctuality is important. There should be ample time before meals for patients to prepare for them, to put their things away, wash their hands and tidy up. Interest can be aroused by talking about food, discussing menus, exchanging recipes. Where possible, or desirable, patients may assist in the cooking of meals and, at any rate, in the laying of the tables. The meal itself should be a pleasurable occasion. It must be unhurried, nobody should disturb the harmony. Patients who may provide a disturbing influence may have to be served before or after the others, or in a separate dining-room. Patients who like each other should find places next to each other and table conversation should be kept at a steady, leisurely flow. Meals should not produce anxiety, arguments should be avoided and any difficult situation which may arise over the feeding of resistive patients should be dealt with apart from others. The atmosphere of the dining-room should be congenial. The aesthetic pleasure of well-laid tables, well-cooked, well-served food cannot be ignored.

The nurse should think carefully about her own role in connection with meals. She may regard herself as the hostess who offers the food, not merely the 'maid' who carries it around. Constant running in and fetching and carrying can have a very unsettling effect on patients. A nurse who remains in the dining-room, who can sit down with the patients at the table, can convey an attitude of relaxation and enjoyment, even if she is not sharing the meal.

It may be of some importance to decide whether meals should be served in the wards, or away from them in a self-service dining-room. The latter method usually has the advantage of providing hotter food, reducing delay between cooking and serving, and also of cutting down waste. Some patients enjoy the restaurant atmosphere of the dining-room, and benefit from a temporary absence from the ward. For other patients the ward for the time being represents 'home', the place to which they return from work. Meals served in a ward dining-room help to draw patients closer to each other and thus to create the group feeling which should exist between patients and staff of the same ward.

In some hospitals attempts have been made to relieve nurses of purely domestic duties and it has been suggested that the work connected with the preparation for meals and the serving of food might be regarded as non-nursing and be delegated to the catering staff. While it may be a good idea to convey to some patients at certain times that they are independent of the nursing staff, that they are free to partake of restaurant meals as they see fit, that they can choose their menu and are free to miss a meal if they want to do so, it would seem quite wrong to believe that all meals should be regarded in this light. The act of serving food and accepting food has such powerful emotional significance that it provides a special opportunity for establishing important relationships between nurse and patient. When the patient is ready for greater independence it would seem advisable that he himself should assume greater responsibility for the provision of meals, rather than that other members of the staff should be drawn in. Facilities should exist for patients to prepare refreshments for entertainments, to entertain each other and their visitors, to go to the hospital canteen for a snack or to go out of the hospital and have tea in a restaurant in town.

Some patients can only gradually be brought into the community at meal-times, e.g. those who eat much more slowly than the rest, and have not finished in time, and those who may have to have their food cut up small, or minced, for example epileptic patients who might have a fit while chewing large pieces of meat. Some patients may gobble their food, not giving themselves time to chew.

THE DIFFICULT PATIENT

By far the greatest skill, tact and perseverance is required when dealing with patients who refuse food. The method adopted to persuade these to eat must depend on the motive for refusing food. Every effort should be made to discover individual problems in relation to food.

Many depressed patients are too apathetic or too morbidly preoccupied to eat. There is no interest in food. The patient just does not want to be bothered, he is not hungry, has no desire for food. He would much rather be left alone and dislikes the nurse's attention. Sometimes, in order to rid himself of the nurse's attention, he may in fact attempt to eat but he is so slow that he may not receive an adequate diet. Only very careful observation will reveal the fact that such a patient (who may perhaps be suffering from a chronic depressive state) has eaten or drunk far too little during the day. Regular weighing, careful attention to physical health, observation of bowel function, attention to the mouth, which may be dry due to lack of fluid intake, and sometimes the drawing up of intake and output charts, will provide an indication of the patient's state of nutrition. He may be merely passive, apathetic, uninterested, but he may not resist spoon-feeding, or it may be relatively easy to ensure adequate food and fluid intake with encouragement.

Some patients, however, are quite determined not to eat. Some wish to commit suicide and believe starvation to be a suitable method. The nurse has to deal with this situation by kindly but firmly convincing the patient that this method cannot be allowed to succeed. Tube-feeding may be necessary once or twice to convince him, but often the nurse's own conviction that he will eat eventually is conveyed to him by word and bearing and makes him realize the futility of continuing to try to starve himself, although it may lead him to plan some alternative method of committing suicide.

Some depressed patients suffer from delusions which cause them to refuse food. (One example which might illustrate this arose in a ward where nurses' uniform dresses could be buttoned either to the right or left. The patient explained after she had recovered that she had always refused to accept food from nurses whose dresses were buttoned to the right.) The patient may have delusions of poverty or of unworthiness. He may believe that he does not have the money for his food, that he cannot eat what he cannot pay for, or else that he does not deserve it, is wicked, that other people are starving and food should be given to them. These ideas, expressed or kept secret by the patient, effectively deter him from eating. It will not help at all to tempt this patient with better or more expensive foods.

The delusion that the patient has 'no inside', that his 'bowels are blocked' or that 'food turns to poison' inside him may lead to refusal of food. It is difficult to persuade the patient to eat and, having eaten, he is likely to vomit in order to avert the terrible consequences he feels would result from having food inside him. It may be necessary to be constantly with the patient after meals in order to prevent vomiting.

However, when caring for a severely depressed patient, who, for whatever reason, is refusing to eat, it may be necessary to include in his nursing care plan a named nurse to supervise his nutritional intake. This should not be interpreted to mean placing a plate of food in front of the patient and going off to do something else, only returning from time to time to prompt him to eat or to comment on his lack of progress or that his food will be getting cold. It should involve drawing up a chair alongside the patient at the table and quietly conveying by words of encouragement, concern and an unhurried attitude that the nurse fully intends to remain until the patient has eaten and drunk (high-calorie drinks may have to be given in place of a dessert) a reasonable amount of nourishment. Most patients respond to this positive approach, though the nurse may initially need to place the fork or spoon in the patient's hand and to guide it to his mouth.

A patient may fear that he is being poisoned and consequently may refuse food from some members of the staff and accept it from others. He may consent to eat if he sees the food prepared or may eat if the nurse tastes the food first. He may insist on liquid or semi-solid food, which can be properly mixed before the nurse tastes the food. This may be repeated at every meal. Some patients may not reveal the reasons for refusal of food until they have recovered, and their unpredictable and erratic behaviour may puzzle nurses for a long time. Later the patient may explain that at times he had olfactory hallucinations which rendered the food suspect, or that he heard a voice telling him not to eat. He may have refused food when offered with the right hand, but accepted it handed with the left, interpreting this as a sign that he should eat. Many bizarre delusions have a direct bearing on food intake.

Manic patients often refuse food because they are too busy and preoccupied with other things to be bothered with it. It may be possible to persuade such a patient to eat by putting food in his hand. He may, for example, eat a sandwich rather than a plateful of meat and vegetables. It may be necessary to leave food about in the hope that it will be picked up and eaten. If it is not eaten, the nurse must direct the patient towards it by making use of his distractability.

Difficulties of neurotic patients are particularly difficult to solve. In a similar manner to the child, the neurotic patient's refusal of food, or excessive food intake, may be an expression of his worry, anxiety and unhappiness.

Some neurotic patients use meal-times in the way children do, as a weapon against authority, or as a means to attract attention. It is essential not only to find out what the patient is trying to achieve, but also why it is necessary for him to defy authority, or to attract notice in this way. Once it has been made clear to the patient, not so much in words but by attitude, that his motives are understood, that his attitude to authority is respected and his need for attention appreciated, he may be able to give up his symptom.

The patient's refusal of food may represent his attitude, not to the nurse, but to some other person whom she temporarily represents. His refusal of food may be a symbolic way of rejecting love, or rejecting care from a female who stands for a mother figure. It may indicate a fear of putting on weight which may be symbolic of a fear of pregnancy. It may be an expression of rebellion against dependence. Often a patient who refuses food can create differences of opinion among nurses, a situation which he can exploit but which makes him feel insecure and unhappy.

It is helpful to know something about the motives for a neurotic patient's problems with food, but often this is not possible because such motives are unconscious. They may become clear only as they are resolved. The nurse can make a guess and then act on the assumption that the guess is right. If she succeeds, the explanation she thought of was probably the right one. If she fails, the guess is rejected and she must try again. The guesses will become more nearly correct as the nurse tries varying approaches, listing those which succeed and those which fail. What is required of a nurse is not that she should know the reason for the patient's behaviour and act according-ly, but that she should be willing to try to find out. This willingness to understand in itself may convince the patient that the nurse is on his side and all problems may vanish.

'Anorexia nervosa' is a condition in which refusal of food, vomiting and active resistance to all attempts to persuade the patient to eat, can lead to extreme weight loss and danger to life. (For further description see Chapter 2.)

The nurse who has failed to persuade the patient to eat

should not regard this as a personal insult or feel that her failure will be regarded as incompetence. She must, of course, guard against interpreting another nurse's failure in this way. She must learn to observe other people's methods, compare them with her own and try to find out why one method or one person has failed and another succeeded. Sometimes she will continue to be puzzled until the patient himself, after recovery, can give her the real explanation.

10
The Significance of Sleep

It is essential for the patient's physical health that he should have adequate, deep, restful sleep.

INSOMNIA

Many patients complain that for a long time prior to admission they have suffered from 'insomnia'. Careful inquiries show that there are many ways in which sleep can be disturbed. Some patients say that they have not slept a wink for many weeks. This is unlikely to be true, but the complaint should be listened to by the nurse, because it is an indication of the patient's suffering and distress. He may attribute his many symptoms to lack of sleep. He is worried, anxious and frightened. This keeps him awake at night. But he believes that he is worried, anxious and frightened *because* he cannot sleep, and expresses fear of going 'mad' if he does not soon find relief. It is useless to point out to him that there is evidence of his having slept for certain periods; it is much better to listen to his complaint and ask him for details of his insomnia.

Insomnia is very widespread in the community as a whole. General practitioners prescribe a large amount of night sedation. However, because of the highly addictive nature of the barbiturates, most general practitioners subscribe to a voluntary ban on their use as hypnotics. The benzodiazapines have filled this gap. Unfortunately it is now known that they too can cause dependency if taken regularly.

Studies of sleep patterns have shown that the amount of sleep people enjoy diminishes with age; complaints of insomnia increase with age.

The satisfaction derived from sleep depends on its length and depth. The electroencephalograph (EEG) shows a variety of brain waves during sleep. The wave pattern in deep sleep is slow. Although only short periods of the night may be spent in sleep with slow-wave pattern, the satisfaction reported in the morning is associated with this type of sleep. When the brain waves are shallow and fast, there is a subsequent feeling of not having slept well. Efficiency during the day appears to depend to some extent on the amount of sleep during which slow brain waves occurred.

During part of the sleeping period the sleeper's eyes move rapidly and the electroencephalograph record shows rapid eye movement. Waking the sleeper at this moment makes it clear that he has been disturbed in the middle of a dream. If people are deprived of the opportunity of dreaming, they also complain of a poor night's sleep.

The patient's own account and complaints may therefore be justified, even when the night nurse's observation indicates that the patient slept for longer periods than he is aware of.

Some patients fall asleep quite easily in the evening, but wake frequently and remain awake for long periods. To the patient, the wakeful periods seem endless, the periods of sleep pass unnoticed or by comparison appear to be short.

Patients who are anxious and frightened find it difficult to go to sleep in the evening. Once asleep, they sleep soundly and do not wake again until morning. But the early hours of the night are agony. The more the patient tries to sleep, the more anxious, and therefore the more wakeful, he becomes. Rather than suffer these dreadful hours, the patient prefers to remain up and dressed, and, like a child, practises delaying tactics in the evening. He may take a long time undressing, go back again and again for something he has forgotten, fold clothes meticulously and repeatedly, fetch water and hot-water bottles and generally make bedtime difficult for all. If he is harassed and nagged, his anxiety increases and his sleeplessness becomes worse. It is better to convince him that his difficulties are appreciated and that the nurse will be near and will help him fall asleep.

There are some patients who find the relaxation techniques they have learned during the day to be of value in overcoming their initial insomnia. However, very anxious patients may require the night nurse's encouragement to put them into practice in the first instance.

Some patients, especially those who are depressed, wake up

very early in the morning and at that time find life quite intolerable. The early hours of the morning might then become the most propitious time for an attempt at suicide.

NIGHTMARES

Many mentally ill patients suffer from nightmares. The patient may wake during the night terrified, in a cold sweat and trembling. He requires someone to be near in order to bring him back gently to reality and to tell him that he had a nightmare, a bad dream, and that he is quite safe. The patient may wish to speak about his dream, or he may just want a nurse to sit by him for a few moments until he has calmed down. Dreams play an important part in the manifestations and treatment of mentally ill patients. It may be very desirable for the patient to remember his dreams and to tell either his doctor or the nurse, who could write it down for him.

Naturally, after a bad night, the patient feels tired all day. He seeks every opportunity to lie down on his bed, lacks energy and inclination for work. He may doze off to sleep, so getting some badly needed rest, but finding it all the more difficult to sleep the following night.

FACTORS INFLUENCING SLEEP

Many sleep disturbances are symptomatic of psychiatric disorders. Often, however, the patient's inability to sleep is caused by conditions in the hospital ward. Most people find it disturbing to sleep in a room with others, especially strangers. Some dormitories in psychiatric hospitals are so crowded, beds are so close to each other, that it is not surprising that patients sleep badly. Patients who in their own home have interior-sprung mattresses or latex-foam beds may be expected to sleep on hard hospital beds. Pillows may be hard or arranged in an unaccustomed manner, coverings too tight or too heavy. Patients who are used to open windows find the ward stuffy, others complain of draught.

Most patients, at least during the first few nights, complain of noise; they are aware of the breathing and snoring of others, of the footsteps of the nurse, the whispered talk in the corridors, the ringing of telephone bells and the clanking noise of crockery in the kitchen. The light is left on during the night, disturbing to some patients although it is subdued, and disturbing to others who would prefer bright lights because they are frightened by shadows and the dim outlines of furniture.

It is the first and foremost duty of the night nurse to minimize disturbing factors in the ward and to realize that these are not the same for all patients.

It is impossible to over-emphasize the importance of silence in the ward, of ventilation and warmth, of comfortable, well-made beds, remade if the patient is restless. Needless to say, the patient should not be allowed to go hungry or lack water to drink. Hot drinks may help, and he may find relief if he gets up to empty bowels or bladder, or merely to change his position.

To the patient it is not only important that all things should be done to ensure a quiet night, it is important *how* they are done. The way in which the nurse offers him a drink, or remakes his bed, is often more important than the actual drink or bedmaking. The presence of the night nurse may be all that is required in order to reassure the patient. If the nurse is not in evidence, he may call out so as to reassure himself of her presence and, having called, he is bound to ask for something. The nurse should understand this need, and be present even if the patient does not require any attention. She should inform patients of her movements, tell them that she will be in the ward, explain how they can attract her attention. If she goes away from the ward to her meal, she should tell the patients about this, and also mention who will be there to relieve her.

In order to ensure that patients obtain a good night's sleep, the routine of the ward must be so arranged that all have adequate amounts of recreation and outdoor activities during the day. The retiring hour should be suited to each ward and ample time should be allowed for gradual preparation for bed. There should be a reduction in noise and excitement before bedtime and a period of quiet relaxation.

Flexible arrangements for retiring are very helpful. Some people habitually retire late and read for a while before switching off the lights. They find this helps them to get to sleep quickly.

It is not always essential that a patient who is wakeful should remain in bed. To sit in the dayroom reading, or to talk to the night nurse for a while may be more helpful than efforts to go to sleep.

It is incumbent on the day staff to read the night report, and to increase activity during the day if it seems indicated by poor sleep at night.

Spectacles should not be taken away from patients. There is nothing more irritating to a patient with poor eyesight than to be without his glasses, unable to read, unable to watch what is going on, and unable to sleep because of the general noise and activity.

NIGHT SEDATION

If, in spite of all these nursing measures, the patient does not sleep, or complains of not sleeping, the nurse should keep a careful record. Every half-hour she should check whether the patient is awake or asleep, and in the report she should not only state the number of hours of sleep, but give an account of sleep rhythm and quality. Temporary resort to a hypnotic drug may have to be considered, particularly during the acute phase of a patient's illness, but the right sedative can be prescribed only if the doctor is fully informed of the patient's sleeping habits and of the effect of the drug. The nurse should know if the sedative prescribed for the patient is quick or slow acting and whether or not it has prolonged effects. This is particularly important with drugs to be given 'if necessary' or to be repeated. She should know how late it is desirable to give any drug, and how long she can delay, in order to give the patient a chance to sleep without sedation.

Hypnotic drugs reduce the amount of 'paradoxical sleep', that is the amount of sleep when rapid eye movement and dreaming occur. What dreams there are, may be less vivid. When sleeping pills are taken over a long period there is also a diminished amount of those sleep phases which are most satisfying and during which growth hormone is secreted. For these reasons, as with the dependency problem already noted, the prolonged use of sleeping pills is undesirable.

One other problem associated with the use of hypnotic drugs

is the fact that the initial dose may soon lose its effect. The body compensates by counteracting the effects of the drug. The brain metabolism changes, so that the previous sleep pattern is re-established in spite of the drug. To obtain a sedative effect the dosage then needs to be increased. It then becomes very difficult indeed to stop taking drugs as the patient would suffer from increased restlessness and insomnia, complain of excessively vivid dreams and feel extremely anxious. Because it is so difficult to revert to normal sleep after prolonged use of sedatives, it is particularly important that the initial prescription is well adapted to the patient's specific needs and that the nurses' observations help to restrict the use of drugs to a minimum.

For the night nurse to lend a listening ear to the anxious patient, to provide a leisurely, soothing and warm bath for the overactive manic patient, to give the patient troubled with hallucinations the last dose of his antipsychotic medication at night, are possible alternatives to the prescription of a hypnotic drug. The presence of the night nurse may be reassuring by itself.

Further reading

Oswald, I. (1984) Insomnia. *British Journal of Hospital Medicine 31* (3), 219.

Tyrer, P.J. (1984) Benzodiazapines on trial. *British Medical Journal 288*, 1101.

11
The Long-stay Patient

The terms 'long stay' and 'rehabilitation' tend to go together. When one thinks of the long-stay patient the question of his rehabilitation often follows automatically. To understand why this should be so it is necessary to look at what has been happening to the patient during his long stay in hospital.

THE EFFECT OF INSTITUTIONAL LIVING

Some patients who have spent many years in psychiatric hospitals behave as if they were suffering from dementia or as if a state of chronic schizophrenic illness had rendered them dull and unresponsive. It has now been demonstrated that their condition is due not solely to the psychiatric disorder which caused their admission to hospital, but to the effect of institutional living itself. The terms 'institutionalism' or 'institutionalization' and 'institutional neurosis' have been applied to this condition. Clearly in future it must be prevented, but patients already suffering from the ill-effects of certain aspects of hospital life need help in regaining independence, initiative and zest for life.

Institutional neurosis is the effect of the patient's resignation to the conditions which prevail in some institutions. Inactivity, idleness and boredom result in a progressive withdrawal by the patient. He sits slumped in his chair or stands about in corners, and walks with a characteristic stooping gait. Facial expression is vacant and the patient takes little interest in his personal appearance. He rarely initiates action and he readily obeys orders and instructions from the staff.

Because the patient appears so inactive, nurses are often unaware of his potential abilities. They act for the patient, speak for him and answer questions on his behalf. They assume that the patient does not understand, and talk about him in his presence. This authoritarian attitude of the nurses, however kind and benevolent, makes the patient even more passive and withdrawn.

Every aspect of the patient's life needs attention when a rehabilitation programme is planned. At first every encouragement is given to him to take responsibility for his own life in the ward. He can make decisions about the clothes he wears and about the choice of food. He needs facilities to attend the hairdresser; he should choose his own clothes and look after his personal belongings. Private possessions are of great importance and the patient should be encouraged to give a personal touch to his own living space, putting photographs or ornaments on his bedside table and having his own belongings on his bed. He should have a key for his own wardrobe or cupboard and keep his property safely locked away. Facilities for self-medication, such as the provision of individual locked containers inside his wardrobe or bedside locker are necessary to increase independence further.

The patient's day should be as full as possible with a realistic programme of work and leisure. It is normal to be up and active for at least 14 hours, preferably 16 hours, out of 24.

VISITORS

The most important aspect of rehabilitation concerns the patient's link with people outside the hospital. If the patient's family can be induced to take an interest, this can be of utmost value, but even if relatives can no longer be traced, the patient can be put in contact with members of the hospital 'league of friends' or other voluntary workers. Many hospitals have found that unrestricted visiting helps to maintain contacts. If visitors can come at any time of the day and join in the hospital activities, they can be helped to a better understanding of the patient's behaviour, and will begin to realize that they need not over-protect or fuss over him when they are alone.

Whenever possible, the patient should go out with his visitors, at least to a restaurant for a cup of tea but, when it can be arranged, preferably to the visitor's house. Practice in living in the confined space of a private home and sharing in normal family life is of great help. The patient and the relatives can be encouraged to keep in touch by post. If contact has been lost over the years, the nurse can encourage the patient to write a letter. Most patients appreciate and enjoy receiving letters and postcards and can often be induced to reply.

During the time when visitors are in the hospital the nurse's help may be required to overcome embarrassment and anxiety. Relatives may become very upset if the patient does not immediately respond and may believe that their visits are not worth persevering with. They may also not realize that it is good for the patient to become involved in the problems of the family. Quite mistakenly, they may believe that they should spare the patient worry and anxiety by not talking about themselves. If the nurse is available during visiting time and gets to know the patient's relatives really well, she can help the visitors to establish contact more easily and keep the patient's interest alive between visits.

In order to re-establish the patient in society it is essential that he should have money to spend. On his visits home he needs to be able to pay for himself, he needs to know how much the fare home costs and how much it costs his family to visit him. If he goes to a café, he should know how much it is reasonable for the shop to charge. He should be able to plan his own personal budget and know how long he must save before he can buy a suit or a coat or a pair of shoes.

WORK IN REHABILITATION PROGRAMMES

Work in hospital can be of great value, provided the patient receives the full industrial rate of pay for the job he does. Even if he is charged for board and lodging and consequently is left with very little pocket money, it helps the patient to regain self-esteem if he receives a full pay packet and disposes of his own money. It is humiliating and harmful to pay the patient only a few pence when he is performing a full day's work.

Patients' money

The patients' ability to manage their own money, however small the amount, to look after it, to spend it wisely or to save up for planned bigger expenditure later, is very important. Patients who have been in hospital for a long time may have difficulty with the changing value of money and with the general changes in the nation's economy and patterns of consumption. Because the patients have difficulties it is easy to relieve them of the problem and to do their shopping for them. This temptation should, however, be resisted. The chance of rehabilitation in the community diminishes if the patient cannot cope with his own financial affairs. Some patients have saved up a considerable amount of money because life in hospital provides them with their basic needs and no one has encouraged them to spend or helped them to do so. Some patients' money derives from their earnings in industrial therapy or from other work in the hospital. Some patients go out to work and earn a full wage. Some patients receive money due to them from a pension fund, from social security or from some investment. Some patients' relatives send them regular sums of money. No patient should be destitute; if there is no evidence of a regular income, the social worker should be informed.

Problems may arise in the ward if patients do not know how to use their money. Safe keeping in the ward is often difficult and the responsibility for banking large amounts of money in the ward is not one nurses should undertake lightly. There is a great deal of book-keeping involved in distributing money and obtaining receipts, especially where personal spending by the patient needs supervision. It would seem that the most valuable contribution the nurse can make is to help the patient to understand his financial position and to learn to plan and control the spending of his money. When the nurse is at the same time the paymaster and the holder of the purse strings, she cannot fulfil the supportive role which could lead to the patient's autonomy and independence.

Industrial training

Some hospitals have been able to give patients a very useful industrial training by opening up industrial workshops and receiving contracts for industrial work for which the hospital receives normal piece rates of pay. Unfortunately, in times of economic decline, outside contracts for work are difficult to negotiate. The hospital may have to employ a manager or other staff to supervise the workshop, but any profit after overheads have been paid is shared by the patients. The value of factory work, when patients come from an industrial area, lies not only in teaching the patient to do a repetitive manual task with which he may be able to earn his own living. The main purpose of it lies in getting the patient used to the atmosphere of a real place of work, away from nursing staff and doctors and reminders of sickness. The patient can develop regular work habits, submit to the directions of the foreman, learn to clock in and out, and become perceptive of unwritten rules about working speed, rest pauses, cups of tea or smoking. He can become familiar with trade union practices and work organization. Most significant of all, he begins to become aware of his own significance in life and this helps to remove some of his submissiveness, even in the ward setting.

For patients who are not likely to return to industrial occupations it is difficult to provide equivalent training facilities. Farms and gardens are appropriate in agricultural districts, but most psychiatric hospitals have now given up running their own farms, and for most patients farm work is inappropriate. Many hospitals have successfully moved patients from wards into group homes so that they can do their own housekeeping, shopping, cleaning, cooking, entertaining friends, sewing and even carrying out small interior decorating jobs; this will all be valuable experience.

The Disabled Persons (Employment) Act of 1944 made it compulsory for certain employers to engage a percentage of registered disabled people. Those suffering from psychiatric disabilities are entitled to register as disabled and consequently may be able to find sheltered employment after leaving hospital. They may also be able to attend an Employment Rehabilitation Centre for assessment and may be accepted for retraining in a Government course. Work in hospital, if well planned and supervised, can prepare the patient for these experiences.

It is not always desirable to discharge the patient from hospital and at the same time expect him to find work. Adaptation to living outside hospital is difficult enough without the additional stress of adaptation to work. Some patients need residence in hospital while they begin to work outside. Others move out of the hospital either to a hostel or to live with relatives or friends, but continue to come to the hospital to work (see also Chapter 20).

Some contact with the hospital, either through a social club or by visits from social workers or community psychiatric nurses, may be necessary for a considerable period of time before the patient can finally accept complete independence.

Further reading

Barton, R. (1976) *Institutional Neurosis*, 3rd edn. Bristol: J. Wright.

Butler, R. & Rosenthal, G. (1978) *Behaviour and Rehabilitation*. Bristol: J. Wright.

Goffman, E. (1970) *Asylums*. Harmondsworth, Middlesex: Penguin.

Morgan, R. & Cheadle, J. (1981) *Psychiatric Rehabilitation*. Surbiton: National Schizophrenia Fellowship.

Watts, F.N. & Bennett, D., eds. (1983) *Theory and Practice of Psychiatric Rehabilitation*. Chichester: J. Wiley.

Wing, J.K. & Morris, B., eds. (1981) *Handbook of Rehabilitation Practice*. Oxford: Oxford University Press.

12
Nursing Disturbed Children and Adolescents

Some general principles underlying the care of psychiatrically disturbed patients have been described so far.

In this and the following chapters some of the principles will be discussed with reference to certain groups of patients for whom special provisions are necessary.

Children and adolescents, for whom an increasing number of hospitals are setting aside wards or units for treatment, are two such groups.

Although not all psychiatric nurses will have the opportunity of nursing children or adolescents, they may be interested to know something about the essential aspects of caring for these patients.

Disturbance in children can manifest itself first at home or at school. All children pass through difficult phases at some time or other and it may be extremely hard to decide whether a child's behaviour necessitates professional help or not. For brief periods disturbed behaviour is usually tolerated, though considerable anxiety may be aroused. Parental anxiety may then in turn result in increased disturbance in the child's behaviour.

When the child's disturbance becomes severe or goes on for a long time parents may feel under increased pressure to seek guidance and help.

Help is available from a number of sources. There are child guidance clinics associated with education authorities, where an educational psychologist assesses the child's problems and either treats the child or obtains psychiatric advice.

When the general practitioner is first consulted by the parents the child may be referred to a child psychiatrist in a paediatric or psychiatric out-patient department. In psychiatric clinics associated with the health services it is usual for a child psychiatrist and psychologist to see the child for diagnosis and treatment and a social worker to help the parents with their problems.

Social workers who in the past only became concerned with disturbed children and adolescents after a breakdown in the home had occurred, are increasingly charged with prevention. Children and adolescents may be referred to them in the first instance, and they may be able to give the necessary support with or without consultation of a psychiatrist.

In-patient treatment in hospital is only rarely resorted to. Treatment as out-patients or in special day or boarding schools for maladjusted children is much more frequent. Even when a period of in-patient treatment is necessary this is only a short episode in a much longer phase of treatment outside. The health of the whole family must therefore always be considered when a child is referred for psychiatric treatment.

In the case of children, psychotherapy sometimes takes the form of indirect interviews. The child finds it difficult to explain his worries and fears but he can talk about them more freely while he is playing, painting or drawing. His use of toys in the playroom indicates the stage of his development, and the nature of his disturbance. Observing the child at play reveals whether he plays constructively or destructively, whether he is relaxed or tense, inhibited or imaginative, friendly or hostile. Playing with dolls may reveal his feelings about various people.

Some of the children seen in clinics are mentally retarded. Often the anxiety of parents about the late development of a child causes emotional disturbances which are the real reason for seeking help. Reassurance and arrangements for special training and special treatment may enable the parents to accept the limitations of the child, and when excessive demands are no longer made on him, he may again settle down.

THE DIFFICULTIES OF DIAGNOSIS

Among the children who show disturbed behaviour necessitating treatment are those who may be suffering from early psychotic illnesses, those whose difficulties are associated with brain damage, epilepsy, or encephalitic infections, and those whose disturbed behaviour is closely related to mistakes in upbringing, to emotional disturbances in the family and to maternal unhappiness and anxiety. Many children come from broken homes, some are orphans, many have suffered separation from the mother during the first few years of life.

It is difficult to diagnose clearly any particular form of psychiatric illness in children. Many of the symptoms which are found in sick children are similar to those found in psychotic or neurotic adults, but some symptoms, which would be serious in adults, may be perfectly normal, at least at some stage of childhood. Withdrawal into fantasy, giggling and posturing, which would indicate a schizophrenic illness in adults, are not abnormal in early adolescence. Compulsive rituals are common in small children and form part of many games played, even by those who are older. Showing off is common, interest in the body, display and exposure are characteristic stages of development in most children, especially girls. No single symptom can be taken as evidence of mental disorder in a child. Even where the child's total behaviour pattern is definitely maladjusted it is difficult to decide if the illness is a reaction to a current emotional disturbance in the parents, evidence of the development of a neurotic personality, or an early psychotic manifestation.

Childhood autism is one of the psychiatric disorders which may be difficult to distinguish from other psychotic disorders of childhood and from mental retardation.

Children are easily influenced by environmental changes. Much suffering among them is the result of reaction to tensions experienced in the home. Children also influence their environment and much parental unhappiness and tension is caused by the maladjustment of a child.

Symptoms in children are as much determined by their age and stage of development, as by the specific disorder from which the child suffers.

At every stage of development the child is capable of only a limited repertoire of behaviour, and disturbance can occur only in such aspects of behaviour. In very young children the most common manifestations of disturbance affect sleep and feeding. Later, difficulties arise with elimination. All these are referred to as habit disorders.

As the child grows older he normally becomes interested in the physical environment. Play is important in the development of physical skills and intellectual progress. At this stage some children manifest their disturbance in apathy, lack of curiosity and failure to play; others play wildly and restlessly with such persistent overactivity that little progress is possible. Speech development is often disturbed and consequently the child's ability to communicate with people is poor.

At the time when the child becomes aware of his ability to make decisions and to influence others, disturbance often takes the form of temper tantrums, or of terror and panic attacks when the child feels overwhelmed by his own failures. Nightmares and periods of withdrawal into fantasy may be expressions of the child's difficulties.

As the child gets older behaviour disorders become more common. At school there may be complaints of bullying, disobedience and truancy, and at home there may be defiance and disobedience.

When the child resorts to destructive or delinquent behaviour parents may become particularly worried and exasperated.

A child's pattern of disturbed behaviour may of course persist beyond the phase of development when it first appeared. Children learn whether crying, whining, bullying or temper tantrums best solve their problems, and characteristic patterns of interaction develop in the families of disturbed children.

THE FAMILY

Even if it is too soon to hope that, in the future, adult mental illness will be prevented by the treatment of maladjusted children, it is necessary and helpful to break the vicious circle which results when the parents feel unable to handle the difficult situation created by the child's disturbed behaviour. The parents feel guilty, they experience mounting anxiety and helplessness and fear of criticism by friends and relatives. The child in turn reacts to the tension at home by becoming more disturbed. It is not usually the severity of the child's disturbance, but the parents' feeling of inadequacy that first causes psychiatric help to be sought.

The child psychiatrist takes the whole family situation into account when treating children. Not only the child's behaviour, but the mother's feelings about him are investigated. During treatment a better understanding of the child's problems is often acquired by the parents, and the child sometimes becomes sufficiently self-confident and adaptable to remain well, even if upsets occur in the family.

Admission to hospital, or even to a child guidance clinic as an out-patient, creates considerable conflict in the parents. It appears to them to be an admission of failure to have to seek help, and often they feel guilty and responsible for the child's illness. The hospital staff is sometimes treated with resentment and hostility as a result of this, and the hospital is criticized. The parents of a mentally ill child require as much sympathy, help and understanding as does the patient.

The doctor always obtains a history from the parents and encourages them to speak freely before asking detailed questions. Later the social worker gives the parents the help they require and interprets to them the approach of the psychiatrist and the hospital. She also helps the parents to understand their fears and to overcome their mistrust of the hospital and in particular of the nursing staff. Gradually they realize that their own failure to help the child is not interpreted as incompetence and that the nurses are not competing with them for the child's love and affection.

TREATMENT OF THE DISTURBED CHILD

Admission to hospital becomes necessary when a crisis occurs in the home and parents and child need a rest from each other, or when insufficient information is available from the parents and additional information is required from hospital staff who are able, by close observation, to assist in the assessment of the child's problem. The child is not always clearly aware of the reasons for admission to hospital. He may believe admission to be punishment for past misdeeds, and may resent the hospital and its staff. On the other hand, he may have very clear ideas about the help he would like but his ideas may not quite coincide with those of his parents. He may wish for some magic to remove his troublesome baby sister, for example, or for some medicine which might make him a good boy or for some operation which might change him into the kind of child his parents would prefer—into a girl, for example, or into a bright boy who is good at school.

It is important that the child's story should be listened to and his point of view respected if treatment is to be effective. If the child believes that doctor and nurses only listen to the mother's side of the story, he may not find it easy to express his own problem and difficulties. The general attitude should convey to the child that the staff are on his side and eager to understand how he feels.

Though children are often admitted after considerable tension at home, separation from the parents is nevertheless frequently traumatic. Homesickness and a period of grief and distress are very common during the early days of hospitalization.

The hospital ward must provide a warm, friendly harmonious background. Daily routine should be normal for the child's age and level of development.

Very young children can establish successful relationships with only a few individuals and all disturbed children have difficulties in making contact with many people at one time. A stable nursing staff is therefore required. Whenever possible the child should have one special nurse whom he can consider to be his own.

The routine must be flexible, according to the child's age and degree of illness, yet it must be sufficiently fixed to give him a sense of security.

The routine of children's wards must, of necessity, be different from that of adult wards because the normal pattern of activity for children is totally different.

The fixed points in a child's day, as in the adult's day, are meal-times. While the adult's day has a pattern of work and leisure, the child's day has a pattern of school and play. Bedtime and bath-time have much greater significance in a child's life than in the adult's.

Small children are sticklers for precise repetition in routine. The fact that the soap is in a different place in hospital from home may greatly distress a small child. The precise order in which dressing, washing or preparation for meals are carried out may be very important to him, just as his stories must be told with specific use of words and the bedclothes must be tucked in in a specific way.

Precise repetition of daily routine is much more important to the child than to the adult, who is usually able to cope with minor alterations from day to day even if he is mentally ill.

Over a period of time, however, the child's pattern of life changes much more than the adult's. An illness, for example, of three months occupies a relatively short space of time in an adult's life. For the small child three months may seem like an eternity. He may have difficulty in imagining the future so far ahead and therefore have difficulty in believing that he has a future life outside hospital. He may be unable to remember three months back, and therefore become more seriously detached from his home and family than the adult does in a similar time span. To be three months older means a lot to a child in terms of knowledge gained and in terms of rights and privileges.

The organization of a children's ward should, therefore, not only be concerned with providing the framework within which the child can learn to deal with his difficulties and problems, but also with the provision of an environment in which the child can grow and develop.

In the daily routine school work, music, handicraft, sports, carpentry all have a definite place in the timetable according to age. Outdoor activities must be arranged. The rest of the day can be spent in free play or games, entertainments, parties, stories or quiet reading.

The weekly routine means that each day is different from the others. Outings and visitors are planned for the week-end, different lessons take place on different days of the week. A predictable pattern emerges from the off-duty arrangements of the nursing staff and the interviews with the doctors. Children need target days for which to prepare and which divide the year into measurable periods. End of school term, for example, like Christmas day or birthdays, helps to measure time. It is always helpful if some specific event is being planned—a sports day, for example, an open day at school, an exhibition of paintings or the performance of a concert or play.

The activities of a children's ward should offer scope for children of all ages. Because the children are all disturbed, difficulties may arise at any time. Although when a child is upset, he may not be able to participate fully in the daily routine, the knowledge that the routine exists is of importance.

He must know what he is meant to do, even if at the moment he is unable to comply. If there is nothing for him to do, boredom sets in and increases the disturbance.

Each group of children may be interested in different pursuits and each nurse should use her own ideas and resourcefulness. One of the few general rules is always to take part in the children's activities. If the nurse is an uninterested, detached observer, she finds it very difficult to influence the children's activities. If she participates, she can suggest changes if the group becomes too wild or control over the game is lost, or if she feels that boredom might disrupt the group.

It is a good plan for the nurse always to have one or two new ideas up her sleeve when she is looking after children. When all are happy the children suggest their own activities. When interest flags it is useful to introduce something new and exciting, quickly and without delay.

The general attitude and approach to disturbed children are determined by the fact that the disturbance is considered to be a symptom of illness, not a sign of wickedness. All the staff are able to treat the child's behaviour with tolerance if they understand that he is unhappy, perhaps frightened, and very much in need of love. When children are mentally ill very few rules of behaviour can be laid down or enforced. This does not mean that antisocial behaviour should be encouraged. On the contrary, the nursing staff should try to make clear to the children what are desirable standards of behaviour. They can do this by example, encouragement, approval of appropriate behaviour, and positive suggestion to the child. Nurses can make it easier for a child to behave well by making few demands. But when uncontrolled, disturbed behaviour does occur it is treated in a matter-of-fact, unemotional manner and without moral condemnation.

The role of the nurse

One of the duties of the nurse is the prevention of physical injury to children or staff and as far as possible the limitation of damage to property. It should be made clear that overtly antisocial acts cannot be permitted and that the child will be prevented from injuring himself or others. This may have to be done by removing the child bodily and if necessary more than one nurse must be available. There is no need for anger to be shown. As soon as possible the nurse must convince the child that her love is not affected. No humiliation of the child should be involved and peace is re-established automatically once the disturbance is over, without any need for the child to 'lose face'.

Children who have lacked love and approval often find it difficult to believe that they really are accepted by the nurses. For a little while they enjoy the approval they receive and behave very well. Gradually they feel compelled to test the sincerity of the staff and their behaviour becomes worse, as if to provoke hostility and force the staff to show their hand. Continued friendliness drives the child to further experimentation. Gradually he becomes anxious and frightened, wondering how far he can go, and eventually forces the issue with a full-blown outburst of aggression.

Calm, quiet nursing staff, who remain in control of the situation, usually reassure him sufficiently for him to settle down in the ward.

Behaviour which may be acceptable because a child is severely disturbed may be imitated by other children who are well enough to go home soon, and who may have to learn to submit to the usual social sanctions. This raises the question of possible punishment. Punishment may be necessary as the child recovers. It is often demanded by the child whose sense of justice may be the best guide when it is difficult to differentiate between naughtiness and illness. No physical punishment can ever be used in hospital. Punishment in the form of exclusion from some activity may satisfy the demand for justice without causing resentment.

Some disturbed children are too frightened and too timid to be naughty at all. A certain amount of defiance, breaking of rules and naughtiness may be the first and very welcome sign of improvement. It would be very wrong if punishment were to frighten such a child back into submission. One of the most difficult tasks is to know what any particular action means to the child and when ordinary social standards should be applied in judging behaviour.

Normally children learn to forego immediate gratification of their wishes and to accept the restrictions of society, in order to retain the love, affection and approval of the person whose approval and love are valued. Usually the close tie with the mother helps the child to learn social codes and to deal satisfactorily with all the frustrations and emotional turmoils which occur in the process. When the emotional upheaval is too great and terrifying, or when the child has not been able to form a close emotional bond with an adult, he may fail to adapt in the normal way.

A child who lacks love and affection can progress only when he succeeds in forming a close relationship with somebody. If the nurse becomes the person whose love and approval are valued by the child, it is sufficient for her to make her standards known. The child will soon learn to conform. Unlimited love and affection are needed by most disturbed children. But the nurse who has successfully become the object of attachment must be careful not to disappoint the child, who would feel badly let down if 'his nurse' were suddenly moved from the ward. Gradual detachment and displacement of affection to another person may be helped by the doctor if it is planned ahead.

Innumerable problems inevitably arise when dealing with emotionally disturbed children. Each difficulty must be overcome as it arises, no general rules can be given, each nurse must develop sufficient self-confidence to make decisions as and when they become necessary. Each must become aware of her own ability to prevent a group of children from becoming uncontrolled. Each must discover for herself how and when it is safe to make demands on children and when to refrain. It is useful to remember how difficult it is to enforce an order given to a child. It is much better not to give it at all if it cannot be enforced. It is usually possible to suggest an activity rather than order it. If the suggestion is not taken, it does not damage the prestige of the nurse. 'Go and have a bath' is a command which may have to be carried out by force if it is not obeyed, but 'How about having a bath?', 'I'll turn your bath water on', or 'It is now bath time', will probably have the desired effect. If it does not, the idea of the bath can be dropped and nobody is the loser.

Many orders given to children and many prohibitions are really unnecessary. The nurse would do well always to hesitate before saying 'Don't', and to decide if she really means to be obeyed. If so, she must be prepared to enforce conformity. If it is not really essential, she might as well refrain from forbidding the action. It is, for example, quite useless to prohibit the use of swear words, as enforcement of acceptable language cannot be achieved. The nurse can indicate her approval of the right kind of language, even reward it, but she should ignore swearing. The child will soon stop using swear words if they fail to have the effect of provoking reactions of the staff.

If the nurse is to feel free to make her own spontaneous decisions in case of difficulty, she must feel secure in her relationship to the rest of the staff. Ward morale in a children's ward requires constant attention. Arguments about children in front of other children undermine confidence and authority. Children learn to exploit differences of opinion among the staff, and become insecure. All staff concerned with the treatment of the child should periodically discuss his progress and try to assess the part each one plays in treatment. Harmony among the staff is as important a factor in the treatment of disturbed children as is harmony in the home in the prevention of maladjustment.

The nursing care of autistic children may at times require that a special effort is made to reward the child when he makes contact with people and to ignore some of the bizarre or distressing behaviour which occurs when the child isolates himself from others. The nurse's spontaneous reactions to the child's disturbed and withdrawn state may be to love and cuddle the child and to give him more attention. Psychologists have shown that this reinforces the child's withdrawal. Nurses may feel unkind when they ignore such behaviour and may feel cruel when they have to insist on eye contact, on verbal response from the child and when, contrary to their own inclination, they may be required to withhold mothering and comfort. To observe how rapidly some autistic children give up rocking, grimacing and other mannerisms when more normal behaviour is reinforced, is, however, very gratifying.

TREATMENT OF THE DISTURBED ADOLESCENT

There is little agreement on what constitutes mental illness in relation to adolescence. An extreme view is that to speak of disturbance in adolescence is simply a euphemism for antisocial behaviour or laziness. Such a view ignores the fact that there are adolescents who cannot cope and are in immediate need of help and sometimes of care in the hospital setting. Over the past 25 years much has been done in the establishment of specialized units for the treatment of disturbance in young people but the nurse may well find that they make up a growing proportion of the patients in the admission, short-stay or disturbed wards of any psychiatric hospital.

Essential to a therapeutic relationship with adolescent patients is an understanding of the physiological, psychological and emotional changes being undergone at this time, so that a distinction can be made between the 'normal' mood shifts and disenchantment with adult values which do not interfere in any serious way with the ability of the adolescent to function, and those inner conflicts which disrupt psychological development to an extreme degree. Attempted suicide (parasuicide), especially by self-poisoning, is very common in adolescence. Girls around 16 years of age are those most commonly at risk. Social psychiatrists have found that these teenagers often come from deprived inner city areas where the incidence of vandalism, rent arrears and juvenile delinquency is high. Among the most frequently quoted reasons for an attempt have been the need to make members of the immediate family realize the girl is desperate for help, or a row with a boyfriend or with parents within the 48 hours preceding the attempt which necessitated admission—usually to a general hospital ward. Some of these adolescents may require to be admitted to a psychiatric unit/ward for treatment if symptoms of clinical depression are present. At all events, the girl and her family are seen by a psychiatrist before she is discharged from the general ward.

Crisis points arise in adolescence in the search for personal, sexual and occupational identity, and much of the disturbance recognized in young people is a result of confusion arising from the difficulties encountered in this search. Many adolescents have experienced so much condemnation and punishment because of their rebelliousness before admission that they expect to be rejected by the staff in hospital, and it is unfortunate if their experience is repeated.

Emotional maturity is not necessarily closely related to age and it may well be that a nurse who is close in age to the adolescent, but also mature enough to accept disturbed behaviour without moral judgement, may succeed in becoming an accepted member of the adolescent group. In this way, she may become an identification model for better adjusted behaviour, just as older members of staff can provide parental authority figures who are acceptable to the adolescent and thus provide a basis for better understanding of his own parents. Nursing adolescent patients requires an acceptance of the symptoms displayed, particularly disturbed behaviour which is likely to intensify in the early days of admission to hospital because of the acceptance and permissiveness shown by the staff, together with a clear understanding of what limits are necessary for physical and social behaviour. The nursing staff should also clarify for themselves that some limits are part of the treatment design, while others are necessitated by communal living, and be articulate on this subject with their patients. By this means the environment will be consistent, secure and supportive, in the sense that the conditions of residence are made explicit from the beginning and consistently enforced. Although the adolescent will almost inevitably rebel against constrictions, a lack of them could contribute to his sense of insecurity. The importance of limit-setting which is clear but non-punitive cannot be over-emphasized.

In essence, the aim of the staff, whether in a specialized unit or in a non-age-grouped ward setting, is to provide an environment in which the disturbed adolescents will be enabled to relate constructively to their peers and to adults.

It will be found that a commonly reported experience of the young people admitted for psychiatric treatment is a profound sense of psychological distance from others. Problems in forming and sustaining relationships, in feeling comfortable with other people, in sharing and communicating their experience and in being able to achieve a satisfactory degree of intimacy, characterize their histories.

Individual treatment and nursing care plans are useful in nursing disturbance in adolescents, their success depending largely on nursing observation of the developmental levels of the individual. Accurate reporting of behaviour and conversation, with staff group interpretation, are nursing functions which contribute greatly to the efficacy of treatment.

It has been mentioned that one characteristic which is most desirable in the nurse who is working with disturbed adolescents, is a thorough knowledge of developmental norms and the problems associated with gaining these. On an emotional level, the nurse should also be aware of her own needs for approval and satisfaction in this situation, which, if not acknowledged, may lead the nurse into the self-destructive position of being a friend without influence. The acceptance of disturbed behaviour which has been advocated may be seen as licence by the adolescent patient unless the nurse can forgo the reward of being liked and indicate very clearly that though she understands the reasons for this behaviour, it is not acceptable in society. Rapport with the adolescent patient is likely to be established most easily through physical care and in an integrated unit, this too can create the same problem. The use of physical and sometimes intimate vehicles for developing a relationship carries implicitly the danger of further confusion for the patient in identifying between the nurse as a mother figure, the nurse as a romantic object and the nurse as a benevolent stranger who is trying to meet some of his needs in a rational and constructive manner. Self-awareness in the nurse can prevent her acting provocatively, even on an unconscious level, with the adolescent patient.

One advantage of having young nursing staff working with disturbed adolescents is the readier acceptance by patients of the nurse who is close to themselves in experience and age rather than a full member of the closed adult world. This closeness, if unaccompanied by a high degree of self-knowledge and professional integrity, may lead the nurse into over-identification with the patients as individuals. It is helpful in this situation for the nurse to attend ward team conferences or any other meeting of professional people, so that her professional identity is underlined and the therapeutic aims of the team are frequently reiterated. Over-identification with young patients may lead to an inability on the part of the nurse to set and to adhere to the limits of behaviour which the patients need and want.

It is helpful in this nursing situation for the nurse to explore her own feelings of anger which will almost inevitably be her reaction at some point in the care of adolescent disturbance, since the disturbance may be expressed in ways which are distressing. Confronted with her own feelings of inadequacy in dealing with some of the situations which may arise, tension and anxiety levels rise in the nurse. This anxiety may be converted into an expression of power with a subsequent feeling of relief which will not harm the nurse but will equally not help the patient.

It may be, however, that the expression of anger will be followed by feelings of shame and guilt which are destructive of the nurse, the patient and the helping environment. This kind of damage can also arise when the nurse represses her angry feelings since anxiety then will continue to impair relationships and environment. There are times when anger can be appropriately and constructively expressed, as long as the nurse explains to the patient the reason for her anger and allows him to validate or correct her feeling. In this way, the patient is being helped to learn how to deal with his feelings, and what is the appropriate behaviour in an anxiety-producing situation.

Although many of the young patients who are admitted to adolescent units or psychiatric hospitals are in a generalized state of developmental turmoil, as already described, there are various diagnostic categories which necessitate in-patient treatment of the adolescent, and two groups in particular should be mentioned since they present particular problems in nursing care.

Solvent abuse ('glue sniffing')

Solvent abuse is not a new phenomenon; ether parties were fashionable during the last century. Its modern abuse, however, dates from the early 1970s—first reports were from the west of Scotland. Concern has been expressed at the increase in this activity in recent years and 81 deaths associated with solvent abuse were reported in 1981.

Children and adolescents are those most likely to abuse solvents—boys between 11 and 21 years and girls between 12 and 21 years have constituted the age range of referrals to a Saturday morning Solvent Abuse Clinic in Scotland since its inception in 1980.

Evostik, happily one of the least toxic, was found to be the most commonly used by the clinic attenders, followed by gas lighter fuel. Other solvents regularly inhaled included cleaning fluids and various aerosols, glues and cements, paint thinners and strippers, and hair lacquers.

Many of the substances used by the young people who abuse solvents can be cheaply purchased, or easily stolen, and anxiety has been voiced at their ready availability to young children. Epidemics of sniffing tend to break out in peer groups of schoolchildren. Most of these outbreaks prove to be transient group experiences for the children involved, but occasionally the more serious and dangerous occurrence of the isolated sniffer is brought to light. Young people who abuse solvent in this way may become habitual inhalers and there is some evidence that these children or adolescents have underlying problems requiring specialist treatment (see below). A few of those addicted to solvents come from deprived and unstable backgrounds. The Solvent Abuse (Scotland) Act 1983 has added the misuse by inhalation of the vapour of a volatile substance, for reasons other than medicinal, to the grounds on which a child may be referred to the unique Children's Panel as perhaps being in need of compulsory care. The Department of Health and Social Security, manufacturers and retailers have recently agreed in principle to voluntary restrictions on the sale of solvents. Legislation is to be introduced to limit sale, and companies are trying to develop non-solvent glues.

There are a variety of methods used to inhale solvent, most are very simple and inexpensive. A saturated handkerchief or a crisp bag containing the solvent is held over the mouth and nose. Initial effects are of euphoria followed by confusion and drowsiness; hallucinations, often vivid and colourful, may also occur. Toxic effects include brain and kidney damage, and respiratory depression and cardiac arrhythmias have been known to occur with fatal results.

'Glue sniffing' though on the increase, is for most young people a short-lived experiment. Nevertheless, parents, school nurses and teachers, the community psychiatric nurse and general practitioner should be alert to tell-tale signs of solvent abuse so that the dangers of this pursuit may be pointed out to the child involved in a counselling session. Repeated episodes of abuse of inhalants can be detected by the smell of the solvent on the young person's breath or clothing. More commonly, the presence of a persistent 'cold', spots or a red ring round the mouth may all be signs of solvent use. Behavioural changes may also be noticed in the classroom or at home. For example, truancy, poor examination performance, an increased tendency to withdraw from the peer group or petty thieving have all been reported. Treatment, if instituted, depends on the individual child and his reasons for abusing solvents. Often the young person's family, with support and guidance from the community psychiatric nurse, can cope successfully with the situation. Referral to a child guidance clinic may be necessary.

Controversy exists over the role of health education in combatting this problem. Advocates argue it is a valuable tool in areas where outbreaks of solvent abuse are known to be prevalent, arguing that it is at least important that children know of the potentially dangerous consequences from certain substances and methods of inhalation. Official policy prefers a low-key approach to avoid drawing undue attention to the problem, while at the same time promoting its early recognition by professionals.

The nurse's role

Specialist treatment for the young person who is habitually abusing solvents may involve admission to an adolescent unit, and should preferably include family therapy, as well as individual psychotherapy.

Habitual use of solvents indicates that the young person has found a method of relieving tension and insecurity and that he will be most unwilling to give this up, adding a further dimension to the nursing care necessity. At first the adolescent patient must tolerate separation from solvents, then exploration of his feelings in order to find out why he first turned to them for comfort, and how he can protect himself against the necessity for them in future. The nurse must be prepared for a great deal of hostility, since she is dealing with someone who is at best ambivalent about being in hospital and at worst completely against any attempt at therapy. It is essential, for any progress to be made, that the nurse avoids a judgemental attitude toward the young patient who abuses solvents and shows a positive approach of genuine interest and understanding of his problems. The distress experienced by the adolescent who is expected to relinquish the prop which he has come to require in order to function requires a high degree of empathic tolerance.

Anorexia nervosa

As with solvent abuse, this condition has increased considerably in recent years. It is found predominantly in girls, and is often related to the problems of puberty and adolescence, so that peak incidence is within the 14–19 year age group. Physically, it is manifested as emaciation from refusal to eat, accompanied by constipation and amenorrhoea, and psychologically there is denial of illness, hyperactivity, sleep disturbance and aggressive negativism against all treatment efforts. It is not merely an anomaly of food intake or weight regulation, but a disorder involving extensive disturbance in personality development.

Nursing care and treatment
It is generally accepted that initially one of the essential ingredients of treatment is to take measures to help the girl to return to her normal weight, and if the loss has been severe, admission to hospital is necessary.

On admission, a nurse may be specially assigned to spend periods of time with the young girl, allowing her to talk about her fears and to foster a supportive relationship. It is often also necessary for the nurse to remain with the patient while she eats her meals, and to reassure her constantly that the aim of treatment is not to make her fat but only to help her regain her normal weight. The nurse should also stay with the girl for a while after the meal is finished, not only to ensure she does not try to induce vomiting, but also to allow the patient to feel that the nurse is interested in her as a person, not just in the amount of food she consumes. If, however, weight-losing behaviours are discovered, these should be discussed openly with the patient.

A nursing care plan is agreed with the patient. This should contain a detailed account of what is expected from the patient, for example a clear statement of the amount of food at each course and the number of courses to be eaten at each meal-time, and also the relevant nursing interventions. This will ensure a consistent approach by all who care for the patient and avoid fruitless discussions and attempts at manipulation by the girl should she sense the situation is ambiguous in any way.

Psychotherapeutic sessions with the psychiatrist should run concurrently with measures taken to reverse weight loss, otherwise the young girl will become increasingly fearful that weight gain is equated with the resolution of all her problems.

Behavioural methods have been used in the treatment of anorexia nervosa. For example, a target weight is agreed upon and a few days later a contingency contract is drawn up, with a full explanation of what is involved given to the patient. Sometimes a hierarchy of desirable events or items is drawn up by the patient and then inverted, making the most desired item the most difficult to attain. Positive reinforcements are discussed and these are contingent on weight gain. Thus, if a target daily weight gain of approximately 0.2–0.4 kg is not reached, certain reinforcers are withdrawn, such as television, newspapers or visitors, until the patient's weight, which is monitored daily, begins to increase towards the agreed goal. It may be necessary for the patient to remain in bed, at least for part of the day, and to use a commode and be supervised during and after meals if there is a failure to gain weight or if on admission the patient's weight is so dangerously low that even the slightest exertion has to be avoided.

As restoration of premorbid weight levels draws near, the patient needs considerable support lest she break off the contract and leave hospital, only to relapse later.

Behavioural techniques must also be coupled with individual psychotherapy, and family therapy is often required to be included in a treatment programme for a patient with anorexia nervosa.

Over two-thirds of patients with this eating disorder return to their normal weight, but self-induced vomiting, laxative abuse, the presence of depression or obsessional features are all indicators of a poor prognosis, as are late onset and a very severe weight loss.

A mortality of 5% has been quoted for sufferers of anorexia nervosa. Suicide is the most frequent cause of death. Acute gastric dilatation and electrolyte imbalance, especially of potassium levels as a result of excessive vomiting and purging, also account for the high mortality rate in this disorder. Anorectic girls from a working-class background are said to do less well than those from the middle classes, from which the majority of these patients come.

Drugs have been tried in the treatment of anorexia nervosa, for example chlorpromazine, which is thought to increase the patient's appetite; antidepressant drugs may be used if depression is also present. None has proved to be outstandingly useful nor to affect the long-term outcome for the patient. Some authorities feel drugs are best avoided if possible.

Anorexic Aid, a self-help group, has published guidelines to help families identify the condition early, and it also gives useful advice on how best to cope with the patient after she has been discharged from hospital.

Further reading

Barker, P. (1983) *Basic Child Psychiatry*, 4th edn. London: Granada.

Claggett, M.S. (1980) Anorexia nervosa: a behavioural approach. *American Journal of Nursing 80* (8), 1411.

Gibson, E. (1983) Body talk. *Nursing Times 79* (7), 60.

Hawton, K. & Goldacre, M. (1982) Hospital admission for adverse effects of medicinal agents (mainly self-poisoning) among adolescents in the Oxford region. *British Journal of Psychiatry 141*, 166.

Hsu, L.K.G. (1980) *Anorexia Nervosa*, SK & F Publications, Vol. 3, No. 4.

McClure, G. (1984) Recent trends in suicide among the young. *British Journal of Psychiatry 144*, 134.

Rogers, H. (1982) Glue sniffing among schoolchildren. *Health Visitor 55*, 236.

Wilkinson, T.R. (1983) *Child and Adolescent Psychiatric Nursing*. Oxford: Blackwell Scientific.

13
The mentally ill elderly patient

Almost half of the patients in most psychiatric hospitals at present are elderly people. In addition a very large proportion of newly admitted patients are over 60 years of age. Of these patients, women are in the majority. Although the patients suffer from a wide variety of mental disorders, it is useful to examine at first to what extent the nursing problems are determined by old age, rather than by the disorder. There are, broadly speaking, three groups of older patients.

1 Those whose mental illnesses resemble disorders occurring in young people, but who happen to be getting on in years. Many of these patients, e.g. those suffering from depressive illnesses, have had previous attacks and may have been in hospital before.

2 Those whose mental illness is an accompaniment of old age. Senile dementia is an example of the disorders of this group. Rather less than 50% of the mentally ill elderly suffer from dementia.

3 Patients who have spent many years in psychiatric hospitals and who have grown old there. Some schizophrenic patients, for instance, may have been admitted at the age of 20 and may still be in hospital at the age of 65 or 70. This last group includes some patients who have partly recovered from the illness which has occasioned their admission but who had no home to which to go when their discharge from hospital would have been possible. Others may have had recurrent attacks of mental illness, returned home slightly less efficient after each attack, and have finally remained in hospital when, owing to their own increasing age, the family no longer found it possible to shoulder the burden of caring for an old and troublesome patient.

THE REACTIONS OF THE ELDERLY

The specific care of each patient depends partly on the nature of his illness, partly on the prospect he has of being discharged. To a large extent it is determined by age alone, and initially it is proposed to examine the problems of nursing the elderly in psychiatric hospitals irrespective of the illness from which they suffer. Later, care of patients suffering from acute and chronic organic psychiatric disorders will be discussed, and something will be said of depression occurring in the elderly person.

All who are sick and admitted to hospital react to their dependence on nurses and doctors in a manner which is in some way determined by their previous experience of similar relationships. Most adult patients, for instance, react to the nurse in a similar way to that in which, many years before, they treated their mothers who provided food, care and comfort. According to the patient's own previous pattern, he treats the nurse, the 'mother figure', with love and gratitude, with adulation, or with hate and resentment. The elderly occasionally adopt the attitude of previous childish dependence. More often, however, they do not allow themselves to accept this position and instead, in the manner of some adolescents, they endeavour to prove their independence, showing militant resentment towards those whose authority they are unwilling to accept.

Normally, particularly in the case of physically ill patients, the nurse can exploit the phase when the patient accepts dependence, use it to build up prestige, and will be grateful for the patient's non-critical submission to treatment. Nevertheless, the nurse should be aware of the abnormal characteristics of this phase and detect the first signs of recovery, when the patient assumes his role of independence and begins to become more critical and impatient. In the case of the elderly, complete dependence is rare and it would perhaps be a bad thing if it occurred. Perhaps the patient's desperate attempt to cling to independence, to assert it and to resist letting himself go, represents the basis on which to build when the nurse tries to help him to rehabilitate in preparation for discharge. But the immediate effect is that old people can be difficult to nurse. They may find it necessary to assert their independence, as if, otherwise, their claim to greater wisdom and experience might be overlooked. Far from manifesting uncritical acceptance of the nurse's endeavour to help, old people often are constantly finding fault and reminding her of her shortcomings. Far from accepting authority in medical matters, elderly patients may be rebelliously antagonistic to all efforts on their behalf, resent being dependent, and particularly being dependent on a young person, someone the age of their granddaughter.

This relationship might create difficulties if, in her turn, the nurse showed resentment and hostility or if she were to react by adopting a patronizing attitude to the elderly patient. These attitudes are quite commonly found in the patient's own family relationships. The daughter, finding the patient rather difficult to manage, becomes hostile and refuses to help or begins to feel ashamed of her elderly relative and becomes patronizing, thereby aggravating already strained relationships. Nurses only too frequently adopt a condescending attitude to elderly patients. Sometimes they show it in their dealings with the patients, sometimes it emerges only in talking about them. It is of utmost importance for the nurse, if she wishes to make a success of her role, to take herself in hand when she discovers such an attitude in herself. The elderly are entitled to regard and esteem by virtue of their superior age alone. To the patient, nurses may be mere children, people whom he considers young, irresponsible and inexperienced. He is paying the nurse a great compliment by entrusting her with his welfare.

Habits established over a period of a lifetime are difficult to change, and, with advancing years, it becomes more difficult to learn new ones. To a young patient, it may not matter greatly that meals in hospital are served at a different time from the one to which he is used; to the older one this may be a continued source of irritation. Hospital routine obviously differs in many respects from the regimen to which each patient is accustomed. It cannot always be made to suit the individual patient's wishes. By making hospital routine fairly constant and rigid the patient may in time accept it. This is a difficult task for the patient and his difficulty should be appreciated. On discharge, he has to make new adjustments in many ways as difficult as the first one. With patience and understanding he can be assisted in adapting himself, but, wherever possible, he should be spared the effort of doing so. Many of the patient's habits could easily be carried over into hospital life if a little effort were made to adapt hospital routine to the patient. Unless his behaviour is decidedly harmful to himself or others, there is no reason why he should not continue to behave in the way he has always done. He is very unlikely, for example, to change his table manners, or his preferences for certain articles of food. Some nurses, while appreciating the patient's difficulties, show their condescension by talking about 'letting the patient have his little ways'. These may be 'little' to the nurse but the irritation caused by unnecessary interference may assume mountainous dimensions in the view of those who are ill, and may seriously impede the nurse in essential nursing matters.

THE PHYSICAL REQUIREMENTS OF THE ELDERLY

The patient's physical health must be considered when the nursing care or routine of the ward is planned. The elderly find stairs very difficult to manage. They become breathless when climbing upstairs, may easily stumble and fall when coming downstairs and are fatigued if required to climb stairs several times a day. This presents a major problem to the planning of psychiatric hospitals and to the allocation of existing wards. Ground floors would be so much more suitable for almost all patients that it is difficult to allocate priorities. Stairs may make it difficult for older patients to participate fully in those social and occupational events which take place away from the wards and may seriously interfere with their use of the garden and enjoyment of fresh air. Those patients who could move about were it not for the stairs, but who are compelled to remain in the ward if stairs have to be negotiated, should be placed in ground-floor wards. Those who are able to go upstairs should be given plenty of time, encouraged to walk slowly and assisted when necessary. A nurse should always be below patients on the stairs. Hand-rails should be provided and stairs kept in good repair. Nurses should report at once when a step is faulty or when patients experience difficulty with sloping steps, or steps which are not clearly visible. Good lighting on staircases is essential and nothing must be left lying about on the treads.

Within the ward nurses should be constantly on the lookout for anything that may contribute to accidents. Highly polished floors are dangerous and the use of small rugs should be avoided. Patients who cannot lift their feet too well are liable to stumble and fall. Needless to say, the floor under a rug should never be polished. Furniture should be firm and fairly heavy. Patients are not likely themselves to move furniture, so that its weight is not a disadvantage. Heavy furniture allows patients to lean on it. The elderly often use the furniture for support when they move or when they get tired, and it would be highly dangerous were it to give way. Any broken furniture should be repaired as soon as possible, or at least moved out of the way. The process of sitting down or of getting up may be most cumbersome for an elderly person, and chairs must give full support when the patient tries to raise himself. High seats and upright backs are on the whole more comfortable for old people than chairs with low seats and reclining backs.

Radiators should be guarded where old people are being nursed. The elderly should never climb a ladder or even stand on a chair in order to reach their belongings. Bathrooms are places of potential danger. Many old people cannot manage to get in and out of a bath unaided and for this reason some old people have not had a bath for a considerable time prior to admission. The patient may resist when a bath is suggested in hospital and the nurse may have to reassure the patient that she will give all the help required. Even with help, however, bathing may be a difficult procedure. A hand-rail on the bath is a help and some modern baths are fitted with one, but old-fashioned baths with very high sides are a problem. The bath should be accessible from both sides. It may be helpful to put a mat into the bath to prevent slipping. Baths of better design, particularly for elderly patients, are needed in many psychiatric hospitals. A thermostatically regulated shower may be an acceptable alternative for some old people, provided they can sit most or all of the time.

The elderly require assistance with washing and dressing. It may become very difficult for them to fasten garments at the back and almost impossible to put on socks and tights. Some patients cannot tie up shoelaces because they cannot bend down without losing their balance or feeling giddy, and they cannot raise their leg high enough to place it on a chair. For the same reason elderly patients have difficulties in washing their feet and cutting toenails. All old people should be provided with the services of a chiropodist. A visit to an outside chiropodist may be a useful reality exercise for the patient who is able to go, if the nursing resources permit. It is also tiring for many elderly patients to raise their arms to brush and comb the hair and, unless assistance is given, the hair may then not receive enough care.

A large variety of aids for the disabled are now available and some of these can be adapted for use of the aged. Nurses should try to keep well informed about equipment as it comes on the market and use their influence and knowledge when new equipment is on order.

Psychiatric patients, when they are old, do not differ from other elderly people in the amount of assistance they require, but they differ in their attitude to those who are able and willing to give help. They are often unable or unwilling to ask for help and accept it grudgingly when it is offered. Much depends on the nurse's approach. If she does not wait to be asked but offers help, anticipating the patient's needs, making it appear that the patient is doing the nurse a favour by allowing her to help, she may succeed. She must, however, refrain from doing too much for the patient. The elderly should be encouraged to remain active to the limit of their capability.

OCCUPATIONS FOR THE ELDERLY

It is generally agreed that the elderly are much happier and healthier if they continue to work and have some interest. Those who continue to work beyond their normal retiring age usually appreciate the fact that they are still able to be useful members of the community, independent by earning at least a small amount of money. After retirement, those with many and varied interests are a great deal more contented than people whose only interest has been in their work. The happiest old people are those who have begun to take up new hobbies before retirement and who have looked forward to the day when they would be able to devote more time to the occupations they enjoy.

The elderly are slower in their actions than are the young, and there are many things they cannot do at all. They should never be expected to lift heavy objects and they must be protected from the risk of physical injury, but if any job can be found within their physical capacity, they should be allowed and encouraged to do it. There are many jobs in psychiatric hospitals which old patients can do quite as well as young ones. They can clean the wards, sweep, dust, polish furniture and brass, but not of course scrub floors. They can prepare meals, wash up and lay tables. According to ability and previous experience, they may sew or help in the laundry. Anyone skilled in these crafts can make rugs, knit, embroider cushions or make toys.

It is desirable that the elderly should work among others of their own age, not in competition with younger and stronger patients. Arrangements may have to be made for more frequent rest pauses or for sitting down where others could be expected to stand. No patient should work beyond the point of fatigue. Half-day occupation is probably enough for old people, because they need more time than others for getting to the place of work and take longer for all their other activities. The slower tempo of the elderly is one of the main reasons why it is desirable not to mix them with young patients in the wards. The routine should be specially designed to take into account their slow movements and their need for more time with everything they do.

The fact that special arrangements are needed for the elderly does not, however, mean that they should be cut off from younger people. The company and stimulation of the young may contribute to keeping the older person interested and active. The judgement and advice of the older patients may be constructively used in the process of discussion and decision-making in the hospital.

Usually elderly patients do not mind rising early. They are often awake from early hours, and prefer to get up. They should be allowed to take their time over dressing and washing and not be rushed. They cannot be expected to be well groomed if they are not allowed enough time. It is much better for the patient to dress slowly than for him to be dressed by a nurse. Plenty of time should be allowed for meals, which should be peaceful, leisurely occasions, looked forward to and enjoyed by all. The patient requires a rest period during the day, probably after lunch, and ample time must be allowed for exercise in the garden, since this entails the changing of shoes and putting on of overcoats and warm clothing.

ENTERTAINMENT

Evening entertainments are better enjoyed by the elderly if they are among themselves, although they appreciate an occasional chance of watching the young ones at a dance. It may be possible to develop new interests, but it takes a long time and the new activity must be started and well established by somebody before it is taken up by those who have never done it before. It is a common experience that there are vogues for certain types of handicraft. One patient may be an expert at knitting bedjackets. If her efforts are suitably admired by all, particularly by the nursing staff, some other patient may decide to try. Soon there may be a third patient trying it and, before long, most patients may be knitting bedjackets. In due course, this activity is replaced by a new one, e.g. embroidery or production of shopping bags, each activity being started and spread in the same manner. Interest in entertainments develops in a similar way. It is no use asking patients if they wish to go to a whist drive. It should be taken for granted that a few will go. Within a few weeks, more and more patients also do so.

Initiative as regards new activities often comes from the nursing staff. The nurse should sit down and play the piano, if she knows how, rather than ask if the patients would like her to, or wait until they ask her. She should be the first to sit down to a game of cards or initiate a singsong. It is unlikely that the patients would ever start without her lead.

Hearing and eyesight usually deteriorate in old age. Many of the activities taking place in hospital cannot be enjoyed by old patients because they are unable to follow clearly what is happening. Plays on the stage are often wasted on them, they cannot understand the jokes and find other people's hilarity irritating. Radio can be enjoyed only if the patient can adjust the set to his own liking; he cannot listen in a group nor can he watch television from the back of the room. In handicrafts he may be able to carry out large movements and distinguish a large pattern, but he may become clumsy and inaccurate if he is asked to do fine work. It should be possible to predict whether a patient is likely to enjoy a particular entertainment and he should not be put into a position where it is brought home to him that his senses are failing and that he is falling off in efficiency.

Failing eyesight and defective hearing may give rise to many misunderstandings between patients and staff. The patient may not understand what is said to him and do the opposite to what was asked. He may think he understood and accuse the nurse of mis-stating the truth. He may know that nurses are speaking, but if he does not hear clearly he may become suspicious and irritable and feel that people are talking about him.

He may become forgetful and mislay his belongings, and then accuse others of having taken them; or he may tell jokes or stories over and over again, having forgotten that he has previously told them. Conversation between old people frequently amounts to two monologues, each one pursuing his own thoughts and paying little attention to the other. In conversation with old patients the nurse should try to follow their thoughts, and, if she wants to make herself understood, to speak in such a way that the patient really attends to her.

PHYSICAL HEALTH

The physical health of all elderly patients must be carefully watched. Coughs should be taken notice of early in order to prevent the development of chronic bronchitis; varicose veins and ulcers should receive attention. The nurse must ensure that each patient receives and takes an adequate, balanced diet and to achieve this the patient must have regular access to a dentist. Dentures, for example, must be comfortable and correctly fitted otherwise the patient will prefer to do without them. Elderly patients may also require some help with elimination problems; constipation, for example, may be troublesome. In old men, it is necessary to ensure that the bladder is properly emptied, and the possibility of enlargement of the prostate should be borne in mind and any early symptoms reported.

Many old people sleep badly and many require some form of sedation. With well-regulated activity during the day, the patients should succeed in getting a few hours' sleep at night. The elderly do not sleep very deeply and if they sleep in dormitories they disturb each other. Small rooms are preferable for elderly patients. Most doctors agree that mild sedation is to be preferred to restless nights and the nurse should observe the effect which the sedative has on the patient in order to ensure that the right kind of drug is prescribed. Restlessness at night is sometimes due to frequency of micturition, and this should be noticed by the night nurse. Sometimes confusion and restlessness at night are the first indications of heart failure. A careful report by the night nurse may lead to earlier diagnosis of heart trouble than would otherwise be possible.

So far, problems affecting all elderly patients irrespective of their illness have been discussed. More must now be said about special aspects of various forms of mental disorder in old age.

The newly admitted patient

Of the three groups of patients, those who are most in need of help are those who are newly admitted. Almost invariably, admission was preceded by a series of crises of increasing severity. Admission to a psychiatric hospital is feared by patients and relatives and resorted to only when no other action is possible. By the time this happens, personal relationships at home have reached breaking point, and are made even worse by the sense of failure and feelings of guilt experienced by those who are ultimately responsible for initiating admission. Young people are so frequently reminded of their responsibility towards the older generation, and so often blamed for the plight of old people, that many will go to any extreme in trying to preserve their aged relative from what appears to them the terrible fate of admission to a psychiatric hospital. The relatives require all the reassurance they can be given that their difficulties are appreciated and they should receive all possible assistance in the struggle with their feelings of guilt and shame. It is often simpler for strangers than for relatives to deal with difficult behaviour in the elderly.

Relatives should be helped to realize that admission to a psychiatric hospital, however late in life, need not be final and that their continued interest is essential if the patient is to return to them after recovery. Often the social worker has to undertake the task of maintaining the relatives' interest in the patient and of giving the former enough support to make them willing and able to take the patient back.

Elderly patients who are newly admitted are often in need of help but reject this with all their might. These are the patients who are often physically below par, undernourished because, living alone, they have been unable to cater for themselves and have not asked for help or have refused it. They may have neglected their appearance for some time, and may be dirty, badly clothed and unkempt, especially if they are also beginning to show signs of intellectual impairment, for example failing memory. They are often very lonely people. As age advances, many friends die, others live too far away to maintain contacts and it is difficult to make new ones. Opportunity does not often arise for meeting new people, and, if it does, the patient may have made himself sufficiently disagreeable to frighten away other possible contacts. The fewer the patient's interests and hobbies, the more difficult it is for him to find satisfaction. Admission to hospital means a complete change in the patient's life to which he may find it very difficult to submit.

The aim in nursing the patient must be to help him to leave hospital in the shortest possible time, better equipped to deal with the problems of old age, which he will inevitably have to face. The nurse can help to do this if she understands as fully as possible just where the patient's particular problems lie, and resists adopting towards him an attitude which might repeat the old situation. While helping the patient to regain better physical health, a routine is established which he should be able to follow after discharge. He is helped to regain self-confidence and self-respect by becoming useful within the hospital, and the way is paved for some occupation to be pursued after discharge. Occupational therapy must therefore take a form which can be continued in the patient's own home. If he can learn to make something with which he might earn a little money, all the better.

While the patient is in hospital he is helped to make friends. This is comparatively easy in hospital where there are fellow sufferers. After discharge, he may be able to maintain his newly formed friendships by joining clubs, either of former patients or other old people's clubs. The community psychiatric nurse can often help by making the necessary introductions to these social activities. During his stay in hospital the patient has been helped to develop new interests and to enjoy leisure-time activities of the kind offered by many clubs. While in hospital he should be encouraged to maintain his interest in the outside world, by talking with visitors about life outside, by conversation with nurses and by keeping directly in touch with the outside world. Elderly patients should be taken out for walks and should do shopping outside the hospital, so that they can manage traffic, deal with money and use public transport. If they are kept too long away from the hustle of the street, they find it terribly difficult to go back. Coach trips and outings are of value, but even more important are such simple activities as crossing the road, paying for bus tickets, handling the money to pay for a cup of tea.

Meanwhile, with help, the patient's relatives examine more dispassionately their own difficulties. They realize to what extent mental illness was responsible for the patient's difficult behaviour. They observe how nurses and doctors handle the situation and how the patient responds. Gradually, first at week-ends, they prepare to take the patient back for short periods and eventually accept full responsibility for looking after a difficult old person, having the reassuring knowledge that the hospital is always willing to give help whenever it is required and that the community psychiatric nurse will call and give continuing support.

It is not always possible to discharge the patient home, but active interest on the part of relatives helps, even if he has to remain permanently in hospital or be transferred to a home for the elderly. A National Health Service nursing home (a new experiment) might be a possibility in the future.

The long-stay elderly patient

In many respects, old age is much less difficult for the patient who has grown old in hospital. For him no change is involved. He is generally in better physical health, well cared for, and in many ways leads a fuller life than many old people normally do. He is not lonely and no retirement problems arise. His job in the hospital can go on indefinitely as long as he can manage it. He has had time to develop many interests because the programme of social events in hospital is quite extensive. Unless the patient is suffering from dementia, or has been allowed to become passive and helpless, the main nursing task is to make his life as rich and useful as his own health and hospital conditions allow.

It should be remembered that the patient who has been in hospital for a long time and who has grown old there may treat the ward or the hospital as his home. He may feel responsible for the place and rightly resent any changes which are introduced without his knowledge and consent. In the course of his stay in the hospital he has met many nurses and he may therefore be uninterested in yet another one who appears in the ward. Especially with a rapid turnover of staff, long-stay patients have learnt to ignore nurses unless they manage to make some unique contribution to life in the ward or unless, by virtue of some special circumstances, their personality or quality of work makes an unusual impact on the patients.

Patients with acute organic psychiatric disorders

One of the cardinal features of acute organic psychiatric disorders is impairment (clouding) of the patient's level of consciousness. However slight, there is an associated reduction in the elderly person's ability to pay attention, accompanied by increased distractability and loss of concentration.

The memory disturbances reflect these deficits and also help to account for the patient's inability to grasp explanations and take in new information. This results in the other predominant clinical feature, disorientation in time, place and ultimately person.

The elderly person, therefore, may look around in a bewildered, dazed and frightened manner, growing increasingly perplexed and anxious; emotional lability is not uncommon.

Speech may be incoherent and disjointed. Illusions may add to his fears—for example an electric flex may be seen as a snake—and terrifying hallucinations may also be present.

Although the nervous system is intact, distorted messages account for many of the patient's responses to his environment, such as bouts of restless overactivity, especially at night, or his apparent unco-operative behaviour and irritable mood.

General aims of nursing care
1   To protect the patient from injury
2   To adapt the patient's environment to his psychological needs
3   To care for the patient's physical needs

In order to escape from his hallucinations, the patient may act impulsively. In the initial, acute phase a nurse must remain with the patient continually. If possible, a close relative may relieve the nursing staff for periods of time. His calm, reassuring and soothing influence on this acutely disturbed patient can be useful. The relative, however, will in turn require considerable support from the nurse.

Primary nursing* is especially suited to meet this patient's psychological needs. Overstimulation is avoided by the presence of only one or two nurses and, in addition, continuity and consistency of approach is achieved. In the face of this patient's excited behaviour, the nurse should try to remain calm and address him in a clear, firm and distinct voice. She must be prepared to repeat explanations, again and again if necessary, using simple and short sentences.

The patient's environment should be adapted to reinforce reality and to reduce excessive stimulation. A quiet side room may be chosen—provided staffing levels permit—with a low bed to avoid injury when the patient is overactive. Good lighting is necessary throughout the 24 hours lest shadows increase the possibility for illusions. Superfluous items of equipment should be removed for the same reason. Large clocks and clearly visible calendars assist orientation; familiar objects such as family photographs can also help.

If the patient is confined to bed for medical reasons, he should be encouraged, if possible, to sit upright. A nurse who leans over a recumbent patient can be perceived as a threatening and frightening figure. Often a hand on the patient's arm or brow can help focus his attention and establish face-to-face contact. This is of value before the nurse begins to explain a procedure she is about to carry out, or to convey, non-verbally, care and concern when the patient is distressed.

If spectacles or a hearing aid are normally worn, the nurse should ensure they are available to the patient; without them the patient's already tenuous grip of reality is further weakened.

---

*Primary nursing in this context is a system of organizing care in which one nurse is responsible for any one particular patient and only a small team is involved.

Any physical care given to the patient should be explained step by step. For example, when bathing the patient in bed the nurse should give a running commentary—'I'm going to wash your face first ...'—and in order to interpret reality further for the patient she should allow him to see and to touch his face flannel. As soon as the patient is physically able, he should be encouraged towards self-care; no matter how little he can accomplish at first, it can be comforting for this patient to discover, for example, that his arms (and legs) can still function as they should.

An elderly patient suffering from an acute confusional state is often physically very ill and may show signs of vasomotor instability, such as flushing or pallor, rapid pulse, raised or lowered blood pressure. In addition hyperpyrexia or hypopyrexia, tremor of the fingers, hands, lips and facial muscles may be seen. Nursing observations should be recorded frequently during this phase, as often as half-hourly if required. During lucid periods the patient may complain of headache and weakness.

Nursing care of a physically ill elderly person includes encouraging adequate fluid intake to prevent or counteract dehydration. It is essential that frequent drinks are offered, the nurse taking full advantage of the patient's lucid periods as they occur. Whenever possible the patient should be allowed to drink by himself and, if the cup is filled only half full, this will avoid spillage from his tremulous hand. It will also lessen distress to the patient. Fine glassware should not be used since it could be bitten through if the patient suddenly became very disturbed. Fluids should include high-calorie nutritious drinks, but strong tea and coffee are best avoided because of their stimulant effect. An accurate fluid balance chart should be kept.

Other aspects of nursing care include assisting the patient with his personal and oral hygiene as well as anticipating his elimination needs or responding to them. Attention to the cleanliness and integrity of the patient's skin is necessary, especially if he is sweating profusely or is incontinent of urine.

Although restlessness is a common feature, it should not be assumed that this is invariably due to the patient's organic psychiatric disorder. The immediate reason for restlessness may be impacted faeces, or, more commonly, the elderly person's wish to go to the toilet. The presence of an indwelling catheter does not necessarily alleviate this problem. A bewildered and frightened patient may be quite unable to understand that he no longer requires to micturate if he has a urinary catheter *in situ*, especially when the feeling of the need to micturate is created by the presence of the catheter.

Patients with subacute organic psychiatric disorders

As the name implies, this state presents a much less florid picture and can be missed in a patient who is already suffering from a chronic organic psychiatric condition. However, the nursing staff, having a thorough knowledge of the patients on the ward, can play a vital role in the early detection of this state. The nurse can observe any sign that a patient's level of consciousness is fluctuating, or that his behaviour is deviating from its normal pattern. Expression of fleeting delusions or unwarranted suspiciousness occurring for the first time should alert the nurse to its presence.

One example which might illustrate this arose in a ward where a patient suddenly and uncharacteristically accused a female staff nurse of making passes at her husband who had visited that afternoon. Clinical examination later confirmed that this patient was suffering from a chest infection giving rise to a subacute organic psychiatric disorder.

Patients with chronic organic psychiatric disorders (dementia)

In a chronic organic psychiatric disorder all aspects of the patient's mental life are eventually disturbed. There is often a history of progressive falling off in mental functioning, beginning with minor memory impairment (short-term memory is affected rather than long term), lapses in standards of behaviour and difficulty in grasping essentials, finally leading to severe memory loss and general disintegration of the patient's intellectual powers. By the time the elderly person is admitted to hospital she might be disoriented in time and place and there is often evidence of a lack of self-care. Emotional responses may be blunted or, conversely, there may be lability of mood. Close relatives occasionally believe the patient to be 'depressed' (more will be said of this later).

A husband may tell of his wife's restlessness, especially at night with consequent periods of sleeping during the day, and of her wandering out of her home and being unable to find her way back. Outbursts of aggression and querulousness may also be reported if this elderly person is thwarted in her desire to leave the house whenever she wishes.

Nursing care

The primary aim in caring for the patient with a chronic organic psychiatric disorder is to improve, or at least maintain, quality of life for as long as is possible.

A carefully drawn-up nursing care plan should help ensure a consistent approach. As with the acutely confused patient, primary nursing is preferable, there being only a limited number of new faces for the patient to get used to at first.

Independence in the activities of everyday living should be nurtured from the day the patient is admitted to hospital. One cardinal rule is not to hurry the patient, but to allow her to carry out tasks at her own pace. The nurse should always give the patient time to answer when a question has been addressed to her. Waiting for an answer and listening to what the patient has to say helps boost self-esteem. The patient may stop reacting altogether if no one is willing to listen. Misinterpretation of surroundings may be worsened if an impatient nurse hurries the patient while washing and dressing, for example. The nurse must resist the temptation to take over the patient's self-care.

Routine should be simple, consistent and supportive. Any necessary change should be made slowly after giving the patient a careful explanation of what is to come. The nurse should not expect responses from the patient that are beyond her capabilities. It may be necessary on occasions to decrease the environmental stimuli by reducing demands on the patient so as to prevent a reaction of undue distress or frustration.

On the other hand, the nurse should assist the elderly patient towards eventually making full use of her abilities, limited though they may be in many instances.

The patient's orientation and sense of identity can be helped by the provision of some private space around the bed area where familiar objects may be displayed. If practical, family photographs, a treasured object and even a favourite chair can help the patient recognize his own territory.

Colour can be used freely as a further aid to spatial orientation. For example, toilet doors could be painted blue, with blue tiled stripes running along the floor of rooms and corridors leading to them.

The nurse must also ensure that information is clearly available to the patient who is disoriented in time. Large clocks with distinct numbers for each hour are essential, as are reality boards and/or calendars with clear figures and letters giving the date and the day of the week.

Despite these measures, some patients, especially in the later stages of dementia, may still be seen wandering about in an aimless fashion. It is important that the nurse copes with this type of behaviour in a non-threatening way. She should go up to the patient slowly so as not to startle, call her by her correct name and then reintroduce herself. It is not helpful to ask the patient where she is going, but rather to walk alongside her for a short distance. The nurse could take her arm and talk in simple, short sentences and in concrete terms about some neutral topic, such as the weather. Both could pause at a window and look out to reinforce what the nurse has already said. If the patient is upset, the nurse should respond primarily to the emotion—rather than to the content of what is being said. The patient's distress should be acknowledged and she should be reassured of the nurse's concern and protection. Should it be necessary to disagree with the patient, this should be done tactfully and gently. Presently the nurse can perhaps guide the patient back to the day room to join the others. It should be appreciated that a patient who abruptly gets up from an activity and leaves the room to go to 'make the family's dinner' may be indicating that she has had enough for the present and this should be acknowledged.

Weather permitting, a short walk in the fresh air can often help to relieve the patient's tension and reduce wandering to a certain extent.

As a result of short-term memory loss, the intellectually impaired patient is not able to process new information efficiently. A nurse's reassurance to the effect that she is aware the patient cannot remember some things but that she will be around to help with this problem can have a supportive effect.

The use of non-verbal communication such as touch, tone of voice and posture can sometimes alleviate a sense of isolation in patients with advanced dementia. Eye contact should be established whenever possible, either by sitting at the same level or sitting on the floor in front of the patient looking upwards. Eyes can be an indispensable medium for effective non-verbal communication. Just as the patient can see in the nurse's eyes a genuine look of caring, the nurse can detect in the patient's eyes any discomfort, pain, anger or fear she may be experiencing. There could be occasions too when the patient is 'telling' the nurse to go away, for example when she pointedly walks away or closes her eyes. The nurse should be receptive to these messages and respect them.

A seriously demented patient may have to relearn some of the basic skills involved in self-care if these have been lost through lack of use prior to admission. Behaviour therapy techniques such as backward or reverse chaining may be used when encouraging the patient to dress, for example. Bladder control may have been lost, but before an attempt is made to restore function, medical causes must first be sought and, if present, eliminated. Some patients can be helped to become continent if, for example, special charts are used over a period of time and carefully analysed to identify the peak times at which the patient should be encouraged to micturate. Positive reinforcers in the form of appropriate and prompt expressions of praise by the nurse can help to maintain the desired response from the patient. Being continent raises self-esteem.

Reality orientation
It is important that the nurse should use all interactions with the elderly demented patient to give him basic information relating to orientation. Firstly, she should call the patient by his correct name and reintroduce herself on approach, then give the time of day, explain slowly and clearly what is happening and later, as appropriate, relate details about the ward and its surroundings. Thus a night nurse, on approaching a restless elderly patient wandering around in the early hours of the morning, might say, 'Hello, Mrs Scott. I'm Nurse Green. It's two o'clock in the morning ...', rather than the more usual questioning approach of 'Why are you not in bed, Mrs Scott? Where are you going? Is there something the matter? ...'. This

is sometimes referred to as 'informal reality orientation' or '24-hour reality orientation'.

A more formal type of reality orientation (RO), sometimes called 'class reality orientation', involves small group sessions and is carried out for patients who, though not severely organically impaired, are nevertheless apathetic and socially withdrawn. Two or three times a week, or sometimes daily, the same group of patients meets for approximately half an hour at the same time of day. A therapist, who may be a nurse or another member of the multidisciplinary team, talks with patients about a variety of different topics such as the weather, food, holidays or past personal events. In essence, the aim is to reinstate existing memories rather than to attempt to create new ones. This orientation towards reality is based on the idea that certain types of basic information are essential if the demented patient is to function at a reasonable level.

For some patients these sessions are the highlight of their day, but not everyone who attends reacts favourably. The attentive nurse should note and report any undesirable behavioural changes in the patients who are members of the group. A patient may have to be excluded if he is observed to show symptoms of overt psychotic behaviour after, say, the second or third week of reality orientation sessions.

Demented patients can also benefit from less formally structured group activities arranged by the nursing staff. These might include gentle physical exercises with musical accompaniment, followed by attempts to increase social interaction and lessen isolation. A session may take the form of familiar music being played with the opportunity of reminiscences afterwards. The recollection of significant events in the patient's life, such as past successes and other positive experiences, can contribute towards enhancing self-esteem and feelings of individuality. Nurses, too, gain considerable job satisfaction from the personal relationships strengthened on these occasions, and patients appreciate being listened to.

It is important for the nurse to appreciate that any activities she plans for the elderly patient should be appropriate for this age group and, if possible, culturally valued. Childish spelling games, for example, should not be included.

Everyday simple measures such as the reorganization of seating arrangements and the provision of small round tables can also be effective in maximizing spontaneous social interactions among elderly patients.

Depression in the elderly patient

Depression is not uncommon in the elderly and, as with many psychiatric disorders, the causes are a complex interaction between social, psychological and biological factors. The precise 'mix', however, varies from one elderly person to another. Social isolation, for example, may contribute towards an elderly person's relapse only a few months after having had successful treatment in hospital for a depressive illness. A traumatic life event, on the other hand, such as the death of a spouse, can give rise to feelings of helplessness and hopelessness and may trigger off a depressive episode, particularly in a person prone to recurrent attacks. Sometimes the depression manifests itself in somatic features, for example anorexia, insomnia, constipation, in addition to psychotic symptoms such as delusions of guilt and auditory hallucinations. A favourable response to one of the second-generation antidepressant drugs may lend support to a possible biological basis for the illness.

Depression in the elderly can be severe; indeed, the incidence of suicide rises with age. The 'young' elderly (65–74 years) are especially vulnerable and men more so than women.

Occasionally patients suffering from dementia may be reported by close relatives to be 'depressed'. While these patients are indeed sometimes dejected and have a tendency to weep inappropriately in emotionless circumstances, they do not usually show the extreme apathy, self-denigration, early morning wakening (late insomnia) and profound feelings of despair found in the truly depressed elderly person.

Pseudodementia (depressive pseudodementia)
Depression in the elderly, especially the very elderly, can, however, present atypically and the observant psychiatric nurse can on occasions be expected to assist in establishing a correct diagnosis.

One such atypical presentation is that of pseudodementia. A close relative may report that prior to admission the patient had become inaccessible and that sometimes his speech had been incoherent. Refusal of food and drink may not be uncommon.

In hospital the patient may show apparent disorientation, perplexity and occasionally diminished awareness, but without any obvious depression of mood, giving rise to the probability that he is suffering from dementia.

Some signs of apparent memory disturbance may be present, but further careful examination may reveal that intellectual impairment is confined to rote learning, whereas in dementia the deficits are widespread (global) and affect all areas of learning. Unlike the patient with true dementia, a patient suffering from pseudodementia is able to cope with a considerable amount of new information provided it is well structured and the patient's full attention is gained. As with all depressed patients, difficulty in concentration is a problem.

Other factors to be considered in the differential diagnosis are the duration and mode of onset of the symptoms. A history of a fairly sudden qualitative change in the patient's behaviour is compatible with a diagnosis of depression, as is a recent traumatic life event. A family or personal history of depression—occasionally concealed initially by relatives—may also point to a depressive reaction.

It is also of interest to note that these patients can often give a clear account of their illness provided they are not rushed and the questions are skilfully phrased to avoid negative replies such as 'I don't know'.

Whereas the patient with true dementia will start to undertake any task and then break down if overstretched, the depressed patient may immediately become distressed and make little initial effort to perform even the simplest task.

The psychiatric nurse should note any occasions when the patient emerges from spells of inaccessibility and incoherence to make such statements as 'I'm not worthy of this food', a remark strongly indicative of a patient who is depressed.

If the patient actually remembers details of his daily routine when he was fully attending to the nurse's words, this indicates a diagnosis of depression rather than dementia. An observant nurse might report, for example, that the patient was able to find his way to the toilet (or the dining room) fairly soon after his admission without her having to give directions over and over again.

It is not known why depression should sometimes present in this atypical way in the very elderly, but some deficit in the neurochemistry of the ageing brain has been posited.

Further reading

Arie, T. (1983) Pseudodementia. *British Medical Journal 286*, 1301.

Holden, U.P. & Woods, R.T. (1982) *Reality Orientation*. Edinburgh: Churchill Livingstone.

Towell, D. & Harries, C. (1979) *Innovations in Patient Care*. London: Croom Helm.

Trochman, G. (1978) Caring for the confused or delirious patient. *American Journal of Nursing 78* (9), 1495.

Wolanin, M. & Phillips, L. (1981) *Confusion: Prevention and Care*. London: C.V. Mosby.

14
Nursing Patients Who Feel Depressed

DEPRESSION

At some time or other, everyone has felt somewhat depressed, has thought that life was just too much of an effort and hardly worth living and felt generally 'under the weather'. Friends have days when, from their actions, appearance and words, it is evident that their mood is black. Most people have seen a friend in grief and sorrow and experienced the urge to express sympathy and yet known the helpless groping for words which would comfort or would convey their real feelings. Conventional words of condolence may then have been uttered but silence soon fell owing to an inability to console. Yet the visit paid, and even the silence, together with a sharing of his grief, gave such a friend some help and comfort.

Moods of depression do not last very long in normal, healthy people. The mentally ill patient, however, may continue to feel depressed for a very long time and the nurse must continue to comfort, well beyond the point when she actually experiences sympathetic grief with the patient.

The right thing is automatically done when a bereaved friend is visited. Anyone trying to give consolation is quiet and not noisy or boisterous. Little is said and there is no joking or looking particularly happy. No reference is made to the good things in life or to personal pleasures and there is intense awareness of an inability to help, but the slightest sign of interest on the part of the bereaved is encouraged by vividly taking up any topic he himself may broach.

In the nursing of depressed patients this is just what needs to be done, but for very much longer and in much more difficult circumstances. The only comfort that can be given to the patient is empathy, interest and appreciation of his mood. The nurse continues this without ever giving the slightest sign of boredom or irritation and she responds to the slightest evidence of the depression lifting.

The symptoms of depression

The feeling of hopelessness, misery and despair experienced by depressed patients is easily communicated to the nurses. Gestures, facial expression, posture, all convey the patient's dejection. He may express in words his feeling of unworthiness and guilt, and experience a desire for punishment which he may even try to inflict upon himself. Voices may comment on the patient's imagined sinful behaviour and he may consider himself too wicked to be in this world, too dangerous to others to be in contact with them.

Some depressed patients feel flat, apathetic and lifeless. They are unable to respond to people, their emotions are dulled and their ability to react to others diminished. Love, hate and affection mean nothing, the patient feels indifferent and the world around him seems changed.

The absence of emotion makes it more difficult for the patient to communicate his depression to others. He becomes asocial, withdrawn and lacks energy. He experiences difficulty in thinking and does not concentrate easily on what is said to him. His speech and movement become slower, his bodily functions disordered.

It is no easy task for the nurse to give emotional warmth and personal care to the unresponsive patient, who yet needs interest and affection and is aware of the emotional attitude of the nurse, but unable to respond to it. He is not helped by being forced into activity, and cannot benefit from contact with too many people. The continued bodily care and personal service given by one or possibly a few nurses may help to re-establish a little emotional response. The nurse should be able to give warmth, even though she does not receive any response, and should be able to assess the patient's ability to receive solicitude without being overwhelmed by even greater feelings of unworthiness. On recovery many patients comment on the fact that attention from a nurse was desperately needed at the time of deepest depression, but that it seemed quite impossible to make this need known. The physical presence of the nurse may be sufficient by itself during the acute phase of a depressed patient's illness; a comforting arm round his shoulder can convey more than words. Any nurse who is able to respond in this way to a patient's need for company at a time when he cannot make the effort to ask for it, is greatly appreciated by the patient.

Physical care

A depressed patient is often physically unwell. Constipation, loss of appetite, skin rashes and boils may occur, and only the most careful nursing can prevent serious deterioration in his physical condition.

Feelings of unworthiness may lead the patient to wish to punish himself by not eating, and the problem of providing food and fluids in adequate amounts is the crux of nursing care (see also Chapter 9, The significance of food). The task of eating may be broken down into minute steps by the nurse, who should indicate that she will carry out her responsibility to provide sustenance although she appreciates the reasons for the patient's refusal to eat. Small meals composed of food the patient is known to prefer, as ascertained from relatives if necessary, may be given. Keeping a record of the amount and kind of food taken at each meal will provide a valuable index as to whether the patient is receiving the necessary variety in his intake. Some foods may interact with drugs, making observation vital (see Chapter 18). Regular weighing and the condition of the skin and mouth are reliable criteria by which to judge the adequacy of nursing measures in regard to food and fluids. Careful attention to the patient's personal hygiene, frequent bathing and attention to the mouth help to prevent skin and mouth infection. Exercise, plenty of fluids to drink and a diet containing an adequate amount of roughage should prevent constipation. However, a laxative may have to be given on occasions owing to the tendency for some antidepressant drugs to cause constipation.

The patient takes little interest in his personal appearance, has no initiative, no energy, and all the effort to maintain his health has to be made by the nurse. In the acute stage of depression, it may be necessary to dress the patient, then as he progresses to help by assembling his clothing, and handing it over, one garment at a time. Large tasks are often overwhelming for the patient in the early stages, so should be broken into achievable units according to progress.

Since circulation may be impaired by the slowing down of bodily processes, patients are particularly liable to feel cold. The nurse should be aware of this, so that an extra sweater or blanket can be provided if necessary. Suggestions as to change of position, elevation of the feet, or the giving of passive exercise by light massage may also be helpful in reducing the effect of sluggish circulation.

SUICIDE

Depressed patients usually improve, although without active treatment this may take a long time. With the help of drugs or electroconvulsive therapy, recovery takes place more quickly. Meanwhile, nursing is aimed at preventing suicide and relieving the intense suffering of the depressed patient. The nurse's approach, her attitude and general understanding assist him in his recovery. Only skilful observation, incessant vigilance and the most intimate knowledge of her patient can help her to prevent suicidal attempts. However resentful the patient may be of being kept alive, the nurse must remember that depression passes. Once he has recovered, the patient may view the problems in a different light and be grateful that he was not allowed to kill himself. As depression deepens a patient may feel increasingly desperate and may fear that he will be unable to resist the impulse to commit suicide. Such a patient may seek admission hoping that he will be prevented from carrying out any suicidal ideas he may have. He puts his life into the hands of the nursing staff and needs the sense of security gained from being under constant observation.

It is not always easy to assess how serious the patient's suicidal intentions are, but all expressions of suicidal thoughts and every gesture the patient makes to take his life should receive full attention. There is a common fallacy that a person who talks about committing suicide will not ever do so; this is completely untrue. Suicide is the action of a person who is desperate. Suicidal attempts may be made to draw someone's attention to the patient's plight. If the patient succeeds in his cry for help and attention is paid to him, he may not need to resort to further suicidal acts. If his attempt is ignored, or worse still ridiculed, he may be driven to more desperate action.

Sometimes a patient improves dramatically after a serious suicidal attempt. This may be because his suffering may be interpreted as atonement for the guilt he imagines himself to carry, or it may be because his relatives or friends have suddenly understood the patient's need for support. Once the patient no longer feels abandoned he can bear to be alive.

If his suicidal attempt fails to bring his relatives to his aid, the nurse has to do the best she can to stand by the patient and provide the motive for living. If, however, the nurse also fails to pay attention to the patient, he feels almost compelled to prove how serious his despair is. Patients sometimes tell one member of the staff about suicidal thoughts, begging the person not to betray their confidence. This should never be agreed to. However convincing the patient's plea may appear, he may in fact wish his intentions to be known. If he did not want the staff to protect him, he would not mention his thoughts to anyone. If the nurse in whom he had confided had agreed to keep the knowledge secret, the patient would have interpreted this as an invitation to go ahead with his plans.

It may be helpful for the nurse to know that one of the most acute danger periods for suicide is when the patient just begins to recover from the despair which engulfed him in the acute stage of his illness. The passivity which then characterized him gives way to the first stirrings of energy which may, in his still very depressed state, provide him with the impetus to attempt to end his life.

This initial 'recovery' period can coincide with the early stages of antidepressant drug therapy or occur after the first few treatments with electroconvulsive therapy. Research has pinpointed certain other danger periods when the patient is liable to attempt to harm himself. These include periods when the ward staff are preoccupied with various other duties and distractions such as meal-times and shift changeover, and times when fewer staff are on duty, e.g. weekends and night duty. It has also been shown that the patient may have an air of serenity in the period immediately prior to the suicidal attempt. It has been postulated that at this stage the patient is no longer in conflict with himself and has finally made up his mind to carry out his plans.

Some psychiatric hospitals used to be so designed that obvious suicidal risks were minimized. Window panes were small, making it difficult for a patient to pass through them. Windows were blocked or locked, opening a few centimetres at the top and bottom only, and usually sufficiently far apart to make it difficult to fasten a rope on to a window frame. Staircases were so constructed that it was impossible for anyone to throw himself over a banister, and were of short flights so there was little danger of a patient throwing himself downstairs. At the top of the stairs there were gates or open doors. If the doors were locked, they were some distance from the head of the stairs. This prevented a sudden dash towards the staircase when anyone entered the ward. There were few projections to which ropes could be fixed. Pipes and radiators were covered in so that it was impossible to hide any articles behind them. Lights were placed high up, close against the ceiling; fires were guarded. The most dangerous articles were kept under lock and key. Such architectural devices, however, are no longer found in most psychiatric wards, and extra vigilance is therefore required in the case of patients who may be contemplating suicide.

Routine precautions against suicide

Some hospitals take routine precautions in wards in which suicidal patients are nursed, so as to reduce the risk of suicide by any of the more usual means. The ratio of staff to patients in these wards is relatively high so that patients can be under constant observation, day and night. Routine varies in different hospitals. Whatever the routine in any particular ward, it is most important that all members of the staff should be thoroughly familiar with the rules and carry them out faithfully at all times. It is relatively unimportant, for example, whether the doors of a ward are open or locked, but very important that all members of the staff should know which doors are open, which locked, and that each should be able to rely on every other member of the team to lock those doors which are meant to be locked.

Dangerous objects

In many hospitals patients' property is listed and checked on admission and certain potentially dangerous articles are removed if a patient is known to have suicidal thoughts. Scissors, nail files, razor blades and drugs are usually taken away and the patient is told that he may ask for these articles when he needs them for use. By removing them in the first instance, and only giving them out when required, the nurse is aware of the number of sharp instruments or tools in use at any time, thus ensuring that they are used only for the proper purpose.

It is advisable to look through the patient's property most carefully on admission, because drugs or razor blades can be hidden in the most inconspicuous places. Linings of pockets or handbags are obvious hiding places but patients may secrete dangerous articles in seams, in tins of talcum powder or lipstick cases, in face-cream jars or about their own persons. If all the patient's belongings are removed on admission and only returned after careful inspection, some danger is avoided. The nurses know of all the articles the patient possesses, and anxiety shown by him for the return of a particular object may lead to a more thorough search and often the discovery of something that has been hidden. This, of course, apart from lessening danger, gives a valuable lead to understanding the patient's state of mind.

The property is examined with the full knowledge of the patient and preferably with his assistance. To most people it is distressing and embarrassing to allow strangers access to their personal belongings. The patient is almost certainly distressed when he knows that the nurse wishes to examine his property on admission. It may, however, be reassuring to him to know that the nurses care for him sufficiently to take the necessary precautions which ensure the safekeeping of his belongings and the safety of his person.

Nurses sometimes find the task embarrassing and for that reason might tend to hurry over the procedure. Half-hearted attempts to look at the patient's belongings do nothing to alleviate distress. If the nurse fails to discover dangerous objects the patient has secreted, the patient feels less than safe with such a nurse and consequently more anxious. The patient's property can never be examined in secret and without the patient's knowledge, firstly because this would be extremely degrading to the patient, and secondly because if any dangerous articles are found, this has to be fully discussed with the patient.

Some precautionary measures are possible without excessive restriction of the patient's activities.

When clothes are marked with the patient's name, belts, dressing gown and pyjama cords can be stitched in, shoelaces firmly secured and the most dangerous articles of clothing kept from him until more is known about him. If no torn linen is ever used in the ward, it becomes possible at once to discover when the patient is trying to tear sheets or blankets, or collect pieces of tape which could be used at some future time to make a rope.

If all beds are regularly stripped by patients and nurses together and if lockers are regularly cleaned out, especially after visitors have left parcels, then any dangerous object the patient may try to hide is easily discovered. Alternatively, visitors may be requested to give anything they have brought for the patient to the charge nurse first of all.

If cutlery is put out only just before a meal is due to be served and if the right amount of cutlery is always laid for each patient and collected from each patient when the meal is finished, special checking of cutlery becomes unnecessary.

If breakages occur, it is helpful if the broken pieces are cleared with all possible speed and if a nurse assumes responsibility for checking that all pieces are accounted for.

It is unusual for patients who are depressed to have baths without a nurse being present. The nurse must always check with the charge nurse before allowing a patient to bathe alone. Actively suicidal patients would not be allowed into the bathroom by themselves. In some hospitals or in some wards, hot-water taps are removable and used only by the nurse, never being handled by patients. Bathrooms, when not in use, are kept locked, as also are kitchens, broom cupboards and sluice rooms. Patients who are acutely depressed usually enter the kitchen only if accompanied by a nurse. The patient's clothing may be kept locked up, clothes either being handed to him by a nurse or he may be allowed access to them only when accompanied. By these means the nurse knows what the patient is wearing, and at any time could give an accurate description of him if the need arose. She also knows if the patient has any money on him, and how much, since she will herself have given it to him on request. Nurses should know which patients wear spectacles and notice at once if they are missing. If any patient is wearing jewellery, wedding ring or watch, this too should be known and noted. Some patients sleep with their dentures in place, a fact which must be pointed out to the night nurse.

Matches and lighters may not be allowed in the ward and the nurse lights the patient's cigarette for him. She then knows when anyone is smoking and is able to make sure that the cigarette is put out when finished and not used to light another. This reduces the risk of fire.

Smoking in bed is usually discouraged, except when the patient is in bed all day.

Poisons

All poisons, drugs and lotions are kept under lock and key and no bottles are ever taken into the ward. If a disinfectant is required for cleaning, the pail of water is brought to the store-room and the disinfectant put into the water there. Medicines are poured out in the room in which the medicine cupboard is kept, and taken into the ward one at a time. Tablets are sometimes given crushed, unless contrary to manufacturers' instructions, so that they cannot be hoarded, or medication may be available in syrup form. No patient ever gains access to an open drug cupboard. Cleaning materials are kept locked, because polish and cleaning powders are potentially dangerous. Sterilizing and clinical rooms are not entered by patients. Once a treatment tray is prepared, it is never left out of sight of a nurse. If any surgical procedure is carried out, one nurse is responsible for the safety of the equipment while another carries out the treatment. Temperatures are taken in the axilla, not in the mouth. Patients should never be left while any treatment is being carried out. The nurse may need to stay with the patient for some time after giving medication.

Observation of suicidal patients

If these precautions are carried out in a ward in which potentially suicidal patients are nursed, they facilitate the special care and observation which are necessary when any individual patient is known to have expressed suicidal ideas. It may be necessary in special circumstances to keep a particular patient under constant observation. Whenever a member of the staff becomes aware of her patient's suicidal intentions, she must immediately report this to all who are concerned in his care. The nurse who is assigned to look after the patient should ensure that her relief is well instructed in her duties. In some hospitals patients under constant observation are always accompanied by a nurse, but any other members of the staff, e.g. occupational therapists, must also assume responsibility.

While a patient is under constant observation, he should never be out of sight or out of reach of the nurse. Whether this can be achieved when the patient is up and dressed, or whether it is necessary for him to remain in bed, depends on the staff available.

It is impossible to keep a patient under constant observation without his knowing that this is being done. The nurse should therefore meet the patient's questions quite frankly, and either herself explain the procedure to him or make sure that his doctor has done this. The patient may ask the reason for the surveillance, but is then merely expecting the nurse to confirm reasons well known to him. With a little tact the nurse can usually manage to obtain from him the explanation of why he is being observed and so avoid the embarrassment of pretending not to know.

Constant observation is an extremely arduous duty. For parts of the day it may be possible to keep the patient occupied. Games of chess, card games, reading aloud, may make his, and the nurse's, life easier, but if he is severely depressed, he may not wish to speak or be spoken to, there may be long periods of silence and complete inactivity on his part, during which the nurse must keep herself occupied, without ever relaxing vigilance. She must not become so absorbed in any work that she will not notice the patient's every movement, yet she cannot just sit and stare at him. The patient has little to do other than to watch the staff, and any carelessness or negligence on the part of the nurse is noticed and use may be made of this knowledge at some later date.

It is often pointed out that the effect of constant observation is that the patient observes the staff more efficiently than the nurses are able to observe the patient. It may indeed be much more dangerous to carry out constant observation negligently than to relax the rules altogether. The more it is necessary to take precautions, the more resourceful must the patient be if he is to outwit the staff. The removal from him of all the usual means of committing suicide may act as a challenge to him to find new and unusual methods.

It is perhaps with this idea in mind that most hospitals have abandoned constant observation, and report no increase in the incidence of attempted or successful suicide. They claim that no patient would abuse the confidence and trust which the staff have placed in him. This, however, appears to some people to represent a somewhat superficial view, even if it is true that statistically the incidence of fatalities does not rise.

The nurse's trust in the patient may prevent his suicide in hospital, but may result only in an earlier discharge, followed by successful suicide. In any case, it seems hardly fair to place the responsibility on the patient, when he may have entered the hospital for protection.

Where life is at stake, statistics seem unimportant. Even a single successful suicide is unforgivable if the nursing staff have to admit that they had taken no steps to prevent it. It is sad if the patient succeeds in committing suicide in spite of all precautions, but to have to admit a knowledge of the patient's intentions which were then ignored would be but cold comfort to a bereaved relative, who may well feel that he could have done better himself.

When a patient in the ward makes a suicidal attempt, or when a successful suicide has occurred, widespread repercussions are usually evident among patients and staff. Nurses feel guilty at what they perceive to be a failure in their task of preserving life. They may resort to 'scapegoating' of each other, trying to attach blame to someone in an attempt to clear their own conscience. They very naturally wish to ensure that no negligence has occurred. Nurses feel despondent and distressed, and however earnestly they may try to spare the other patients' feelings, their own emotions inevitably affect ward atmosphere.

There are usually at least a few patients who share in the self-reproach and guilt feelings of the nursing staff and who believe they might have been able to prevent the tragedy had they been more observant or more ready to confide in the staff that they knew of the patient's suicidal intentions.

The general depression in the ward is often aggravated by the anxiety patients begin to feel for their own safety. Many patients become uncomfortably aware that they may find themselves unprotected should they succumb to suicidal impulses.

Free discussion of the incident often relieves anxiety far better than an attempt to maintain secrecy. Patients often put forward constructive and practical ideas on how future attempts could be prevented and often suggest methods of co-operation designed to protect each other. When patients feel able to share responsibility for each other, close observation by nurses becomes less important and the restrictive aspects of supervision can be more easily relaxed.

The importance of teamwork

To sum up, it may be said that the nursing of suicidally depressed patients is the acid test of a good nurse and of teamwork and co-operation. Opinions differ as to the best method to be employed. Some feel that every conceivable precaution must be taken to prevent suicide. Others believe that constant observation increases rather than relieves depression, and that in order to help the patient over his depressed mood certain risks must be taken. Those who are in favour of stringent precautions point out that the reasons for depression are unconscious, not related to the present, and that good nurses can carry out constant observation without it becoming irksome to patients. Those who prefer to give the patient a maximum of freedom point to the success of their method.

All, however, are agreed that if risks are taken, this should be done deliberately and that, while calculated risks may be justifiable, negligence is not. All are agreed that it is essential for all staff to work as a team, to be fully aware of whatever rules are in operation, and to carry out any agreed procedure with 100% efficiency. With this in mind, the most stringent care has been described here. Every nurse must ensure that she is fully aware of all the rules which apply to the ward in which she is working.

Further reading

Cormack, D. (1983) *Psychiatric Nursing Described*. Edinburgh: Churchill Livingstone.

Gray, E.G. (1983) Severe depression: a patient's thoughts. *British Journal of Psychiatry 143*, 319.

Rowe, D. (1983) Helping the depressed patient. *Nursing Times 79* (43), 62.

Taylor, C.M. (1982) *Mereness' Essentials of Psychiatric Nursing*, 11th edn. London: C.V. Mosby.

15
Care of Disturbed and Violent Patients

Most visitors after their first tour through a psychiatric hospital express surprise at what they have seen. Some of them ask if they could be shown real patients, those who are violent, noisy or abusive. When the few noisy patients in the most disturbed wards are indicated, visitors feel cheated and presume that something is being kept from them. The popular idea of mental illness is that of violence, aggression and danger. This idea is also often expressed by new nurses, who inquire about the 'dangerous patients' and ask to be instructed as to how these may be controlled and as to how they may protect themselves from those who are violent.

The experienced nurse knows that violence is extremely rare. Impulsive behaviour sometimes occurs, but there is little real danger of physical injury to herself. She may forget, however, that her own competence, self-assurance and tactful handling of patients are factors in preventing violence and excitement, and that this would occur much more frequently if the nursing staff were less competent, or more tactless, aggressive or insecure. The new nurse experiences fear and misgivings, and this very insecurity is communicated to the patient, who, in the presence of one inexperienced member of the staff, may become frightened. Because he is frightened he may become aggressive. It is therefore very often the new nurse who has to bear the brunt of the violent patient and who requires some reassurance and support.

Even though excitement and violence are rare and usually appear during a short phase of the illness only, the nurse should know what to do with the patient during this phase. The reasons for disturbed and violent behaviour should be investigated in order to be better able to prevent it or to calm the patient as rapidly as possible when he becomes excited.

Aggressive or violent behaviour can nearly always be traced to disturbances in the relationships between people. Aggression is not an attribute of a person, but a response to a frustrating or frightening experience. It is a feeling most people experience at some time or another.

Children often express their aggressive feelings quite openly. When they are very young they kick and scream or have temper tantrums. As they grow older they learn to express their aggression more in speech and less in action, and later still, they learn to control their aggression. There are times when they give no overt indication of it at all.

In our society considerable value is attached to this process of control.

In order to succeed in controlling aggression it is necessary, in the course of growing up, to experience it openly and to practise various methods of dealing with it. Children who are made to feel guilty about their aggressive impulses may lack practice in the process of control. Eventually they may succeed in hiding their aggression from everyone, even from themselves. They may appear meek and mild, gentle and placid. Behind this appearance may lurk the fear that to feel aggressive is dangerous and that any show of aggression might get out of control.

It is possible that unconscious fear of their own aggression is to be found in nurses too. Possibly the fear many nurses express, of being attacked by a patient, is caused by anxiety that their own aggression might be aroused by a violent patient.

It is a necessary stage in the control of aggression that one should be consciously aware of its existence. Children who have never been allowed to say that they felt angry with their parents are much more likely to have difficulty with their repressed aggressive feelings than those children who in an angry moment can safely say to their mother, 'I hate you'.

In psychiatric wards patients and staff sometimes have problems in controlling their aggression. In the relative safety of a psychiatric ward patients' control may give way. Aggressive behaviour may occur in patients who had previously been unaware of their aggressive impulses. This is referred to as 'acting out'. In some respects it may be helpful in the treatment of the patient that unconscious aggression should become overt by acting out. The effect of it is, however, so disturbing to the patient himself, to the other patients and to the staff, that the aim of treatment often consists in helping the patient to 'verbalize', i.e. to talk openly about the difficulties rather than to act out.

Nurses sometimes believe that it is wrong for them to experience anger or aggressive feelings. Nurses cannot, of course, 'act out' when they feel angry. If a nurse tries to hide her feeling, some of it may nevertheless manifest itself in actions; she may break things, make unnecessary noise, be rather rougher in carrying out physical treatment than she would otherwise be, forget some attention she has promised a patient or avoid altogether speaking to a patient to whom she feels aggressive. It is as necessary for nurses as it is for patients to feel free to talk about their frustrations and anger.

Sometimes it is appropriate for the nurse to tell a patient how angry she feels. Failing this opportunity, open discussion with colleagues at regular staff meetings is necessary to ensure that difficult patients can be dealt with without nurses losing control over aggressive feelings.

EXCITABLE MANIC PATIENTS

Some patients suffering from mania are in a highly active and excitable state. They feel on top of the world, full of energy, able to shoulder the greatest burdens. Their self-confidence is supreme. They feel happy, are capable of quite unusual feats, have extraordinary strength and feel able to work or keep active for long periods without tiring. They are full of ideas, but ideas occur to them so rapidly that they have no time to put any of them into operation. Everything they see or hear suggests a new line of thought. The patient is delighted with his own performance.

Those who watch such a patient know that he is badly in need of rest, food and drink, but he has no time for any of these essentials. A course of action must be planned which will enable the patient to sleep, so that he may recover from his excessive energy output. It would be desirable that he should wash, eliminate urine and faeces in the proper place, but all this means nothing to him. He cannot understand such preoccupation with what seem to him to be trivialities. He is busy with greater things and finds people slow, dull and rather annoying. He resents interference with his activities and may become most aggressive and angry if he believes that he is not getting sufficient support.

The manic patient is easily distracted and his interest can be roused and changed by a word or gesture from a nurse. Provided the nurse has the presence of mind to detect danger before it arises and to distract the patient's attention, no one need ever be hurt by a patient suffering from mania.

Empathy with the patient's feelings is essential. His anger when frustrated is very similar to the annoyance everyone experiences when people move unnecessarily slowly or fail to understand what appears a very simple matter. The difference between the normal person and the patient is that normal people can control their anger, whereas the manic patient may be unable to do so. To help the patient, the nurse should find out what has aroused his anger and avoid irritating him.

DISPLACED ANGER

The anger of an individual patient may not be directed against nurses. It may be aimed at his wife or mother and may arise whenever anyone unconsciously reminds him of the hated person. The nurse may represent a 'mother figure' to the patient, whose hate and aggression are then vented on the nurse. It helps a great deal to remember that in these cases the nurse 'stands for' someone else. If she learns not to take the patient's aggressions any more personally than his affection, she can usually deal with the situation sufficiently calmly and quickly to pacify him. Frequent multidisciplinary team meetings for all those dealing with the patient are necessary in order to understand his attitude and so to be able to modify it.

DELUDED PATIENTS

Some patients are angry about delusional frustrations. If the patient thinks he is being poisoned, he very understandably wishes to protect himself. If he feels threatened, he may defend himself. It may not always be possible to predict impulsive behaviour if it arises from a delusional system or if it occurs in response to the command of voices. But though it may not always be possible to predict when a patient will become angry, if the nurse knows him well it may be evident to her that impulsive behaviour may occur. In order to help a patient who suffers from delusions the nurse must know about them and allow the patient to tell his story without contradicting or ridiculing him. If she shows interest and tries to understand how things must appear from the patient's point of view, the patient's behaviour assumes a meaning. When one realizes that he acts as if his delusions were true it is easier to help him.

A patient who feels that people are against him becomes easily angered, suspicious and tense. While the nurse tries to convey to him that she is on his side, and will protect him from any enemies he may believe he has, she may be able to pacify him. If she becomes involved in his delusional system, if he feels that she, too, is in league against him, she is no longer in a good position to help. But at least she knows when this is happening and can be prepared if and when an attack is made.

FACTORS INFLUENCING VIOLENT BEHAVIOUR

In any ward in which potentially aggressive patients are nursed, there are occasional outbursts of violent or destructive behaviour. The better the general nursing and management, the fewer these outbursts. When they do occur, they must be dealt with quickly and effectively. When it is all over, nurses should try to find the reason for the disturbance, try to reconstruct the situation in order to see if better observation might have allowed them to predict and so prevent it. The nurses should try to be quite frank in their discussion of the causes of the outburst and should seriously examine their own actions in order to discover to what extent they may have themselves unwittingly provoked it. It is easier to point out to each other where each has gone wrong than to realize personal attitudes. Other people's evaluation of the part each has played should be accepted. This should be done, not in any spirit of criticism, but in an attempt to co-ordinate the approach to the patient and to prevent recurrence of the incident.

It has been shown that outbursts of violence happen most frequently when the staff are not in agreement about the best approach to the patient or when they do not get on with each other. Possibly their own anxiety and tensions are transmitted to the patient, and he, being less completely in control of his emotions, shows his anxiety in aggressive behaviour.

The really constructive work in a ward of disturbed patients is done when the patients are quiet, for it is at those times that there is an opportunity of building up therapeutic relationships with them. It is only at moments of relative calm that it is possible for the nurse to convince the patient of her interest and ability to help and support him. He can be guided to channel his energies acceptably. Energetic games and occupation, for instance, can be organized if the patient is physically strong enough to enjoy them.

If the patient is helped to sleep better, he may be more relaxed and later more able to tolerate frustrations. On the whole, the atmosphere of the ward depends on the presence of sufficient numbers of efficient, self-confident, calm nurses who convince the patient that they are his friends.

Nurses can only feel calm and self-confident if they are well prepared for their responsibility and feel secure in their status and position in the hospital. Good, responsible management by senior nursing staff has, therefore, an important part to play in the prevention of violence.

DEALING WITH VIOLENT BEHAVIOUR

However calm and competent, however understanding and tactful nurses may be, they may still at times encounter aggressive and violent behaviour. In order to be able to help the patient, the nurse must know how to deal with any combination of circumstances which may arise. In dealing with the patient she must act in such a way that:

1 The patient does not suffer physical injury
2 The patient does not become exhausted
3 Other patients or visitors are not excessively disturbed by the incident
4 Other patients are not injured
5 The nurses involved are not hurt
6 Property is preserved as far as possible
7 The patient calms down again quickly after the disturbance

The last point should be kept in mind throughout the incident. When the disturbance has subsided, the patient feels guilty and frightened, and nurses must do all they can by their attitude to show him that they bear him no ill-feeling. They must convince him that they do not judge his behaviour as being 'bad' or 'wrong'. Their duty is effectively to prevent him from doing harm to himself or others but, having ensured this, they continue to show their liking of the patient and their interest in him, and make efforts to understand him. It must be made as easy as possible for him to calm down without feeling that he has 'lost face' in any way.

Everyone knows from experience how difficult it is to 'climb down' after a quarrel or argument and to take back what has been said. Pride forbids being the first to make a peace offering and so arguments and hostilities are perpetuated, because both parties consider it humiliating to cease. When dealing with a disturbed person, it would be quite unreasonable, therefore, to expect him to take the initiative in making peace. Nurses lose nothing by offering every conceivable opening to the patient to return to peaceful behaviour.

Weapons used by violent patients

The aims in dealing with violent, excited patients have been listed in the order of importance. But it is useful to deal with them also in reverse order. For many reasons, nurses should ensure that property is not excessively damaged. First, an outburst of destructive behaviour leaves the patient more frightened at the effects he has produced. Second, once furniture and glass are broken, the patient is able to arm himself with dangerous weapons, and inflict injuries upon himself, on other patients and on staff. It is then more difficult later to treat the incident as if it were unimportant. It is therefore sometimes thought advisable that the ward should be suitably equipped for patients who may become violent. Single rooms may be used to isolate a patient if necessary. In these rooms windows should be unbreakable, or shutters could be available to protect the windows and glass panes on doors. The side-room doors should open outwards so that the patient cannot barricade himself in and should be wide enough to allow furniture to be removed quickly. A few hospitals prefer rooms which have padded floors and walls to protect the patient from injury if he bangs his head or falls. Furniture in the ward should not be easily broken. It may be wise to remove ornaments which could be thrown or broken; nothing should be left lying about which could become dangerous. Brooms left behind doors and unnecessary occupational tools are all potentially dangerous weapons. In spite of reducing the amount of furniture and the number of ornaments, the ward can be made to look pleasant and comfortable, for example by using soft furnishings, embroidered cushions and covers and having pictures fixed to the wall.

Controlling the violent patient

Injury to staff can be prevented only by the most careful teamwork. Adequate numbers of nurses are essential, but numbers alone are not enough. Each nurse must know that she can rely with a hundred per cent certainty on the help of the others. She must be able to call for help and obtain it without delay. Each nurse must be prepared to go to the aid of others with the utmost speed.

No nurse should ever attempt to enter single-handed into a struggle with a patient. It is much safer always to leave the patient alone for a moment while getting help. If he should succeed in injuring the nurse, she might then be unable to obtain help. Whenever force is resorted to, there is danger of injury to the patient. The nurse should ensure that she has a witness whenever there is any possibility of her being likely to cause injury or bruising to a patient. The latter may attribute bruises to a nurse when she has not in fact caused them. The hospital is obliged to investigate any complaint against a nurse made by the patient or his relatives, and, even if she has acted with the utmost restraint, she may find it difficult to prove her case without a witness. It is obvious that every injury sustained by a patient or nurse in the course of a struggle should be reported at once and that a written statement should be made by all nurses concerned in the matter.

In order to protect other patients, it is necessary to know which patients do not get on well with each other and, if possible, to separate them before friction arises. The nurse may be able to sense tension in a group of patients and by tactful intervention may prevent major upsets.

Isolation of violent patients

Occasionally, but with good nursing only in the rarest circumstances, it may be necessary to lock the door of the patient's room for a while until some better method of dealing with a particular situation can be found.

If the nurse, in an emergency, has locked the door of a patient's room on her own initiative, she must immediately send for the doctor. Some people consider that to lock a patient in is never justified. Others feel that in the defence of other patients it may occasionally be necessary.

The disturbed patient himself very rarely benefits by this in any way. On the contrary, he is likely to become extremely resentful, and this can only increase his aggression, not diminish it. The nurse's attitude can convey to the patient that her action is not meant to be punitive, that it is an emergency measure carried out with regret but with no ill-feeling, and that it will be discontinued at the earliest possible moment.

The patient may feel profoundly humiliated by the experience of being locked in and may find it very difficult later to establish any satisfactory relationship with the nurses responsible for this. On the other hand, he may be grateful that he was prevented from causing bodily harm to others and may not harbour resentment against the nurses. Occasionally a patient asks to be locked in his room when he is aware that he is losing control over his actions. He may feel safe in a small, protected room, or he may consider that he is receiving just punishment if he is locked in and then be able to feel less guilty about his actions.

Manual restraint

In order to prevent the patient from injuring himself, it may be necessary to resort to manual restraint. This is as unpleasant for nurses as it is for the patient and he should be aware that the former are reluctant to impose it. If there were the slightest suggestion that nurses enjoyed using force, their position would become quite intolerable. When it is necessary to use restraint, several nurses should be available and act in a co-ordinated effort. They should approach the patient simultaneously, if possible from two sides, and should quickly put him on the bed in the position which will make it easiest to hold him without causing him any discomfort. No more force must be used than is absolutely necessary to keep his movements under control. Nurses should decide beforehand how to approach the patient, so that each knows exactly what to do. It would be folly to take hold of one arm only, because the patient would then hit out with the other. Both arms should be taken at the same time. Movements are best controlled if the large joints are held, i.e. shoulder and hips, rather than wrists or ankles. In order to avoid bruising, a blanket should always be between the nurse's hand and the patient's skin. As soon as possible, the nurses should relax their grip, though they should remain in position to strengthen it if necessary. The fact that they relax almost at once may help to prove their peaceful intentions to the patient. Usually, when there are enough nurses, the patient quickly gives up the struggle. The nurses' attitude should make this easy and as little humiliating as possible. Immediately he has become calmer, the difficult task of building up his shattered self-esteem should begin.

To summarize, it has been shown that violent behaviour in psychiatric wards can largely be prevented by good hospital and ward management and in a therapeutic atmosphere. It has also been shown that it cannot always be prevented, especially where patients with a criminally violent history are admitted. When aggressive incidents do occur, a high degree of skill and co-operation is necessary to control the patient's behaviour with minimal force. Because such incidents are rare it is difficult for nurses to acquire the necessary experience and skill in the management of violent behaviour, and consequently some nurses feel unsure of their own competence, should it be put to the test. Successful prevention is of course difficult to demonstrate. Newspapers and the public at large hear only those instances when prevention failed and in particular when some staff member is accused of ill-treating a patient.

Though rare, incidents of ill-treatment are profoundly disquieting, not least because of the damage to staff morale and because of the conflict of loyalties they create. Prompt, impartial enquiry into allegations of ill-treatment is essential. When disciplinary action against some member of staff is necessary it should be clear to all that the patient's interest and the integrity of the staff are protected. Many employing authorities issue printed guidelines to all staff.

Further reading

Campbell, W., Shepherd, H. & Falconer, F. (1982) The use of seclusion. *Nursing Times* 78 (25). 1821.

Department of Health and Social Security (1976) *Management of the Violent and Potentially Violent Patient*. H.C. (76) 11. London: HMSO.

Moran, J. (1984) Aggression management: response and responsibility. *Nursing Times* 80 (14), 28.

16
Nursing Epileptic Patients

Epilepsy is a condition in which episodic transient periods of disturbed behaviour or consciousness accompany abnormal electric discharges of the brain. Manifestations of epilepsy vary according to the site and cause of the brain's abnormal functioning. The sign of this condition, sometimes called a seizure, can be elicited in anyone by the administration of a controlled electric current, for example ECT, so epilepsy can only be regarded as pathological when it occurs spontaneously or in response to stimuli to which most brains are inert. Thus it can be said that everyone has a 'convulsive threshold' and the epileptic is a person whose threshold is so low that he has a recurrent tendency to these attacks. The two commonest forms of epileptic attacks are known as major and minor epilepsy.

Major epilepsy

Major epilepsy, or *grand mal*, is characterized by definite stages, beginning with the aura or warning, which is peculiar to each patient and heralds the onset of an attack. The fit is divided into three stages, beginning with the tonic stage in which the patient falls to the ground unconscious and with all his muscles, including the respiratory muscles, in spasm. This stage lasts about 30 seconds and is succeeded by the clonic stage when there are regular jerky movements of the limbs in which the tongue may be bitten by the contractions of the jaw. Incontinence of urine and occasionally of faeces may occur. This stage usually lasts from 1 to 2 minutes. The final stage is called the post-ictal (recovery) state, which often passes into sleep lasting for several hours. After an attack the patient's mental state may be one of confusion and he may be irritable, violent and aggressive without having any realization of his actions. This is known as 'post-epileptic automatism'.

Minor epilepsy

Minor epilepsy, or *petit mal*, is characterized by momentary breaks in consciousness without convulsive attacks. The patient ceases any activity in which he is engaged, stares vacantly and may sometimes fall to the ground. These may also be known as 'absence' attacks.

EPILEPTIC PSYCHIATRICALLY ILL PATIENTS

Most people suffering from epilepsy are able to lead a normal life, but a few are admitted to psychiatric hospitals, often for reasons not directly related to their epilepsy. Typical epileptic seizures as described above are rarely observed. Accurate description of each individual patient's seizures is a valuable help in diagnosis and treatment of the condition.

It is often suggested that the nursing care of epileptic patients differs in some respects from that of other psychiatric patients. This is true in so far as observation of fits and the care of the patients during and after fits are concerned. Apart from fits, however, epileptic patients probably have no more symptoms or characteristics in common than other mentally ill patients. In order to give epileptic patients all the care they require it is necessary to know why each patient was admitted to a psychiatric hospital.

Some patients are in psychiatric hospitals because they suffer from some such mental disorder as schizophrenia or depression as well as epilepsy. The nursing care of these is determined by the nature of the mental disorder, although the occurrence of fits creates additional problems. Patients in whom epileptic fits may be due to birth injury may also, for the same reason, suffer from mental handicap or from an organic psychosis. Both the epilepsy and the mental illness require appropriate treatment.

Confusional states

Some patients, after fits, undergo periods of confusion when they require skilled supervision lest they come to harm. These periods vary in length and frequency, and between them some patients are able to be discharged from hospital. The intervals may always be of the same duration and the patient may be able to arrange to come into hospital when he himself realizes the need. During confused periods he may have difficulty in recognizing familiar people or objects, or may become noisy and destructive. He may be unable to attend to his own toilet or elimination and may become incontinent. He may become ill from undernourishment, exposure, injury to the skin and lowered resistance to infection. The patient's physical health requires attention, and, provided he can be nursed successfully during the period of disordered consciousness, he may be able to continue his usual occupation when the confused phase is over.

Some patients' confusion is obvious. Others, however, behave in a manner which gives the impression that they are fully orientated and quite conscious. Later it becomes clear that the patient has complete amnesia for periods during which his consciousness seemed to be complete. The patient's actions during the confused period were carried out automatically and he cannot later be held responsible for them. Occasionally during these periods he may injure himself or others and he needs protection from the consequence of his actions during these phases.

Emotional states

Some epileptic patients, at the time of fits, or even at other times, find it increasingly difficult to control any emotional reactions which may perhaps unwittingly be aroused by people in the environment. The patient may be irritable, experience hate or anger and, not being able to keep himself under control, may become violent, abusive and dangerous. Moreover, if he feels that he is losing control, he may become extremely frightened. Tension mounts until it becomes intolerable, and an uncontrollable outburst of violence occurs. Nobody enjoys violence, least of all the patient, who afterwards feels guilty and ashamed. He hates himself and hates others for causing him to lose control over himself. Such a patient requires someone who understands him and so can prevent an outburst before it reaches a peak. In a psychiatric hospital this is quite possible. When the nurse knows the patient really well she can usually detect when he is becoming more irritable and tense, and can persuade him to relax. He can be left undisturbed by other patients and the nurse can foster a quiet atmosphere by postponing making any demands on him and refraining from any comment which might upset his control. Sedation well before the storm breaks may be used, or any method of reducing tension known to have been effective on past occasions. The most important of these methods is for the nurse to remain calm, not to show anger or hostility and not to become frightened. This is only possible if she knows the patient well, realizes that he is ill, and treats his aggression as a symptom of his illness. Outside psychiatric hospitals it is not always possible for calmness to reign in the face of a patient's aggressive behaviour, but if community care can effectively be arranged, the nurse or social worker who visits the family can help to prevent serious disturbance.

Some epileptic patients, who have been taking anticonvulsant drugs for some time, begin to show mental symptoms, often resembling those of mania, or they may occasionally display the features of confusional illness or of dementia. It is sometimes necessary to withdraw the drugs in order to establish to what extent symptoms are due to drug intoxication, and also to what extent drugs are really necessary to keep the fits under control. During this period the patient requires continuous observation and very careful nursing, and therefore in-patient treatment.

Behavioural disorders

By far the greatest number of epileptic patients are in psychiatric hospitals because of behaviour disturbances. Over a period of time, the patient's behaviour may have become so difficult that it is impossible for him to remain in the community. It is possible, though no conclusive evidence exists, that some forms of epileptic illnesses lead to a progressive deterioration in behaviour and to a characteristic kind of personality disorder.

Patients suffering from 'temporal lobe epilepsy' sometimes show a characteristic form of disorder which often responds well to surgical removal of the epileptic focus in the temporal lobe. Restlessness, irritability, slow circumstantial speech and episodic outbursts of aggressive behaviour are common.

Often, however, behaviour disorder is not the result of epileptic illness, but a reaction to the way in which the patient is treated by society. Whatever the cause, the nurse will find it much easier to remedy the patient's behaviour if she assumes that it is the result of environmental influences. It used to be believed that epileptic patients were people whose personality showed antisocial characteristics. If, before she ever approaches the patient, the nurse believes that epileptics are hypocrites, schemers, liars and generally untrustworthy people, her attitude will show diffidence and suspicion of their every action, which may then result in bringing out in them the very characteristics she has expected. If, however, she assumes that the patients are kindly disposed, pleasant and likeable people, her approach to them will be much more natural, spontaneous and friendly, and they may respond by differing very little from other groups of patients.

It is very easy, if one is suspicious of people, to create a situation which is self-verifying. The way in which one approaches a person of whom one is suspicious creates in that person hostility and aggression he had not previously felt. The moment these feelings emerge they serve to confirm that the suspicions were justified.

It is possible that in the past nurses created among epileptic patients the behaviour and personality traits of which they were afraid.

EPILEPTIC CHILDREN

Nurses who do meet an epileptic patient who is sly, treacherous, deceitful and untrustworthy should try to think of the kind of social life people suffering from epilepsy are liable to lead. From the moment fits occurred, be it in childhood or later, the patient has been prevented from leading a normal life. Fits are very terrifying to witness. Undoubtedly the child's parents are most upset when they first discover that he has had a fit. They communicate their anxiety to the child, who is disturbed by the sudden inexplicable attacks and feels that something is happening over which he has no control. Once the diagnosis of epilepsy is made, the parents are in a greater dilemma than ever. They are worried, feel guilty and responsible and seek in the child's antenatal history, or in heredity, an explanation for the illness. They become over-solicitous, restrictive and at the same time over-indulgent. They may wish to protect the child from injury by keeping careful watch, but at the same time they prevent normal activity in sports and games, and never let the child out of their sight. They may feel frightened, possibly even repelled by the fits, and will probably be a little resentful about the difficulties created in their lives by the fact that an epileptic child must be cared for. It is a great strain to bring up an epileptic child, especially where there are several children in the family, and, however devoted the parents, the child must sometimes realize how much inconvenience he causes.

School represents a problem. If the child has frequent fits, ordinary schools will not admit him. Even if they did, the child would soon fall behind in his work as a result of repeated absences, or because, even between attacks, there is often disruptive activity in affected brain areas which may erase newly laid memory traces and cause him to be inattentive. If he has minor epileptic fits, the position may even be worse; the fits are often not recognized and the child is thought to be lazy, absent-minded and clumsy, and is subjected to criticism and ridicule. Since he cannot control the fits, he becomes despondent and gives up trying, or may become resentful, angry and aggressive. If an epileptic child goes to an ordinary school, he probably feels different, an outsider, an oddity. He may be excluded from many activities and soon realizes that the other children are frightened of or amused by his fits and shun his company on their parents' advice. If the child goes to one of the special boarding schools for epileptic children, he benefits educationally, but family life is disrupted and this may give rise to many of the patient's later difficulties.

The National Society for Epilepsy has recently produced a comprehensive educational package for the use of nurses in the community working with epileptic children and their families.

THE EPILEPTIC IN SOCIETY

As an adult, the epileptic finds life just as difficult. Many jobs are out of the question for him. It would be most unwise for anyone who is liable to have fits to drive a bus or a car, or to choose any occupation which requires climbing ladders or handling dangerous machinery. The number of occupations from which he can choose is limited, but even if he selects one which is well within his powers, he may meet with fear and prejudice on the part of his potential employer. If he tells the employer that he has fits, he may not be accepted. If he does not tell him, he may be dealt with even less sympathetically when his employer discovers the situation. It is not really surprising that some epileptic patients, because of their experiences, become asocial, if not actually antisocial. Some feel that the world is against them and see no reason why they should consider themselves as being a part of a society which has rejected them.

The epileptic in hospital

Even in a psychiatric hospital, although the epileptic's plight is understood and appreciated, there are difficulties in deciding on how to treat him. If all epileptic patients are placed in one ward, an entirely arbitrary criterion is used for selection. Patients who have fits may have very little else in common. Some are severely psychotic, some mentally subnormal, some disturbed, others normal most of the time and merely in need of short periods of supervision. It is unlikely that the patients can form a group, or benefit from psychiatric hospital treatment in the way other patients do, if they are in the same ward merely because they have fits. If, on the other hand, the epileptic patient is admitted to any other ward, he again finds himself an outsider, an object of pity and curiosity, not an accepted member of the group. He is again restricted in his activities and barred from certain occupations. In view of all this, it is not surprising that epileptic patients are sometimes difficult people to manage. It is much more surprising that they lose their temper so rarely, and fit in as well as they do, sometimes becoming some of the most efficient and the most reliable members of the ward community.

NURSING EPILEPTIC PATIENTS

The nursing care of the epileptic patient may be considered under two headings:

1 The general management of the patient within the hospital
2 The special care required in view of the occurrence of fits

The general management should be planned with regard to the patient's mental and physical condition. The patient should share as fully as possible in the life of the community. If his fits are well under control, there should be little difficulty in finding suitable work and arranging a full occupational and recreational programme, although it must be remembered that a certain amount of supervision is always necessary and the patient should not be allowed to work in any place where a fit might endanger the lives of others.

So far as fits are concerned, the following nursing aspects should be considered.
1 Observation and investigation of fits
2 Prevention of fits
3 Care and management during fits

These three aspects are closely connected and dependent on each other. Fits are more easily prevented if they have been carefully investigated and described. Management during a fit is similarly dependent on accurate observation.

Observation of fits

An informed eye-witness account of the seizure can be extremely useful in establishing the correct diagnosis of the type of epilepsy.

From relatives it may be impossible to obtain an accurate description of what has actually taken place during fits they have observed. This is due to the following reasons: first, it is impossible for those who are upset and worried to observe accurately, and relatives are invariably upset by the circumstances. Second. it is impossible to remember accurately what has been observed unless observations are at once committed to writing, before any distortion has taken place, and unless it is realized at the time of observation that a report will later be required. Third, it is impossible accurately to remember every detail. Selection is determined by what the observer considers to be of importance. The popular idea of what is of importance may not always correspond with the actual requirements of the doctor.

The nurse's observation can be more accurate because she acts as the trained observer, who bears these points in mind and systematically sets out to provide what is needed. At first, even the nurse may be upset and excited and the first reports are therefore not always very accurate. They serve a useful purpose if the nurse tries to compare her observations with those of another nurse who has also witnessed the fit and attempts to find out whether her own observations were biased.

After the first experiences, the nurse should be able to remain calm and her observation should improve. The main reason for inaccurate reporting after the first few occasions may be the fact that fits occasionally occur when the nurse is not prepared, and that at times she is taken by surprise. She may feel that she should have been prepared, that she has not been sufficiently vigilant. She may feel guilty because she has failed to observe the onset of the fit or the circumstances which have led up to it. She should resist the temptation of reporting what might have been, and should adhere strictly to facts actually observed. A few fits really well observed are a much better guide to the doctor than a large number of reports which are inaccurate.

As soon as possible after the fit, the nurse must find time to write down her observations. While the fit is actually in progress she should give a verbal running commentary to herself of what is happening. This helps the later writing of the report. A series of headings under which a report is to be made should be memorized in order to have a reply to each question.

As soon as she observes a patient who has a fit, the nurse should note the time, because she should report accurately on the total length of the fit and the length of each stage. Time may seem very long when she is helplessly watching a patient and the period during which the patient is not breathing may seem endless, when in fact it may last only 30 seconds. Some hospitals use charts for reporting a seizure, a useful measure for the nurse who has had little experience of epilepsy, since the observations are listed systematically.

The nurse should prepare a summary of the condition of the ward as she finds it and remember what the patient had been doing just prior to the fit. Fits may occur more frequently when a patient is upset. There may be some relation to the intake of

food and it is a help if the existence of some recurrent
antecedent activity can be established. Some patients, for
example, are most likely to have fits when there has been some
quarrel or unpleasant scene in the ward. Others regularly have
fits during hospital concerts or in the ward when someone plays
the piano. Sometimes it is even one particular tune which is
associated with the onset of a fit. Some patients have fits at
regular times, such as on wakening in the morning, and it may
be worthwhile to rouse them a little earlier than usual with a
cup of tea and biscuits. Any precipitating factors in the
environment should be noted as well as the patient's own mood
or activity just before the seizure.

If the patient is regularly irritable immediately prior to an
attack, this may be an expression of his own awareness of an
impending attack. The irregular electric discharge of the brain
may occur from the onset of irritability. Noticing this may help
in foreseeing an attack and in better management of future
seizures. Any warning the patient may have should be noted.
He may communicate this in words at the time or later, or he
may indicate it by some specific action which always precedes
an attack.

Loss of consciousness or disturbance of consciousness should
be reported. The nurse should practise making the necessary
observations swiftly and in the correct order, to establish the
level of consciousness and whether the unconscious state is
deepening or becoming less deep. She should call the patient's
name, noting any utterances which may give evidence of his
having heard or observed the nurse. She should report posture
or the succession of postures, the movement of the head and
eyes, the direction of movement. The direction of the fall
should be noted. The exact length of time of each stage of the
attack is important. Muscle tone should be observed, whether
the tonic or rigid stage is unilateral or bilateral, whether
twitching starts simultaneously throughout the whole body, or
on which side or which part of the body it appears first.
Twitching may start at one particular point and spread from
there, and the order in which various parts of the body are
affected may be important. Muscle tone at the end of the attack
should be noted. The eyes should be observed. The reaction of
pupils to light, corneal reflexes and eye movements must be
mentioned.

As soon as the attack has ceased, pulse and respiration are

recorded, colour is noted. Biting of the tongue and incontinence are reported, knee jerks and extensor plantar reflexes are tested. A positive extensor plantar response is an upward movement of the big toe when the sole of the foot is stroked. (Normally the toe moves downward.) After the attack it is necessary to note the depth of the sleep which follows, how easy it is to rouse the patient, and the duration of sleep if the patient is left undisturbed. Any complaints made by the patient are reported, e.g. headache or vomiting, so is any evidence of confusion in speech or action. It is very important to establish the length of time during which the patient remains confused because during it he requires supervision and is not responsible for his actions. The patient may appear to be fully conscious, but later questioning may reveal a period of amnesia at a time when confusion was not evident.

Diagnostic investigations

Electroencephalography. Observations of the kind described may give an indication of the localization of a brain lesion which may cause the fits. The observation of fits is usually supplemented by the investigation of the electrical discharge of the brain under a variety of conditions. Electric brain waves have been widely discussed in the popular press, and many patients now arrive in hospital with some vague notion about the tests which are performed. They approach the investigations with preconceived ideas of the purpose of the test. Some patients fear that electricity is being used on the brain, having confused electroconvulsive therapy (ECT) and electroencephalography (EEG). The use of abbreviations adds to the mystery of the subject and many patients are terrified of the technique. It is bad for the patient to worry unnecessarily if a few words of reassurance and explanation can allay his fears. Worry may interfere seriously with the result of the test because the patient may be restless when he arrives at the electroencephalography department, or in some instances may even refuse to have the test done. The patient who is struggling and restless may require sedation prior to investigation, and this may be undesirable. Some patients have exaggerated ideas of the efficacy of the EEG test and believe that their most secret thoughts may be revealed. Not unnaturally, these patients may be reluctant to have the test done. The nurse can find out how much the patient knows about the test, and should then correct misconceptions.

Miscellaneous investigations. The EEG is not always diagnostic of epilepsy; it may be normal between attacks.

Opinions differ as to the extent of the investigations required. Most authorities agree that at least a skull x-ray and an EEG are required. Additional investigations, if specially indicated after a careful history has been taken, include routine haematological and biochemical tests and lumbar puncture. Diagnostic imaging (e.g. CT scan and contrast radiology) is indicated if focal symptoms or signs are present. The age of the patient is also important. If the patient is over 25 years of age, a full investigation is necessary; idiopathic epilepsy rarely occurs after this age.

Prevention of fits

Accurate descriptions of the fits, together with reports of the electroencephalogram, give guidance to the doctor in his prescription of drugs. As the drugs take effect the characteristic features of the fits may change. To assess the efficacy of the drugs prescribed, continued careful reporting of the incidence of fits and a description of them remain important.

Fits are often found to be related to emotional disturbances. Their incidence may be reduced if the patient is well adjusted to his environment, happy in his personal relationships with other patients, doctors and nurses, and if the ward atmosphere is generally congenial to him. A sudden increase in the number of fits may be an indication of the patient's unfavourable reaction to changes in staff or routine, and it may be possible to readjust his environment if this possibility is borne in mind. If the patient's fits are to remain controlled after discharge, it is important that he should have the opportunity of testing his adaptation to work and home life while still under the supervision of the hospital.

Diet and fluid intake are sometimes found to be related to fits. If it is found that these occur with fluid retention, diuretics may be ordered, or the patient may have his fluids restricted. If fits occur frequently during the night, it may be necessary to restrict fluid intake in the evenings. Slight hypoglycaemia may bring on fits. Frequent small meals during the day and a milky drink late in the evening may reduce their incidence. While prevention of fits is not always possible, careful nursing and attention to detail can considerably reduce their number and consequently enable the patient to lead a more normal life.

Precautions against injury

During a fit the most important duty of the nurse is to prevent injury. Epileptic patients in hospital are kept under fairly constant observation day and night. Certain obvious dangers are avoided. The patient may sleep on a low bed so that he would not be injured if he fell out, but this is seldom necessary. He has a hard pillow, in order not to suffocate if his face happened to be covered by the pillow during a fit. Meals are supervised in case a fit occurs, and the patient is encouraged to cut up his food into small pieces because he might choke if a fit occurred while large pieces of food were in his mouth. If the patient is alone in the bathroom, there is some risk of drowning. He should have no opportunity to climb heights. The dangers of traffic are obviated if the patient goes out only when accompanied.

Ward furnishings should be so arranged that the risk of injury during falls is minimized. Low, well-upholstered armchairs and rugs on the floor may help. There should be plenty of loose cushions which can be used especially if the patient falls to the ground. Patients frequently help each other, and should be encouraged to do so, at least to move the patient to a place of safety, or to guide or break his fall. Each patient will feel more secure if he sees that accidents are few and that his fellow patients are cared for and safely attended to during a fit. The patient needs to judge for himself how great the risk of injury is and how far it is advisable to take calculated risks in order to prepare for discharge.

Risk from drugs

Since most epileptic patients are taking drugs of some kind, nurses should be familiar not only with the method of administration of drugs but particularly with the possible toxic effects of each. Nurses who know that excessive drowsiness may result from phenobarbitone will be more alert to changes in the patient's behaviour, and will report his reluctance to go to occupational classes or to join in social activities. If the patient is having phenytoin, the nurse will keep a special watch for spongy gums, and attend more carefully to the patient's oral hygiene. Ataxia and confusion are also associated with phenytoin. She must bear in mind that the noisy, talkative, excited patient may be suffering from the ill-effects of the drug. Some drugs given to epileptic patients cause occasional visual hallucinations. Skin rashes are common, and blood counts may be necessary because certain drugs, for example carbamazepine, cause a reduction in the number of white blood cells and this would predispose the patient to infection. Toxicity of antiepileptic drugs is thought to be reduced if only one drug, rather than a combination of drugs, is used.

After discharge, sufferers from epilepsy continue to take anticonvulsant drugs, for many years, sometimes for the rest of their life. Knowledge about the drugs is therefore as important to the patient as it is to the nurse. The patient should know the names of the drugs he is taking, the dosage which has been prescribed for him and the importance of taking the drugs regularly. He should understand that regular medication is necessary to maintain the required drug level in the blood. Some patients mistakenly believe that they can take a double or treble dose one day if they forget to take the drugs on other days. The danger and uselessness of this procedure should be made clear to the patient. Though prolonged taking of drugs on medical prescription is not only safe for the patient, but necessary, the same drugs may be dangerous if taken by other people. The patient should be fully aware of his responsibility for the safe keeping of his drugs when he leaves the hospital.

There is danger in the hospital care of epileptic patients that nurses retain full responsibility for too long.

The patient suffering from epilepsy needs to be fully involved in the planning of his life after discharge. He must be prepared for the harsh reality of the difficulties of obtaining suitable employment, the embarrassment of meeting tactless or unhelpful people, the problems of preventing injury. The hospital should offer him every opportunity to learn how to do without its support.

Further reading

Scott, A.K. (1984) Management of epilepsy. *British Medical Journal* *288*, 986.

Trimble, M.R., Birdwood, G. & Russell, J. (1982) *Current Themes in Epilepsy*. Horsham: Geigy Pharmaceuticals.

17
The Patient Who is Dependent on Alcohol or Drugs

Alcoholism is a disorder which is common in many countries. The extent to which it is recognized as a social problem depends on the prevailing attitude of the community.

It has long been recognized as a medical problem when people who have taken alcohol regularly over a long period of time come to suffer from brain damage and accompanying mental deterioration or from other bodily damage. Increasingly, psychiatrists and psychiatric nurses are becoming aware, not only of body damage caused by alcohol, but of the difficulties of people whose lives are largely dominated by thoughts about drinking. Such people are addicted to alcohol. How many people have alcohol-related problems is not known exactly, but it has been estimated that at least 2% of patients on a general practitioner's list will be, or have been, suffering from alcoholism.

There has been an increase in alcoholism among women in recent years, which has been reflected in the increase in cirrhosis of the liver in women. Women are more vulnerable to this physical consequence of alcohol abuse than men—they need to drink only a quarter of the amount taken by men to be in danger of liver damage. The fetal alcohol syndrome, i.e. low birth weight, retarded mental development, and skull, face, limb and cardiovascular defects, may occur in infants born to women who have taken alcohol to excess during pregnancy.

Alcohol consumption in the elderly has risen by almost a hundred per cent in the last three decades. Elderly women are more liable to drink too much alcohol than elderly men; social isolation has been suggested as one reason why a third of elderly alcoholic patients drink an excessive amount.

Action on Alcohol Abuse (AAA) is a new organization. It is a small, medically supported, enthusiastic pressure group, established to campaign politically to reduce Britain's alcohol problems. Its aim is to work to combat society's apparent indifference to the growing levels of alcohol consumption.

By contrast, drug addiction was, until a decade ago, thought to be uncommon in the United Kingdom. In recent years, the incidence of drug addiction has increased to alarming proportions, and many, including members of the nursing and medical professions, government ministers and the pressure group MIND (National Association for Mental Health), express growing concern about this. Recently published figures show a sixfold increase in drug abuse in Scotland. A major English city is experiencing a virtual drug epidemic; police seized 5 g of heroin in 1981, and 1000 g in 1983.

Discussions about this problem are, however, confused because no clear definition is used for the concept of addiction. Some people, for example, make no distinction between alcohol addicts and heavy drinkers; others believe that a distinction can be drawn. Some people make no distinction between 'habituation' to drugs and drug 'addiction'; others distinguish between habituation, i.e. the need for increasing dosage of drugs to achieve the same effect, and addiction, i.e. the craving for the drug and the inability to do without it.

In order to remove some of the difficulty of definition and in order to make possible international comparison of the incidence of the disorder and of the effectiveness of treatment, the World Health Organization recommended in 1964 in a technical report (No. 287) that the word 'addiction' should be replaced by the term 'drug dependence'. This term describes much better the central preoccupation of the patients who are totally dependent on a regular supply of their drug of addiction, be it alcohol or any other drug. A decade later, in 1974, the WHO introduced its definition of drug dependence as: 'A state—psychic and sometimes also physical—resulting in the interaction between a living organism and a drug, characterized by behavioural and other responses that always include a *compulsion* to take the drug on a continuous or a periodic basis in order to experience its psychic effects, and sometimes to avoid the discomfort of its absence' (Technical Report No. 551). The use of the term 'dependence' encourages one to concentrate on the patient's needs rather than on the pharmacological characteristics of the drug or on legal definition. In the current definitions, addiction and habituation are no longer used and 'drug abuse' has taken their place. The person who abuses drugs is now sometimes referred to as a 'drug user' or a 'problem drug taker', rather than as a drug abuser.

Patients suffering from dependence on alcohol or drugs have certain problems in common.

1   By the time dependence is established the patients are able to take much more of the drug without showing any ill-effects than would be possible for other people. Patients dependent on alcohol, for example, can sometimes drink two bottles of whisky without showing signs of being drunk. Patients dependent on sedatives take doses so large that others would be made unconscious. Patients dependent on heroin need ever-larger doses to give them the sensation which they hope for. This phenomenon is known as *tolerance*. The ability to acquire tolerance to drugs such as morphine and heroin has always been known. No drugs, however, are entirely safe—tolerance to dexamphetamine, aspirin, barbiturates and alcohol is as common as tolerance to opiates.

2   Patients who are dependent on drugs or alcohol usually experience intense *craving* when the next dose is not immediately available. A patient suffering from the later stages of alcoholism wakes up in the morning feeling shaky, restless and nauseated. He is unable to start the business of the day until he has had a drink. Periodically throughout the day this feeling comes over him again. When the addiction has progressed further, to obtain his drink quickly he keeps a secret stock of alcohol in his office and from time to time, all by himself, he takes a drink. As soon as he has had a drink the shaky, trembling sensation leaves him. Because he knows he can make himself feel better by drinking, the patient's social life tends to be dominated by his need to obtain a drink. He arrives at parties early, to have one drink before the others start; he drops in at a pub on his way home from work. Many patients who suffer from alcoholism are never able to be entirely without alcohol in their circulation. For some alcoholics, known as *bout drinkers*, the craving is only intermittent. They are able to go for weeks or months without a drink, but when a drinking bout starts the craving is paramount.

Craving for other drugs is relatively more difficult to satisfy than craving for alcohol. Unless the drugs are prescribed by a doctor at a special clinic, the patient finds he can obtain his supply only through illegal activities. In order to ensure a supply he must then make contacts with the people who are able to get access to such supplies; consequently he quickly finds himself at the mercy of unscrupulous people who can ask for ever-increasing amounts of money for the drugs, or blackmail the drug-dependent patient into participating in criminal activities. What may have started as an experiment to see if some 'kicks' could be obtained, may end in a life of crime, revolving round the problem of obtaining supplies of drugs.

Many people believe that participating in illegal trafficking of drugs is a greater evil than drug taking itself. They would wish to see drugs, particularly 'soft' drugs such as cannabis, more freely available, as is the case with alcohol, so that people need not resort to crime to obtain them. There is, however, a considerable danger that, in a free market for drugs, drug dependence is becoming as common as alcohol dependence. It is one of the most worrying aspects of the problem of drug taking that many young people appear to start with the relatively harmless drugs which are more easily obtainable, e.g. the smoking of cannabis, and find themselves pushed by the people whose company they keep into dependence on hard drugs, like heroin.

3   The most serious symptoms which may arise occur when the patient is no longer able to obtain the drug on which he depends. These symptoms are referred to as the *withdrawal state*. The shakes and tremors described above constitute withdrawal symptoms. Withdrawal symptoms are very similar in patients suffering from alcoholism and from drug dependence. Restlessness, agitation, terrifying hallucinations, often visual, are among the most prominent symptoms. When the delirium is gross, the patient may be disorientated: he may be quite unable to remember where he is and how he got there. He may mistake people in the hospital for relatives or friends, and may restlessly carry out activities which may be quite exhausting and damaging in view of his poor physical health. Epileptiform fits may occur, especially after abrupt withdrawal of barbiturates or alcohol.

In patients suffering from alcoholism these withdrawal symptoms are referred to as delirium tremens. When a patient who is a habitual drinker is admitted to a general hospital after an accident or for an operation, delirium tremens occurs because the withdrawal of alcohol is sudden. It is a particularly dangerous condition when it occurs as a complication to an already serious surgical condition. For patients commencing treatment for alcoholism or for drug dependence, the withdrawal symptoms are equally severe and sometimes prove to be so insufferable that the patient prefers to discontinue treatment and to discharge himself from hospital. Withdrawal symptoms can be kept under control by the use of one of the benzodiazapines; chlormethiazole may be used but it is more addictive. Very careful nursing attention is required to deal with the restlessness and confusion and to guard against injury. Dehydration and intercurrent infections are possible complications of withdrawal symptoms (see Chapter 13).

Because alcohol is readily available, while the sale of other drugs of addiction is legally restricted, it is easier to become addicted to alcohol than to other drugs, and easier to reach an advanced stage of dependence before the need for medical aid is recognized.

In 1965 a committee, under the chairmanship of Lord Brain, recommended that the right of prescribing certain specified drugs should be limited to a number of doctors working in special clinics. These drug-dependence clinics came into being in April 1968.

In 1973 the Misuse of Drugs Regulations were issued. These regulations define the classes of persons who are authorized to supply and possess controlled drugs (i.e. drugs listed in the Misuse of Drugs Act 1971). In addition they list fourteen opiate drugs and cocaine and state that any person addicted, or suspected of being addicted, to these substances has to be reported to the Home Office Drugs Branch by the medical practitioner treating that person. It was originally thought that this would make it easier to monitor the magnitude of the problem, but there is evidence that any list of registered drug addicts is a gross underestimation of the actual numbers due in part to a failure by doctors to comply with the notification procedure.

There is, however, considerable evidence of illegal supplies reaching drug users. Such supplies may be all the more dangerous for being unofficially produced, packed and marketed. It is often impossible for a drug user to know how big the dosage is which he is taking, how pure the drug is (i.e. whether or not it has been 'cut'), or how 'fair' the price he has been charged.

Research is necessary to find out how serious is the danger of dependence on 'hard' drugs for those who have taken 'soft' drugs such as cannabis. Many people dependent on heroin are known to have started with 'soft' drugs, but it is not known how many people experiment with cannabis or lysergic acid diethylamide (LSD) without proceeding to 'hard' drugs. It appears that among students, experimentation with soft drugs is fairly common. Young people often have the desire to extend their experience. The effects of some drugs such as LSD on perception and feeling have been extensively described. To many people these experiences are pleasurable and even awe inspiring. To some they are a welcome escape from the tedium of everyday life, to others they represent a more positive, almost mystical, awareness of a reality worth exploring for its own sake. The effect of LSD is very unpredictable. Occasionally there is extreme restlessness and terrifying hallucinations may lead to suicide. If judgement is impaired, in what is often referred to as a 'bad trip', dangerous actions may lead to serious accident. No one should embark lightly on experiments with LSD and never when alone. Occasionally LSD is associated with prolonged psychotic symptoms lasting from a week to several years.

There appear to be many people who grow tired of the experience and give up drugs without any difficulty. Others may not find it so easy and may need help. For this purpose it is necessary that they should feel free to discuss their problems and should know where to turn for help.

While the taking of all drugs is regarded as blameworthy, wicked or degenerate, and while all of it is illegal, it is difficult for drug takers to disclose their need for help early enough. There is no means of spotting those who take drugs in the early stages. The need for help must be made known by the drug taker himself or by his friends.

TREATMENT AND NURSING CARE

Treatment of patients suffering from drug dependence can rarely be successfully undertaken unless the patient wishes to be helped. Many patients agree to see a psychiatrist in order to satisfy their employer or their spouse, or they enter hospital under pressure from friends or from a magistrate. Such patients are unlikely to persevere with treatment when the withdrawal symptoms become troublesome or when they experience craving for the drug. When the patient himself has come to the conclusion that he must seek help, such help is more likely to be effective. Unfortunately, many people who are dependent on drugs require the sensations of euphoria, heightened confidence in themselves, emotional upsurge and enlarged perception which the drugs bring about. They may also value their place in the circle of friends into whose company their drug dependence brings them, and they are not able to make a change. It used to be said by 'Alcoholics Anonymous' that it is only when a patient reaches rock-bottom, when he is financially ruined, when his family have left him or when his physical health is seriously impaired, that he genuinely sees the need for treatment. Even then and with the best will in the world, some patients find it impossible to persevere with treatment, and succumb time and time again to the temptation of another dose.

Patients suffering from drug addiction and those suffering from alcoholism increasingly attend day units or drug-dependence clinics for treatment. Often regular attendance at these clinics gives them the necessary support, especially when an interested social worker can assist in solving the financial and social difficulties into which their addiction has led them. Group psychotherapy is often available.

Some patients are, however, admitted as in-patients, some into psychiatric admission wards where they are treated alongside patients with other psychological problems, some into special units for the treatment of their addiction. On admission the patient may sign a contract which gives details of the treatment strategy, and of the way in which staff will respond to specified desirable or undesirable behaviour by the patient. A time limit may be imposed on the duration of the treatment. It may be the policy that a drug-free ethos must be maintained once the initial drug therapy for withdrawal symptoms is discontinued.

In special units patients find support from other patients. They can help each other to explore their difficulties and can develop a common culture within the unit. They can benefit from the feeling of being understood and they can examine their reactions and attitudes in the presence of others like themselves. Staff in such units work there because they have special interest in patients suffering from addiction and are more able than others to understand the patients' difficulties. Some special units and day care facilities are organized and run by voluntary organizations. These include Phoenix House and Alpha House, which are residential; Lifeline offers a day programme to help in the rehabilitation of drug users.

Patients who are in wards with other in-patients often feel that they are misunderstood by staff and patients alike. Where the demands made by other psychiatric patients have priority, the nurses may find patients suffering from drug dependence a nuisance. The craving for the drug and the patient's occasional failure to remain abstinent may be interpreted as non-cooperation.

The advantage of being treated in a ward alongside other psychiatric patients may lie in preventing isolation from society as a whole. It may also be easier to control the supply of drugs from outside the hospital, especially if only one drug-dependent patient is admitted to the ward at any one time. Where a number of patients suffering from drug dependence are treated together it is easy to find some means of having supplies brought in without the knowledge of the staff. Some patients in fact may leave hospital having been put in touch with better sources of supply than had been available before admission.

The aim of group therapy, however, should be to bring such problems into the open for discussion: this is much less likely to happen in a ward with patients suffering from other psychiatric disorders.

As a possible adjunct for the patient suffering from alcoholism who is about to be discharged from a special unit or a general psychiatric ward, a deterrent drug, either disulfiram (Antabuse) or citrated calcium carbimide (Abstem) may be prescribed. These drugs have proved useful for the patient who requires help to maintain sobriety in the early weeks of his return home. Both drugs interfere with the breakdown of alcohol in the body and cause the patient to experience extremely unpleasant and distressing reactions should he take alcohol within 24 hours of his having had the deterrent drug. These reactions include palpitations, flushing, a feeling of choking, pounding headache, nausea and vomiting. The greatest danger for the patient lies in the possibility of a sudden steep fall in blood pressure; patients with cardiovascular disease are, therefore, not given this form of therapy. Before this treatment is instituted the psychiatrist must be entirely satisfied that the patient fully understands the implications of its use.

In the nursing care of patients suffering from drug dependence, all the skills described in earlier chapters are required.

1 The first stage of treatment is concerned with the withdrawal of drugs or with 'drying out' from alcohol. Much of the nurses' contribution consists of physical care. Drugs have to be administered and the patient's nutrition needs attention—often the patient is unwilling to take adequate food or fluid because he feels so sick and is so restless. Vitamin deficiency is one of the complications which result from prolonged existence on inadequate diet on which many patients relied prior to admission. Large doses of B complex and C vitamins intravenously or intramuscularly are given during the early phase of alcohol detoxification.

2 The intense amount of physical nursing care required by the patient during this phase facilitates the creation of an interpersonal relationship between nurse and patient which may be helpful. Patients who have been using drugs or alcohol for a long time often feel that no one trusts them and that they can trust no one. It is helpful to the patient to find a nurse who really listens to him and who is willing to try to understand his side of the story. Some patients have serious personality difficulties and the opportunity to talk about these to a sympathetic nurse may be very valuable. The patient may benefit, not so much from the reply which the nurse offers, as from her continued accepting response even when she learns of the priority he gave to drinking, his sexual problems or his neglect of his family. Many patients feel intensely remorseful and need the opportunity to sort out their feelings by talking about them. The nurse who listens may make it easier for them to do this. It should be remembered that suicide is common in

patients who suffer from drug dependence. Evidence of a suicidal impulse may be detected by the nurse who knows how to listen.

3   The most important aspect of treatment may be the creation in the ward of a new environment in which the patient can make friends and find other satisfactions. To give up drinking or drugs may mean cutting oneself off from the people with whom one previously had social intercourse. The nurse's contribution to the patient's treatment may lie chiefly in helping to create the ward atmosphere in which the patient can feel free from tensions. Interest in work and in hobbies can be encouraged: a new purposive way of living can be established. Ward meetings can be used to help the patient discover his social skills or he may attend a social skills training session. Group psychotherapy helps him to see his specific personality problems and share these with his fellow sufferers.

Many patients who suffer from drug dependence feel that they are outcasts from society. They create for themselves a defence against 'them', i.e. all the people who are against them and who do not understand. In the right kind of therapeutic milieu this attitude can be avoided or overcome.

It is often difficult to achieve the amount of understanding which the patient needs in order to regain his self-respect. Often when the patient speaks of the people who dislike him and who are against him, there is more than a grain of truth in his complaint. The patient's behaviour prior to admission may have strained relationships to near breaking point. His overriding need for his drug or for alcohol while in hospital may result in behaviour which appears to the nurses and to other patients as unreliable and deceitful. It is part of the characteristic pattern of the disorder that these difficulties arise, and part of the treatment that one must persevere in spite of setbacks and disappointments.

When the patients leave hospital they may still be faced with formidable problems. Membership of Alcoholics Anonymous, or of similar lay groups of drug addicts, may help them to obtain the necessary support. It is often possible to put the patient in touch with such organizations while he is still in hospital.

There may be many social and interpersonal problems which

contributed to the patient's becoming dependent. The patient's job may, for example, be such that alcohol cannot be avoided, or the patient's wife may be a competent, managing person, who really feels happier when her husband is ill than when he copes well with his affairs.

It may be useful to involve other members of the patient's immediate family in treatment. During the patient's stay in hospital, group meetings in which members of the family participate may help everyone to understand mutual problems more clearly and to see how far complaints made about each other are valid and realistic. Fellow patients may help to bring the problems of the spouse forward. The patient's relatives may come to accept drug dependence as an illness and may become more able to give sympathy and understanding in spite of all their trials and tribulations. AL-ANON and AL-ATEEN are both voluntary support groups for spouses and teenage children, respectively, of patients with drinking problems.

The continued support and interest from the treatment team may be necessary if the patient is to continue a life of abstinence after leaving hospital.

This support may be offered by the social worker who may continue to visit the patient. It may be given by the doctor in the form of supportive psychotherapy. Some hospitals encourage patients to continue attendance at group psychotherapy sessions for some time after discharge.

It may be that the nurse who has gained the patient's and the relatives' confidence during his stay in hospital is the person to whom the patient can turn again later for supportive counselling.

Further reading

Edwards, G. (1982) *The Treatment of Drinking Problems*. London: McIntyre.

Edwards, G., Arif, A. & Jaffe, J. (1984) *Drug Use and Misuse*. London: Croom Helm.

Report of the Advisory Council on the Misuse of Drugs (1982) *Treatment and Rehabilitation*. London: HMSO (DHSS).

Statistics of the Misuse of Drugs in the UK (1983) Home Office Bulletin.

Watts, F.N. & Bennett, D., eds. (1983) *Theory and Practice of Psychiatric Rehabilitation*. Chichester: J. Wiley.

Part 3
Special Forms of Treatment

Introduction to Part 3

The third part of this book is concerned with various forms of therapy currently practised in psychiatry and with the nurses' function in these therapies.

Over the years, physical therapies have assumed greater and then lesser importance. Psychotherapies have been used more or less effectively depending on the kind of patient selected for such treatment and on the specific treatment style favoured by the psychiatrist or the institution in which he works.

The purposive use of the patient's social milieu to modify his experience of his disorder and to enable him to learn new and better coping strategies has been tried in a variety of forms.

While research has demonstrated the effectiveness of drug treatment for many mental disorders, it has nevertheless been found that other factors, for example the attitude of nurses and a congenial ward environment, enhance the efficacy of drugs. In spite of extensive research into various forms of psychotherapy, no conclusive results about their effectiveness have been demonstrated. That patients may be happier and more active in hospital wards in which attempts are made to create a therapeutic community, than in wards in which the atmosphere is custodial and institutionalized, has been demonstrated. The distinctive therapeutic role of the nursing staff in connection with any of the forms of treatment described in this chapter has so far been very inadequately researched. There is, however, fairly widespread agreement among psychiatrists, health service managers and social scientists who have studied psychiatric settings, that it is the nurses who are responsible for creating the therapeutic milieu in which others can work effectively, and that nurses themselves fulfil a therapeutic role in interpersonal relationships with patients. Where psychiatric hospitals or wards have come in for criticism, for example when enquiries have been instituted to investigate complaints of abuse or ill-treatment of patients, nurses were found to be lacking in interpersonal skills. As long ago as 1955, the WHO Expert

Committee on Psychiatric Nursing pointed out that whatever technical skills were used in psychiatric nursing, the interpersonal and social contexts within which these skills were employed were of utmost importance.

Sociologists have described two types of roles nurses fulfil; an expressive and an instrumental role. In their instrumental role nurses are themselves carrying out therapeutic functions for the patient; in their expressive role they enable others, for example psychiatrists, to fulfil their role.

It is easier to describe what nurses should do in their instrumental role than to identify and enable nurses to learn the skills necessary in their expressive role.

Nurses' values and beliefs, their attitudes and prejudices, their assumptions and feelings are constantly influencing not only their own behaviour, but also that of the patients and of the members of other professions working with them in a team.

It is important that all these personal attributes which nurses contribute to the patients' environment be regularly discussed and examined in the team, as, of course, must be the attributes of all the other team members. For many nurses the openness of peer evaluation and criticism is one of the most difficult aspects of psychiatric nursing to learn and to accept. It should be realized, however, that in the care and treatment of the mentally ill, people are the most valuable resource. The Americans have coined the expression 'the therapeutic use of self' to emphasize the need for all staff, and for nurses in particular, to examine the effect they themselves have on others.

Nurses can convey, by language or without words, the extent to which they care about, to which they are interested in, approve or disapprove of what others are saying or doing.

People often become aware of other people's feelings in a direct way. There are nurses who seem to be able to do this intuitively. There are patients with whom it is easier to share feelings than with others. The ability to feel what others are feeling is referred to as empathy. Nurses who are usually able to have empathy with others may be able to give useful clues in the diagnosis of patients; their difficulty in experiencing empathy may be an indication that the patient suffers from schizophrenia rather than from a depressive disorder.

Patients too have the ability to detect the feelings of staff in a direct, intuitive way. For patients it is not therapeutic to have nurses around with whom they are unable to have any empathy.

Though intuitively shared feelings are to be encouraged, it is possible to acquire skills in developing empathy and conveying this to patients. Empathy with patients who are experiencing emotional turmoil is a painful experience for nurses, one with which they must learn to cope with the help of supportive colleagues. For patients, empathy with staff members and with each other should be a positive therapeutic experience. Individual supportive psychotherapy can help patients to explore their interpersonal relationships; participation in groups can help patients and staff members to gain insight and to develop their coping skills.

Good communication skills, the ability to establish rapport, to listen and to express oneself clearly are fundamental prerequisites for all the forms of treatment described in this third part of the book.

18
Drug Therapy

In the last three decades the introduction of new drugs has transformed psychiatric treatment.

Much research is going on in all countries into the effect of new drugs on the function of the nervous system. The fact that some drugs are found to have specific effects on certain psychological processes has given impetus to research into the nature of mental illness itself. Some drugs, for example, cause hallucinations, others have specific use in diminishing hallucinations. It seems logical to link research into the effect of such drugs with research into the causation of hallucinations.

Some drugs have specifically beneficial results in states of depression, others in manic excitement. This knowledge leads to research into the chemical changes taking place in depressive or manic states, and into the possibility of biochemical causation of these disorders.

Some psychiatrists are interested chiefly in the specific action of drugs they use. Other psychiatrists regard social and psychological methods of treatment as more important. They readily agree, however, that patients who are excessively anxious or disturbed are not amenable to psychotherapy or to sociotherapeutic influences. They use drugs to enable the patient to participate more fully in the activities of the hospital.

Drug treatment is based on scientific research. Such research is only possible with knowledgeable contributions from nursing staff. Prescription of drugs is dependent on reliable observation of patients' behaviour and accurate reporting of change of behaviour.

DRUG TRIALS

Research into the effect of drugs is often initially carried out on animals. When a drug has been found safe for use on human beings, drug trials are necessary to measure the effect, if any, the drug has on patients.

It is necessary to find a group of patients all of whom have a particular set of symptoms and who could be expected to benefit from the drug if the claims made for it were found to be true. Detailed reports must be available for all these patients as regards the history of the illness, the severity of the symptoms and the degree of incapacity. A careful record must be kept of all the therapeutic influences brought to bear and the patient's reaction to them. Some of the patients are then given the drug while the remainder of the group are treated in exactly the same manner in every respect except that the drug is withheld. Progress is carefully recorded over a considerable period.

This is the pattern employed in every trial of a new drug, and an attempt is always made as far as possible to match the two groups of patients, so that the difference in result can be fairly attributed to the drug, rather than to other factors, e.g. age, differences in the duration or severity of illness, or differences in treatment other than the drug itself.

In psychiatric treatment it is particularly difficult to standardize the general treatment of patients, and it is here that the nurse's observations and accurate reporting can make all the difference when results are compared.

It must be taken into account that the giving of a drug may have considerable psychological significance for the patient. The very fact that the doctor has prescribed a drug for him may convince him that something is being done to help him. He may feel that the doctors have discovered the real cause of his trouble. He may believe that only if the cause of the trouble is known can a remedy in the form of a drug be given. The patient may also believe that this cause is physical, since it appears reasonable to him that a physical disorder should respond to drug therapy. To a certain extent this may make him feel that his complaint is more 'respectable', that it can be talked about like other illnesses.

There are usually certain physiological effects, e.g. palpitations or increased pulse rate, observable both to the patient and the nurses. The patient may observe himself closely once he realizes these manifestations. He may discover signs and symptoms in himself which he had not previously noticed but which he now interprets as changes in the course of his illness.

Nurses, having been warned of the possible ill-effects of the drug, observe the patient more carefully and with greater concern, and this closer relationship between the patient and his nurse may have some beneficial effect on him.

All this may mean that the actual administration of a drug introduces a significant difference in the treatment of the patients. It is, therefore, the usual practice to give all patients some drug—a placebo to one group and the drug to be tested to the other group. Sometimes the drug is dispensed by the pharmacist in such a form that neither the nurse nor the doctor knows which patients receive the drug and which patients the placebo. Changes can be made later; the patients who have received the drug can be given the placebo without their own knowledge or the knowledge of the nurses.

The doctors' and nurses' reports can then be independently assessed and some progress made in the proper use of drugs for the patient most likely to benefit.

Some nurses feel guilty about their part in drug trials. It is generally understood that honesty and truthfulness are the correct approach to the patient, so that the administration of a placebo appears deceitful to the nurses. Occasionally it seems unkind to deprive the patient of the drug which might help him and to allow his symptoms to continue while administering only a placebo. It must, however, be remembered that some psychiatric disorders remit without specific treatment, and that the psychological significance of taking tablets is very great.

Extravagant claims are frequently made for new drugs, which later turn out to have been quite unwarranted. To protect patients from possible harmful effects and to ensure that systematic knowledge of the effect of drugs on different mental disorder is obtained, controlled drug trials are indispensable. No patient is ever submitted to harmful treatment and doctors will see to it that no patient is deprived for long of the best available form of treatment.

If the nurse conveys to the patient that she feels dubious about the pill she is offering, she is not only hindering progress but also depriving the patient of the benefit which derives from an enthusiastic and positive approach.

ADMINISTRATION OF DRUGS

Whatever the drug in use, it is the nurse's duty, as soon as it has been ordered, to acquaint herself with all that is known about its action and potentialities.

She must know the following.
1   The prescribed dose, and the maximal dose that can be given under any circumstances.
2   The method of administration and any special points arising from it.
3   The expected effects of the drug.
4   The side-effects which can occur.
5   The possible toxic effects the drug may produce.

The following recommendations should be observed in the prescription of drugs.
1   The name of the medicine should be printed in CAPITAL letters.
2   The dose should be written clearly in the metric system.
3   The route of administration and times of dosage should be unambiguous.
4   The official or the approved name (where available) of the medicine should be used.
5   The signature of the prescriber should be clearly legible.
6   Abbreviations such as SOS, prn, should not be used.

It is also the practice of most employing authorities to have clear policies and procedures laid down and issued to staff in the form of guidelines or codes of practice. (The Royal College of Nursing has also issued a booklet on drug administration.)

The nurse whose reading of the prescription sheet leaves her in any doubt whatsoever regarding drug dosage or administration should seek clarification, because of the dangers of even an intelligent guess at what the prescription may mean.

The nurse is responsible for the safe keeping and storage of the drug. When administering a drug to a mentally ill patient, she should remember that identification of the patient may present more difficulties than in the case of patients in general hospitals, since the former himself may be incapable of confirming his name and unable to remember that he is having any medicine.

A patient's behaviour during drug administration can sometimes reveal important clues as to his present mental state. The patient who is paranoid may question his drugs and may require to be shown the label on the bottle and have it verified against the doctor's prescription on his medicine sheet. The patient secretly harbouring suicidal thoughts may leave the room hurriedly, immediately after being given his medication, to hoard unswallowed tablets for future use. Giving a full glass of water, engaging the patient in conversation, crushing the drug (unless contrary to manufacturer's instructions) or using a liquid form, if available, are some of the measures that can help towards ensuring drugs are swallowed. Urine tests have shown that 19% of medication prescribed in psychiatric hospitals is not in fact taken.

TRANQUILLIZERS

These are groups of drugs which produce a calming effect without causing drowsiness or acting as hypnotics (unless prescribed as such). When the first of these drugs was introduced into psychiatric hospitals in the fifties, they produced dramatic effects and hope was expressed that some hitherto intractable and chronic conditions might be cured.

The beneficial results of these drugs are manifold. Because patients are calm and quiet, the ward atmosphere has in many cases improved. Struggles and restraint are avoided. It is easier to establish active programmes of occupational therapy and rehabilitation and to build up relationships of trust between patients and nurses which help in later treatment.

Extensive research has resulted in so many drugs now being on the market that only a few details on the most commonly prescribed can usefully be given. Most produce some unpleasant side-effects and are toxic to a greater or lesser extent. Research has been directed to finding those drugs which have the most specific therapeutic effects and the lowest degree of toxicity. Most drugs are produced by more than one firm under different trade names. It would be futile to attempt to learn the details of all of these. When the doctor prescribes a drug which is new to the nurse she should request from the pharmacist the relevant information and ensure that she memorizes the essential facts about the drug for as long as it is in use.

Tranquillizers can be divided into two broad groups: major and minor.

Major tranquillizers

These drugs are also called neuroleptics; they produce a state of 'neurolepsis', or calm indifference, without loss of consciousness. They are also known as antipsychotic drugs because of their use in treating patients suffering from psychotic disorders, e.g. schizophrenia.

It is convenient to divide the major tranquillizers into three subgroupings according to the chemical 'family' to which they belong: (1) phenothiazines, (2) thioxanthenes, and (3) butyrophenones.

Phenothiazines

Chlorpromazine (Largactil), the standard phenothiazine, was first synthesized in 1950 and is the best known of this group. It has a pronounced calming effect on acutely disturbed psychotic patients when given by intramuscular injection. It also has a marked hypotensive action given by this route, and the nurse must not allow the patient to get up too soon afterwards. Perphenazine (Fentazin) is another well-known phenothiazine.

Long-acting (depot preparation) phenothiazines, e.g. fluphenazine decanoate (Modecate), have proved to be valuable as maintenance drug therapy for the chronic schizophrenic sufferer who is able to live in the community but is known to be erratic in taking regular oral medication. Phenothiazines do not cure schizophrenia in the sense that an antimicrobial drug can cure an acute infection; they require to be taken on a long-term basis by many people to prevent a return of their psychotic symptoms, and possible re-admission to hospital. Depot preparations are given by deep intramuscular injection, at approximately monthly intervals, by the community psychiatric nurse or another member of the primary health care team. If geographically convenient, the injections may be given at a depot injection clinic.

Nursing staff in some hospitals who give long-acting (rather than oral) preparations routinely in the treatment of patients with chronic schizophrenia, cite as advantages of this practice a resultant reduction in time spent administering drugs and an increase in the time devoted to patient–nurse interactions. However, early favourable reports of recent research state that certain long-acting *oral* neuroleptics (belonging to the chemical 'family' of the diphenylbutylpiperidines) require to be taken only at weekly intervals, e.g. penfluridol (Semap), and another is administered on four days only per week (pimozide/Orap). These drugs may prove a possible solution to the disadvantages of giving drugs by the parenteral route and to the time-consuming thrice-daily administration of drugs.

Thioxanthenes

The best known compound in this group is flupenthixol decanoate (Depixol). It is an injectable long-acting neuroleptic also used as maintenance therapy in chronic schizophrenia. It is said to be as effective as fluphenazine decanoate, but whereas the latter may cause depression in some individuals, this is less likely with flupenthixol decanoate. In fact the allied oral preparation, flupenthixol (Fluanxol), is claimed to have actual antidepressant properties.

Butyrophenones

Although also valuable in the treatment of schizophrenia, this group, of which haloperidol (Haldol, Fortanan) is the most commonly used, is now acknowledged to be particularly effective in the treatment of manic disorders.

Haloperidol (as decanoate) is also available as a depot preparation. It is given by deep intramuscular injection and its effect lasts for four weeks.

Unwanted effects of major tranquillizers

Most of the drugs used in psychiatry produce unwanted (as well as therapeutic) effects, and only some general comments on the more common of those associated with the major tranquillizers can usefully be given in this book.

The severity and frequency of the adverse reactions depend on a number of considerations. Of these, individual response, age of patient, route of administration (injectable depot preparations are often implicated) and type of drug used must be taken into account when side-effects of the major tranquillizers (neuroleptics) are being assessed.

Extrapyramidal effects. This group of side-effects of the major tranquillizers is the most manifest; as the name suggests, it is the extrapyramidal pathways of the nervous system which are involved. These adverse effects are the result of the neuroleptic drugs blocking the action of the chemical neurotransmitter, dopamine, on post-synaptic cells in the corpus striatum (part of the extrapyramidal system). This blockade creates a functional deficiency of dopamine, the effects of which may be seen in a variety of disorders of motor activity (see below), because the corpus striatum is involved in regulating involuntary movement and muscle tone.

However, it is postulated that the therapeutic action of the major tranquillizers in the psychoses rests on essentially the same cellular mechanism, but their beneficial antidopaminergic activity is concentrated mainly in the limbic system in the brain. The limbic system is associated, in part, with a person's emotional behaviour.

The disorders of motor activity due to dopamine depletion may be considered under four headings: (1) acute dystonic reactions; (2) pseudoparkinsonism (drug-induced parkinsonism); (3) akathisia; and (4) tardive dyskinesia.

Regarding the first three of these groups, symptoms diminish if the dose of the offending drug is reduced or stopped. The nurse should observe and report signs of the slightest tremor in the hands of a patient having major tranquillizers. This may be the first sign of adverse effects. If it is not advisable to discontinue the drug, some of the symptoms may be counteracted by the oral administration of an antiparkinsonian agent, e.g. benzhexol (Artane) and procyclidine (Kemadrin).

In the fourth group, tardive dyskinesia, discontinuation of the drug has been known to worsen the symptoms. Attempts to find an effective treatment for this reaction are the subject of much current research.

The butyrophenones and, particularly, the depot preparations, are especially prone to give rise to extrapyramidal side-effects. Recent reports have been published suggesting that clopenthixol decanoate (Clopixol) has a lower tendency to produce extrapyramidal reactions than the other injectable long-acting compounds.

1 *Acute dystonic reactions*: The nurse's role in the early recognition of this distressing condition is vital. It appears early in treatment and is commoner in the younger male patient. It should not be mistaken for schizophrenic posturing. Involuntary contraction of the skeletal muscles, particularly of the head and neck, resembling opisthotonus or torticollis, may be observed; the eyes may be turned upwards in an oculogyric crisis. Any of these adverse reactions should be reported immediately. Relief may be obtained by the administration of procyclidine (Kemadrin) 5–10 mg (approximate dose) given either by slow intravenous injection or intramuscularly.

2 *Pseudoparkinsonism*: This unwanted effect of the major tranquillizers is said to be more common in the older age group

of patients and it usually appears after two to three months of treatment. The patient shows signs of true parkinsonism, e.g. shuffling gait, muscular rigidity, mask-like facies and sialorrhoea.

3 *Akathisia*: Patients affected by this side-effect are often middle-aged. They are unable to sit or stand still and are continuously on the move, and may complain of feelings of inner restlessness as well. This apparent 'fidgetiness' may also cause the patient to have difficulty in getting to sleep at night. Accurate observation by day and night staff is necessary lest this reaction is interpreted as emotional agitation and treated with further medication.

4 *Tardive dyskinesia*: This serious and potentially irreversible condition is recognized to be a danger associated with the long-term administration of the major tranquillizers, and efforts are concentrated on minimizing its incidence. These include regular annual reviews of all patients who receive these neuroleptic drugs over a prolonged period, with a view to a gradual reduction in dosage until the drugs have been stopped or the patient's mental state worsens. In tardive dyskinesia there is an excess of involuntary motor activity. Tongue and neck muscles are especially affected, but the arms and hands may be involved. Body-rocking movements of the whole trunk have been described. Facial symptoms range from occasional movements of the jaw from side to side, and lip and tongue movements which result in mild facial distortions, to those which are incessant and disfiguring. Some of the excessive involuntary movements may be so severe as to interfere with the patient's ability to chew, and his diet may have to be adapted by the nurse to take this difficulty into account.

Hypotensive effects. Postural hypotension, noted particularly with thioridazine (Melleril) and neuroleptics given by intramuscular route in an emergency (see above), is observed, for example, when a sitting patient gets up quickly. The elderly patient is particularly vulnerable in this situation.

However, thioridazine given in an average dose of 100 mg thrice daily is unlikely to produce extrapyramidal reactions.

Metabolic effects
1 *Endocrine*. By way of the pituitary gland, some neuroleptics exert certain hormonal influences such as an increase in

prolactin levels in the blood. High levels of prolactin may give rise to menstrual irregularities and milk secretion in non-pregnant female patients, and to many this is very worrying. The nurse should be able to explain that this is a common and harmless side-effect of their medication.

2 *Body weight.* Patients receiving phenothiazines have a tendency towards obesity—partly due to increased appetite (exception: prochlorperazine (Stemetil) which reduces appetite) and partly to decreased activity in the previously agitated patient. Dietary education by the nurse as soon as the patient begins to show signs of overeating will prevent the need for a strict low-calorie diet later.

Haematological effects. Leucopenia, which may lead to fatal agranulocytosis, is fortunately extremely rare, but, because of its acute onset, may be missed on routine blood testing. It is necessary for the nurse to know the early signs of this potentially fatal condition, especially when caring for a patient who is receiving a phenothiazine, such as chlorpromazine, for the first time, and who may be too acutely disturbed and preoccupied to complain of physical symptoms.

A sore throat may be the first sign. Suspicions may be aroused when the nurse notices the patient holds his throat and grimaces each time he has to swallow. Fever is another early sign and again it may be the nurse who observes the patient shivering, though the ward is well heated. Although both symptoms may, more commonly, herald a mild upper respiratory tract infection, they must be reported and a full blood count should be carried out immediately.

Miscellaneous effects. Patients receiving antipsychotic drugs are liable to develop a light-sensitive skin reaction if exposed to direct sunlight. Barrier creams may be of help, but it is best for the patient to seek the shade if possible. Other sensitivity rashes have also been reported.

Drowsiness is not uncommon at first with neuroleptic medication, particularly chlorpromazine and thioridazine, but usually lessens as tolerance develops.

Dryness of the mouth, constipation, difficulty with micturition and blurred vision may also occur initially.

Minor tranquillizers

Benzodiazepines

Since the introduction in 1960 of chlordiazepoxide (Librium) and in 1963 of diazepam (Valium), the benzodiazepines have overtaken and replaced almost all of the other traditional minor tranquillizers, such as the barbiturates and the propanedioles (meprobamate/Miltown). It has been said that between one in ten and one in five of all adults in the Western World are prescribed a benzodiazepine when they visit their general practitioner.

This group of drugs, of which there are a large number of generic compounds marketed under a wide variety of trade names, is used mainly for the relief of anxiety and insomnia in psychiatric hospitals.

Benzodiazepines may be given to treat all degrees of anxiety and tension, from mild to moderate feelings of anxiety to severe anxiety states and panic attacks. They are also of value in situational anxiety and phobias as an adjunct to behavioural psychotherapy so that relearning can take place.

The benzodiazepines may be used in the treatment of withdrawal symptoms associated with alcohol and narcotic abuse.

This group of minor tranquillizers has anticonvulsant properties and may be discontinued before a patient commences a course of electroconvulsive therapy. Conversely, a patient suffering from epilepsy can benefit from treatment with a benzodiazepine.

Although all benzodiazepine compounds have a hypnotic as well as an anxiolytic (antianxiety) effect, only those drugs which are quickly absorbed to achieve rapid induction of sleep, and quickly eliminated to avoid drowsiness the next day, are used as night sedation.

The elderly patient is especially likely to have residual effects the next day and the nurse should look for evidence of undue drowsiness, confusion and unsteadiness of gait, even when a short-acting hypnotic is used. It has been suggested that half the adult dose should suffice.

Nitrazepam (Mogadon) and triazolam (Halcion) are examples of some of the more commonly prescribed benzodiazepine night sedatives.

Unwanted effects. Physical and psychological dependence on the benzodiazepines has been reported. It is recommended that if a benzodiazepine drug is used in anxiety, it should be as a first-aid measure and not for longer than two months.

Another unwanted effect of these drugs is a 'hangover' of the hypnotic effect the day after the drug has been given. Symptoms include motor inco-ordination and minor degrees of drowsiness, impairing the patient's ability to perform a number of tasks, for example driving a car. Diazepam is thought to be particularly prone to cause this reaction, whereas with clobazam (Frisium) it is said to be less likely to occur. Recent attention has focused on a residual impairment of short-term memory in the morning following night sedation with certain hypnotic benzodiazepines, such as nitrazepam (Mogadon). This is especially deleterious in elderly patients whose cognitive abilities are beginning to deteriorate with age.

Withdrawal fits following long-term administration of benzodiazepines have been described. Patients should be instructed not to stop these drugs abruptly but to 'tail' them off gradually over a period of time.

It is not advisable for pregnant women to take benzodiazepines. Untoward reactions, such as lethargy and weight loss, may occur in breast-fed babies whose mothers have been prescribed these drugs.

Beta-blocking agents

Many of the somatic signs and symptoms of anxiety are thought to be due to increased adrenaline release from the adrenal glands and the autonomic (sympathetic) nervous system. Therefore drugs capable of modifying these effects by blocking adrenaline output are of value in reducing these predominantly autonomic anxiety symptoms, such as palpitations, sweating and tremor. Propranolol (Inderal) is one example; oxprenolol hydrochloride (Trasicor) and sotalol hydrochloride (Sotacor) may also be used.

The beta-blocking agents may be used in combination with benzodiazepine compounds.

Unwanted effects. The patient may complain of fatigue and cold extremities, and also of vivid dreams. Because of their tendency to cause bronchospasm, the beta-blockers are never used to treat anxiety associated with asthma. As with the benzodiazepines, they are contraindicated in pregnancy.

Antidepressant drugs

In some types of clinical depression there appears to be a depletion in the availability of certain chemical neurotransmitters in the brain, e.g. the monoamines, 5-hydroxytryptamine (5HT or serotonin), and noradrenaline—the so-called monoamine theory of depression. Thus it is widely held that the therapeutic effects of antidepressant drug therapy rest on their action in increasing, by whatever means (of which there are many, depending on the drug used), the availability of one or both of the above transmitters at the synaptic cleft of certain receptor sites in the brain.

Three broad categories of antidepressant drugs will be considered briefly: 1. tricyclic antidepressants; 2. 'second generation' antidepressants; 3. monoamine oxidase inhibitors (MAOIs). Some details of lithium therapy will be given separately.

Tricyclic antidepressants. Introduced in the second half of the fifties, imipramine (Tofranil) was the original tricyclic antidepressant. It was followed by amitriptyline (Tryptizol); as effective as imipramine but more sedating and of value, therefore, should agitation accompany the depressive state.

A disadvantage of these early antidepressants—and one not yet fully overcome—is the slow onset of any therapeutic effect. The nurse must know of this time-lag, which may be as long as 14 to 21 days, before the patient's depressive symptoms are alleviated. It could be that a severely depressed and potentially suicidal patient, hitherto immobile (retarded), acquires the necessary energy and drive after a few days on antidepressant therapy to carry out his intention to commit suicide; his mood not yet having shown any improvement.

The 'tricyclics' are sometimes known as the classical antidepressants and are used as a standard against which other drugs are compared.

Clomipramine (Anafranil), though classed as an antidepressant, is said to be useful in treating patients with obsessional and phobic states. As with amitriptyline, clomipramine is available in syrup form and can also be administered if necessary by the intramuscular or intravenous route.

'Second generation' antidepressants. This rash of newer antidepressant drugs is in part the outcome of the concern over the cardiotoxicity of their forerunners, the tricyclics, though their therapeutic effects have not been established as being significantly greater. While distinct from one another and from the classical antidepressants, and differing in the details of their action on the brain, they are thought to have similar therapeutic properties regarding ultimately increasing monoamine availability.

Some of the claims made for products included in this second category of antidepressants are as follows.

Maprotilene (Ludiomil)—a tetracyclic or quadricyclic compound—is said to have a more rapid antidepressant action, but it is more likely to precipitate epilepsy (epileptogenic) in vulnerable patients.

Viloxazine (Vivalan)—a bicyclic compound—is prone to cause nausea, but fewer of the other adverse reactions.

Nomifensine (Merital) is thought to be comparatively free from cardiotoxicity and is not epileptogenic. However, there have been reports of nausea, sleep disturbance and restlessness with this drug.

Trazodone (Molipaxin) is reported to be free of side-effects, including cardiotoxicity, and to act more quickly. Trazodone and another tetracyclic compound, mianserin (Bolvidon; Norval), are said to be of particular use in the treatment of the elderly depressed patient.

Monoamine oxidase inhibitors (MAOIs). Inhibition of intracellular monoamine oxidase—an enzyme which destroys monoamines in certain presynaptic cells in the brain—is thought to bring about an increase in the availability of 5HT (serotonin) and noradrenaline at the synaptic cleft. This is thought to result in a therapeutic response in those depressed patients in whom there is a depletion of these chemical neurotransmitters.

Although there has been a decline in the use of this group of drugs since their introduction in the fifties, a number of authorities attest to their usefulness for patients suffering from atypical depressive reactions. These patients may show other features in addition to a depressed mood, such as anxiety, phobic symptoms and depersonalization. 'Non-endogenicity' is said to be a salient feature in patients who respond to MAOIs. Additionally, depressed patients who do not respond to any other group of antidepressants may show a favourable reaction to one of the MAOIs, e.g. phenelzine (Nardil).

Unwanted effects of monoamine oxidase inhibitors
1   *Liver damage*: Apart from the general side-effects associated with most antidepressant drugs (see below), this group may cause liver damage, but it is said to be uncommon.
2   *Hypertensive crises* ('cheese effect'): Hypertensive crises are said to be five times more likely to occur with the MAOI, tranylcypromine sulphate (Parnate).

One of the substances implicated in this serious, and potentially fatal, reaction is tyramine—a potent hypertensive agent which is found as a naturally occurring amine in the diet. Normally, most of this dietary tyramine, once ingested, is rapidly destroyed by the monoamines in the intestinal mucosa and the liver. In a patient taking a MAOI, however, there is a reduction in the level of these intestinal and hepatic monoamines; his dietary tyramine is therefore not destroyed as it should be, but is absorbed intact. Absorbed tyramine may subsequently release noradrenaline which is present in large amounts in storage sites due to the inhibition of monoamine oxidase (i.e. the enzyme which normally destroys it—see above). Noradrenaline in turn may stimulate receptors in the heart and blood vessels before it is de-activated by the depleted enzyme. This stimulation causes a sudden steep rise in the patient's blood pressure.

Cheese, containing as it does a high level of tyramine, was the foodstuff originally isolated as causing this chain reaction and has given it the name the 'cheese reaction' or 'cheese effect' of the MAOIs.

Any patient who takes a monoamine oxidase inhibitor as an out-patient must always carry a special card with him to remind him of the other substances, as well as cheese, he must avoid. These include Marmite, Bovril and other yeast and meat extracts, broad bean pods (commonly eaten in some cultures), pickled herrings and some animal livers. Alcohol intake must be moderate; Chianti wine, which may contain up to 0.25 mg of tyramine per bottle, must be avoided completely.

Everyday cough and cold 'cures' may contain similar sympathomimetic amines. If taken unwittingly as a simple remedy by a patient taking MAOIs, they could precipitate a hypertensive crisis.

Signs and symptoms of a hypertensive crisis. The patient affected may initially complain of a headache and this must be reported immediately by the nurse. Blood pressure increases of over 50 mmHg systolic and 30 mmHg diastolic have been recorded. The headache may worsen, becoming very severe, and is accompanied by sweating, flushing, nausea and vomiting, or neck rigidity and photophobia. Occasionally a cerebrovascular accident has occurred. This crisis is treated with a receptor blocking drug, such as phentolamine, 5–10 mg given by intravenous injection.

Efforts by researchers to discover effective MAOIs free of the 'cheese effect' have claimed some successes.

Other specific drug interactions. Drug interactions associated with some of the more common drugs used in psychiatry are listed later in this chapter. Those associated with the monoamine oxidase inhibitors are included here because of their specificity.

Pethidine and certain other narcotic compounds must not be given to patients receiving MAOIs; serious, and occasionally fatal, toxic reactions have been reported.

If the prescription of a patient who is receiving a tricyclic antidepressant drug has to be changed to a MAOI, or vice versa, it is recommended that a two-week drug-free period be allowed before the new drug is commenced. Theoretically, the MAOI might be expected to complement the action of the tricyclic drug, but in fact serious reactions have been described when a combination has been used.

General unwanted effects of antidepressant drugs. In addition to the specific unwanted reactions, there are a number of general side-effects, occurring especially in the early stages of drug therapy, which are common to most if not all antidepressant drugs. The atropine-like (autonomic) action of these compounds gives rise to dryness of the mouth, difficulty in visual accommodation, and constipation. A further side-effect, urinary retention, calls for special vigilance from the nurse caring for the elderly depressed male patient who may have existing difficulty with micturition due to an enlarged prostate gland. Other unwanted effects include drowsiness, dizziness, unsteadiness of gait and postural hypotension—all also potential problems in the elderly patient.

Long-term administration of antidepressant drugs. As with any drug, each patient varies in his or her response to an antidepressant compound. Quite a few different drugs may have to be tried in succession before a favourable outcome is eventually obtained. Should the patient suffer from recurrent depression, the psychiatrist may decide, on the patient's recovery from his present depressive state, to continue with the successful drug for some considerable length of time after discharge. It has been found that if this drug is discontinued prematurely, resulting in the patient's relapse, there is no guarantee that its reinstitution will prove to be therapeutic for this patient on a second occasion.

Lithium therapy

Since the introduction of lithium salts in 1949 as antimanic agents, hundreds of reports have been published covering all aspects of lithium therapy. Today, lithium enjoys an established reputation as an effective and valuable drug in the prophylaxis of recurrent affective disorders, especially in the depression of manic–depressive psychosis.

Though still sometimes used for patients suffering from a manic episode, it has the disadvantage of taking about a week before any improvement is effected, and compares unfavourably with some of the quicker-acting neuroleptics, such as haloperidol, chlorpromazine (used intramuscularly if required) and pimozide. Occasionally, lithium may be given in combination with a neuroleptic; some clinicians prefer not to give haloperidol or fluphenazine with lithium because of reports of adverse effects.

Claims have been made for the use of lithium in the treatment of certain types of depression, but current evidence does not support its use in preference to a classical or 'second generation' antidepressant drug.

Preparation of the patient before lithium therapy. In addition to a physical examination and routine laboratory investigations, such as checking the patient's blood urea levels (the principal route of excretion of lithium by the urinary system) and thyroid function because this may be affected during lithium therapy, the patient may also undergo a lithium clearance test to obtain some indication of his lithium excretion rate. The results can help when an appropriate initial dose of lithium is being calculated. Irrespective of the product used, some doctors prefer to give lithium in divided daily doses rather than in a single one. This is thought to reduce the possibility of high postabsorptive lithium peaks. Such peaks result in high concentrations in the glomerular filtrate, which may contribute to the nephrotoxic effects associated with this drug.

Lithium is marketed as lithium carbonate, either as the preparation known as Camcolit, or as sustained release tablets, e.g. Phasal or Priadel.

Monitoring serum lithium levels. To avoid the potential dangers associated with lithium therapy, the dosage required to obtain an appropriate serum lithium level must be calculated for each patient. Thus it is necessary for the patient to have blood samples taken at least weekly during the first few weeks of treatment.

Many authorities recommend that the serum lithium level should be between 0.6 and 1.2 mmol/l and should not exceed 1.5 mmol/l. A lower level of 0.4–0.8 mmol/l has been suggested by some workers as a safer, but still effective, range for prophylactic therapy.

At least 12 hours must have elapsed between the ingestion of the last dose of lithium and the blood sample being taken from the patient. The nurse must know of this interval and ensure that the patient's medication is stopped at the appropriate time.

Once the acceptable dose of lithium has been established for the individual patient, the interval between serum estimations may be increased to monthly, provided he remains well and shows no evidence of untoward reactions to the drug. The age of the patient should also be considered. Elderly patients receiving lithium therapy require more frequent monitoring because of the inherent reduction in renal functioning as a person grows older. Other patients may ultimately require to have their blood checked at 4–8-weekly intervals only, though not less often than every 12 weeks. The patient's thyroid function is also checked from time to time.

Unwanted effects of lithium therapy. Pregnancy is a contraindication to the use of lithium. Lithium is said to have teratogenic effects on the fetus, particularly if given during the first trimester; the cardiovascular system is especially vulnerable to malformation. A woman is not advised to breast-feed her baby while taking lithium. The drug passes into the milk causing such adverse effects as hypotonia and hypothermia in the baby. Alternatively, the mother may discontinue lithium medication during the breast-feeding period, but this may not be advisable. A person prone to recurrent depressive episodes is especially vulnerable in the puerperium.

In view of the relatively narrow therapeutic range for lithium, it is important for the nurse and the patient to be aware of the signs and symptoms of impending toxicity. It is useful to distinguish between (a) side-effects which are relatively common initially, though some may persist beyond the initial phase of treatment and are upsetting for the patient, but are nevertheless harmless, (b) later side-effects, and (c) prodromes of lithium intoxication.

Initial side-effects. Initial feelings of anorexia, nausea or a metallic taste in the mouth are not unusual. The patient is usually in hospital when lithium therapy is first instituted and it is helpful for the nurse to know that these symptoms can be minimized if tablets are given during or after food.

The patient may complain of a fine tremor of the hands; loose stools are often reported in the early stages of treatment. The nurse should ensure that the patient knows the difference between loose stools and diarrhoea (see below). Some patients may find constipation, a dry mouth and thirst troublesome side-effects. Skin eruptions and an exacerbation of existing skin conditions have been reported.

Later side-effects. Weight gain may be noted and oedema may be present. Hypothyroidism has been known to develop and is treated with supplements of thyroxine. Persistent polyuria and polydipsia (known as reversible nephrogenic diabetes insipidus) may interfere with the patient's sleep. The night nurse may be the first to note and report this side-effect if the patient is still in hospital.

Chronic renal damage has been reported as a long-term reaction to lithium therapy. It is claimed that this has been due to the higher level of lithium used in the past and should not occur now that more is known about the drug.

Patients receiving lithium therapy should be advised to avoid situations which give rise to prolonged sweating. The salt lost is replaced in the cells by lithium, with a consequent reduction in lithium clearance. This in turn gives rise to high blood levels of lithium and a risk of toxicity. A period of exceptionally hot weather can have this effect. Similarly, a bout of food poisoning, which also causes electrolyte imbalance, could have serious consequences and should be reported at once.

Prodomes of lithium intoxication. Impending toxicity is associated with symptoms such as excessive thirst, vomiting and/or diarrhoea. Medical help should be sought immediately. Neurological signs which may occur include a coarse tremor, slurred speech, sleepiness, sluggishness, ataxia, dizziness and mental confusion. The drug is withdrawn and blood is taken for serum lithium estimation. If prompt action is not taken in this medical emergency, the patient's condition will deteriorate rapidly. Sodium depletion is again a potential danger in this situation and an intravenous infusion of saline may be set up for rapid replacement, especially if the patient is vomiting and not able to take fluids orally. Patients with severe lithium poisoning may require peritoneal dialysis.

Drug interactions with lithium therapy. Increased sodium chloride intake, in one form or another, can lead to increased lithium clearance with a resultant drop in serum levels (i.e. the opposite effect of sodium chloride loss).

Other compounds known to interfere with lithium clearance are diuretics, indomethacin (Indocid) and certain antiobesity drugs, which cause lithium levels to rise. Some published reports have found that lithium may potentiate the action of muscle relaxants.

Miscellaneous drug interactions

Apart from the special drug interactions already described, a number of drugs, particularly those used to treat the psychiatric patient who has a physical condition, interact adversely with some of those commonly used in psychiatry.

For example, it is now well recognized that if a patient is receiving an antidepressant drug, this may reduce the therapeutic effect of the antihypertensive drug he is concurrently taking for his hypertensive condition. Both drugs are thought to be in competition for the receptor sites; the phenothiazines and the butyrophenones may also interact in this way.

A patient who is taking benzodiazepines, phenothiazines or butyrophenones should be advised to drink alcohol with caution; these drugs can potentiate its action and increase central nervous system depression. Other central nervous system depressant drugs must only be prescribed with caution for patients receiving minor and certain major tranquillizers.

Further reading

Barr, M. & Kiernan, J. (1983) *The Human Nervous System*, 4th edn. London: Harper & Row.

British Medical Journal (1981) Leader: Tardive dyskinesia. *British Medical Journal 282*, 1257.

David, J.A. (1983) *Drug Round Companion*. Oxford: Blackwell Scientific Publications.

Royal College of Nursing (1983) *Drug Administration. A Nursing Responsibility*. London: Rcn.

Silverstone, T. & Turner, P. (1982) *Drug Treatment in Psychiatry*. London: Routledge & Kegan Paul.

Snyder, S.H. (1980) *Biological Aspects of Mental Disorder*. Oxford: Oxford University Press.

Subhan, Z. (1984) Benzodiazepines and memory. *Psychiatry in Practice 3* (19), 15.

19
Electroconvulsive Therapy

Electroconvulsive therapy is a technically simple treatment, but the patient requires support and reassurance from tactful and understanding nursing staff.

It is a treatment which, because it is relatively safe, quick, cheap and frequently effective, was used somewhat indiscriminately and uncritically in the past. It has been employed in out-patient departments, clinics and hospitals and has proved beneficial in certain psychiatric disorders.

The first therapeutic use of an electrical current applied to the human brain was by Ugo Cerletti in 1938; ECT (its commonly abbreviated name) has been used continuously since then and has survived as the only physical treatment, apart from drug therapy, still in regular use in psychiatry.

INDICATIONS FOR ELECTROCONVULSIVE THERAPY

As a result of recent research trials, ECT is now agreed to be maximally effective in treating patients with severe depression, particularly if psychotic symptoms, such as delusions and/or auditory hallucinations, are present.

This therapy may be life saving in certain circumstances. If, for example, the patient is severely depressed and is expressing suicidal ideas, or has just made a serious attempt on his life, a course of ECT may be started in preference to the risk of waiting for a week or so until drugs take effect.

Sometimes patients do not respond to or are unable to tolerate antidepressant drugs; ECT may be beneficial on these occasions.

Electroconvulsive therapy was used for patients suffering from mania but has been supplanted by drug therapy. However, it may still be given to patients with severe mania who respond adversely, or too slowly, to drugs.

Although ECT does not effect a cure, it can often cut short a patient's suffering.

PHYSICAL CONTRAINDICATIONS FOR ELECTROCONVULSIVE THERAPY

Opinions vary about the contraindications for ECT. Some doctors claim that there are almost no absolute contraindications if the patient is likely to suffer more harm if his severe depressive state is allowed to continue. They point out that depressive illness carries a significant mortality (5% at 5 years) and that sudden deaths have been reported with certain antidepressant drugs (Zimelidine (Zelmid), a new antidepressant drug, was withdrawn from general use in 1983 because of fatalities associated with its use).

However, where deaths have been associated with ECT (1 death in 2594 courses of treatment—Royal College of Psychiatrists Report, 1981), they have tended to be cerebrovascular or cardiovascular in nature, and many psychiatrists regard raised intracranial pressure (confirmed or suspected), the presence of an aneurysm or a brain tumour, a history of a recent cerebrovascular accident or myocardial infarction, and the evidence of cardiac arrhythmias, as contraindications for electroconvulsive therapy.

These specific contraindications have been chosen because the passage of the electric current is known to produce certain cerebrovascular and cardiovascular changes. These include: (a) a considerable, though brief, increase in cerebral blood flow, and (b) initial bradycardia (counteracted by atropine, see below) followed immediately by a short-lived but sudden tachycardia. There is also a steep, sharp increase in blood pressure (systolic).

Neither patients with epilepsy nor those with an indwelling cardiac pacemaker need be precluded from receiving ECT.

Old age itself is not a contraindication for ECT but post-anaesthetic recovery time is longer in the elderly patient. This is measured by the time taken for their return to normal respirations, consciousness and orientation.

THE THERAPEUTIC EFFECT OF ELECTROCONVULSIVE THERAPY

Electroconvulsive therapy can be described as a therapeutic dose of electricity applied to the patient's head. The amount of current used varies slightly but is usually about 36 joules lasting from 1 to 1.5 seconds. The desired result is a generalized seizure lasting approximately 30 seconds.

However, not only is an electric current passed across the patient's head, but he is given atropine beforehand and receives an anaesthetic and muscle relaxant drug. The patient also 'experiences' a brief period of unconsciousness and has a grand mal seizure. Before, during and after 'treatment' the patient receives considerable attention from the nursing staff. Some patients attach psychological significance to the treatment. Thus, in theory at least, the beneficial effect on the patient could be a result of any one, or any combination, of these component parts of the treatment.

Results of research over the past quarter of a century have, however, convinced many psychiatrists that the induction of the generalized seizure activity in the patient's brain is possibly the crucial element in the procedure.

It has not been established why this activity should be therapeutic, and a number of theories have been put forward. Chemical changes occurring in the patient's brain as a result of the fit is one of them.

Number and frequency of treatments

The number of ECT sessions required to produce this therapeutic effect depends on each individual patient's response. This varies considerably from one patient to another.

A course may consist of approximately four to eight treatments, though some patients will require fewer and others more. The treatment is usually repeated two, or occasionally three, times a week.

Electrode placements

Bilateral ECT is the term used when one electrode is placed on each side of the patient's head, over the temporal lobe, 4 cm above the midpoint of a line drawn from the lateral angle of the eye to the external auditory meatus.

These bilateral placements are still sometimes used in Britain, and those who favour this method claim that fewer treatments are required and that a more rapid initial improvement is produced—a vital consideration if a patient is in serious danger of committing suicide.

Unilateral ECT, as the name suggests, is when both electrodes are placed on the same side of the patient's head. These placements were first introduced in 1942, and have been more widely used from the sixties onward in the hope of reducing the memory disturbance associated with the after-effects of ECT. The stimulus should be applied to the patient's non-dominant hemisphere. It has been shown that dominant unilateral ECT produces greater memory disturbance than bilateral. Therefore if a patient's handedness is in doubt, bilateral ECT is the method of choice.

'Unilateralists', while in agreement about the preferred method of electrode placement in order to minimize confusion and memory impairment in the period immediately following ECT, offer a bewildering variety of placings for the second electrode. The first is usually placed on the conventional site over the temporal lobe.

It is important, however, that at least the electrodes are spaced widely enough to allow sufficient current to penetrate the patient's skull and cortex and not simply to pass round the skin.

Psychiatrists in favour of unilateral electrode placements also state that headache, if it occurs at all, is less severe than after conventional bilateral ECT. They also claim that, overall, the therapeutic action of unilateral ECT is as effective as the traditional bilateral ECT.

STAGES OF TREATMENT

Treatment can be divided into four stages.
1   Physical and psychological preparation of the patient.
2   Care of the patient immediately before ECT.
3   Care of the patient in the treatment centre.
4   Care of the patient following ECT.

Physical and psychological preparation

Physical preparation

A thorough physical examination is carried out to make sure the patient is physically fit for the series of general anaesthetics involved in a course of ECT and for the treatment itself. Treatment is postponed if the patient has a respiratory infection.

The nurse may be required to take and record the patient's temperature, pulse, respirations, and blood pressure, the evening before treatment is given, and again the following morning. The patient's weight is also recorded.

The doctor also gets written consent from the patient to carry out the treatment. The question of giving a patient treatment without his consent has been debated at length in recent years and the required procedure is now laid down in the new Mental Health Acts (see Appendix). If the patient withdraws his consent at any point, the medical staff should be contacted at once and treatment will not be given meantime.

Psychological preparation

One of the results of the very widespread use of ECT is that it is now rare to meet a patient who has never heard of this form of treatment; television has given it wide coverage and over the past decade it has been the subject of considerable controversy and adverse publicity.

Often patients have known someone, or heard of someone, who has been treated with ECT. The patient's attitude is therefore coloured by the experience of his friends. He will eagerly demand this treatment if he knows of someone who was helped, or fear it if his experience has been unfavourable.

Even if the patient has not heard of electroconvulsive therapy prior to admission, he will almost certainly meet in hospital those who are undergoing this treatment. Patients can often be heard discussing their treatment with each other and comparing notes, and the nurse can easily discover how the patient is likely to react to the news that he is to have electroconvulsive therapy by observing him while other patients talk about it.

Relatives may be initially apprehensive when told that the patient is to have this treatment. They should be given an explanation of what is involved and the opportunity to ask questions; the patient may be too morbidly preoccupied and uncommunicative to broach the subject. Continued support and reassurance should be given to the relatives until the patient begins to show some improvement from the course of treatment.

Psychological preparation of the patient for a course of electroconvulsive therapy should begin with an explanation of what to expect, given in the first instance by the doctor, usually while he is obtaining consent. This part of the preparation is most important. Studies have shown that almost half of patients who had had a course of electroconvulsive therapy felt that the explanation given beforehand was inadequate.

After the doctor has explained the treatment, the nurse is often approached by the patient, who asks questions about it, hoping to have the doctor's words confirmed. The nurse should therefore know what form the doctor's explanations have taken and should also ask the patient what the doctor has said. Nothing could be worse for the patient's fears than apparent contradiction between doctor and nurses.

A patient who is severely depressed may, because of poor concentration, retain little or nothing of what the doctor has told him. It can be helpful if the nurse takes advantage of the patient's diurnal mood variation (worse in the morning, slightly better towards evening), if this is present, to repeat the doctor's explanation later in the day.

Although there are variations in the details of the explanation given to the patient, with some points stressed more than others, the general principles are similar.

Often it is reassuring for the patient to know that a nurse from his ward will accompany him for treatment and will remain with him throughout the session. He is told that a light anaesthetic is given to put him to 'sleep' and it may be added he will 'not feel a thing'—that it is a painless procedure.

The patient is told that on wakening from his short 'sleep' he will probably feel 'fuzzy' and light headed and will remember nothing about it. This is the very thing which some patients worry about, if they happen to have heard about the loss of memory which follows ECT. In this case the doctor will assure the patient that loss of memory is only transitory and that there is no danger of important things being forgotten.

Some patients about to have ECT for the first time require

special attention from the nursing staff on the evening before treatment. A nurse should be available to spend some time with the apprehensive patient, repeating if necessary what is involved and allowing the patient ample opportunity to ask questions. A fellow patient on the ward who has benefited from this form of treatment may be willing to talk with the patient. This unique reassurance can be very helpful.

Immediate care before treatment

However carefully the patient is prepared the evening before, on the day of his first ECT he will experience some apprehension which the nurse must try to alleviate. If ECT is given in the morning, the patient may require to fast from midnight. At any event, the anaesthetist will usually require the patient to have had nothing by mouth for 6 to 8 hours before treatment is due. As is the practice before any general anaesthetic is given, the anaesthetist's instructions must be strictly adhered to. If, by any chance, the patient is given food or drink by mistake, this must be reported. Treatment will be postponed.

It is difficult for the patient to be occupied until the last moment. The best thing is to tell him at approximately what time he will be having treatment and to attempt to be as punctual as possible. The worst of the waiting time comes after the original appointment.

Half an hour before the patient leaves the ward, he may be given a premedication of atropine (0.6 mg approximate dose) intramuscularly, prescribed by the anaesthetist. Atropine not only dries up the secretions but, more importantly, it prevents marked bradycardia when the current is passed, by its partially blocking the vagus nerve supply to the heart. If this drug has been ordered and for some reason not given, it is essential that the nurse accompanying the patient informs the nurse in charge immediately she enters the treatment room. The anaesthetist will give the atropine intravenously.

After the atropine has been given on the ward, the patient has to be closely observed in case he unwittingly drinks to relieve the unpleasant dryness in his mouth caused by the drug; some anaesthetists prefer to give the atropine routinely by intravenous injection, before anaesthetizing the patient, to avoid this risk.

The severely depressed patient is particularly liable to break his fast. He may forget he has been asked not to eat or drink or may be too depressed to be concerned about such restrictions.

Final ward preparations before treatment include making sure the patient has removed tight clothing so that breathing is not restricted, and the female patient should not wear any make-up or nail varnish which might mask cyanosis. Any metal objects which might deflect the current, such as earrings and hairgrips, are not worn. A depressed patient who has lost weight before admission may require to have her wedding ring strapped in position. All other valuables are put in safe keeping, and prostheses, if worn, are removed and placed in labelled containers. Patients who wear dentures and/or spectacles should be given the choice of wearing them until they are about to enter the treatment room. The patient wears a special ECT identity bracelet on the day of treatment. If a smoker, the patient is asked to try not to have a cigarette before ECT. The nurse should explain that smoking increases the production of mucus in the respiratory tract. The patient is asked to empty his bladder and, if possible, his bowels immediately before leaving the ward.

The nurse who accompanies the patient is responsible for collecting the relevant documents: the patient's TPR and BP charts, medicine prescription and recording sheet (or a note of current medication), ECT record form, consent to treatment form; the patient's case notes are sometimes included in this list.

Electroconvulsive therapy is usually carried out in a central treatment unit to which all patients are taken. If this arrangement is not possible, it is important that the waiting area is completely separate from the treatment room. The recovery area must also be separate from the other two rooms. There is a trained nurse in charge of the treatment centre and she is responsible for ensuring that the special equipment is available and in working order. This equipment includes oxygen cylinders and special equipment to assist breathing, for example Brooke's airways and Ambu-bags, and equipment for intubation. A defibrillator is also needed. A special electrolyte fluid may be required to soak padded electrodes. This prevents burning of the patient's skin and also aids conduction of the current. The nurse is also responsible for re-ordering drugs for anaesthetic and emergency use, as required. Other duties include in-service teaching of all nursing and support staff attending or working in the centre. She also plays an important role in informing the ward staff of the approximate time of the treatment session and of any untoward delays. This information can be quickly passed on to the patients involved. (If ECT is carried out in various locations throughout the hospital, a nominated nurse should be responsible for the nursing contribution in each area.)

Care during treatment

While in the waiting room, a nurse should always be present, guiding conversation and providing distraction from the topic of ECT. The patient's dentures and spectacles, if still worn, are removed and put in a place of safety before treatment is given. The anaesthetist is told of the distribution of any loose teeth or crowns the patient may have; this determines the most suitable mouth gag to use. A tooth may come out or break if the patient were to bite too forcibly on a hard part of a gag during the convulsion.

In the treatment room the patient is asked to remove his shoes before lying down on the trolley. The covering blanket should leave his feet exposed so that any twitching of the toes during the fit can be clearly seen.

The accompanying nurse continues to give the patient reassurance and support until the anaesthetic takes effect. Her role is to attend to the patient; she may be asked to exert gentle pressure on the patient's major joints. The anaesthetist gives the patient a light anaesthetic, e.g. methohexitone, followed by a muscle relaxant, e.g. suxamethonium, to modify the muscle spasm during the fit. This is followed by 100% oxygen administered by mask—the anaesthetist has to ventilate the patient's lungs because of the paralysed respiratory muscles. The psychiatrist then places the electrodes on the patient's head and induces a convulsion by the passage of the electric current from the machine. After the convulsion, oxygen is again given by the anaesthetist and is continued until the patient is breathing spontaneously. When the anaesthetist is satisfied that the patient can breathe independently, the patient is turned on to his side and taken to the recovery room to regain consciousness.

After-treatment

The immediate after-care of the patient follows the same principles for anyone recovering from a general anaesthetic. A trained nurse is in charge of the recovery room. She must be fully competent in recovery techniques and procedures. She is responsible for the equipment in the recovery room; this includes spare airways, vomit bowls, an Ambu-bag and suction apparatus. The patient is placed in bed in the semiprone (or three-quarters prone) 'recovery' position, and must be carefully observed to ensure that his breathing is not obstructed. The nurse, who must always be close by until the patient is fully conscious, should note—and record if instructed—the patient's colour, pulse rate and volume, the quality and rate of respirations, and, in certain circumstances, blood pressure may be measured.

When the patient regains consciousness he is often restless and may try to get out of bed too soon. The nurse may have to remain with the patient in case he should harm himself. At first the patient may be unsteady when he tries to walk and it is better if two nurses escort him to the post-recovery room. The patient will be confused, not knowing where he is or how he arrived where he is, and will certainly not remember having had ECT. It may be necessary to speak slowly but clearly, in short sentences, using the patient's name when addressing him. The nurse should mention her own name, and that of any other nurse with her. It saves embarrassment and worry to say 'Nurse Smith will give you a cup of tea now', rather than to leave the patient to try to remember Nurse Smith's name, by merely referring to her as 'Nurse'.

For some hours after ECT the patient, particularly if he is elderly, may have difficulty in remembering, and to many patients this is very worrying. Over and over again the patient may approach the nurse and ask the question. 'This is Thursday, isn't it?' or 'Is it supper time yet, nurse?' or 'Is this my bed?'. Time and time again the patient tries to reorientate himself in the ward and, so long as he is not snubbed, he comes to the nurse for confirmation that he remembers correctly. He needs reassurance that this is only a temporary side-effect of the treatment. Careful observation during the confused period is necessary because the patient may enter someone else's bed, use someone else's belongings or wander off through any doors accidentally left open, possibly even out into the road, where he might meet with an accident. Not until the patient has fully recovered his orientation can he be safely left out of sight.

BEHAVIOUR AFTER TREATMENT

The patient's mood and behaviour undergo considerable change during the course of convulsive treatments and these should be carefully observed and reported. Usually, after the first few treatments, the patient becomes more active and his appetite and physical condition improve gradually. It may be, as he becomes more active, he is more able than before to put into practice any suicidal plans he has made during his more retarded period; vigilance should not be relaxed until the mood has ceased to be depressive.

A few patients may show an upward mood swing towards an abnormally elated (manic) state after perhaps three or four ECTs. The next treatment is postponed but may have to be restarted if the patient should revert to his depressive state. If the patient's elation does not subside spontaneously, it may be necessary to discontinue ECT and institute antimanic drug therapy.

Any improvement shown by the patient should be fully utilized by the nursing staff, not only in raising his morale, but in attending to any physical symptoms which may be present, increasing food intake, providing exercise and generally building up his physical condition. Gradually the patient can be helped to form satisfying social relationships with other patients and start to attend group meetings and other ward and outside social activities.

OUT-PATIENT ELECTROCONVULSIVE THERAPY

Electroconvulsive therapy is occasionally given to patients as out-patients. Preparation is the same as for in-patients, and relatives, as well as the patient, are given specific information. It is not usually hospital policy to allow any patient who has had out-patient ECT to leave the treatment centre unaccompanied.

If, for some reason, this cannot be arranged, the nurse in charge of the centre is responsible for ensuring that the patient has fully recovered from his treatment before being allowed to leave. At any event, the patient should use a taxi; he must not be allowed to drive himself home.

Further reading

Carr, V. et al. (1983) Use of ECT for mania in childhood bipolar disorder. *British Journal of Psychiatry 143*, 411.

Fraser, M. (1982) *ECT—a Clinical Guide*. Chichester: J. Wiley.

Kendall, R.E. (1981) The present status of ECT. *British Journal of Psychiatry 139*, 265.

20
Work, Recreational and Diversional Therapy

To a large extent, the patient's progress can be judged by his eagerness and ability to work. Work is an essential therapeutic tool in psychiatry. This fact has long been recognized by psychiatrists and nurses alike, and in all psychiatric hospitals provision is now made for a large variety of occupations, designed to suit different people at various stages of their illness. Although many hospitals employ industrial and occupational therapists and craftsmen to instruct patients and supervise work in the workshops and occupational therapy departments, it is nearly always the nurse's task to ensure the success of the arrangements in operation at the hospital.

Two functions in particular should be carried out by the nurse; first, to ensure that the patient has both knowledge and conviction that the occupation is truly therapeutic and, second, to provide him with sufficient incentive to undertake work. Her ingenuity added to any special talent she may possess are often invaluable in stimulating interest. The nurse co-operates with psychiatrist and occupational therapists in making sure that the right kind of occupation is found for each patient.

WORK AND SOCIETY

It is well to remember the importance of work in normal life. For many people it occupies the greater part of every day. The majority have to work to a regular time-table, arriving in the morning at the correct time and carrying out a full day's work. Most people have to mix with others during their working day. They work side by side with colleagues, co-operate with them on a single job, or compete with them in doing what has to be done. They have to take orders from superiors, submit to criticism, sometimes unjustified, and accept correction. They may have to give orders to others, and criticize or correct the work of those in subordinate positions.

People do all these things in order to earn their living, to take responsibility for their families and to enable them to devote the rest of their time to the enjoyment of their leisure in pursuits such as sports, games, theatre, music and travelling. Many people require special incentives in their work: wages, shorter hours, better working conditions. Many others, however, derive pleasure from work itself. They have chosen their occupations in such a way that work provides them with full satisfaction and few extraneous incentives are needed. Others, again, care little for money incentives, they work best when they know that their efforts are useful and appreciated by others. Whatever the main incentive, the working man is making a very difficult and complex adjustment, not only to the work situation as such, but to his family who benefit by his work, and to society which expects him to work in return for the benefits it bestows upon him.

Work has for long been so highly regarded in Western society, and especially in Protestant countries, that unemployment may cause considerable distress and contribute to the development of mental disorder.

WORK IN MENTAL ILLNESS

For one reason or another, a patient who is mentally ill may find it no longer possible to cope with work. An individual may fail in many ways in adaptation, but society takes the most serious view of the person who is incapable of working.

Very frequently the history of a patient reveals an unsatisfactory adjustment to work. Some patients have a very poor work record, frequent changes of jobs having been made, always for trifling reasons. Some have gradually deteriorated in efficiency and attendance over a period of time. Some have broken down when faced with new responsibilities, others have held jobs too simple and monotonous for their intelligence. Some housewives have neglected their families and simply stayed in bed, refusing to do anything at all. People who behave like this suffer financial loss, lose the esteem of their family and friends, and their prestige vanishes. They are criticized, exhorted and advised; they are made to feel the consequences of their behaviour.

When the patient comes into hospital, he is accepted as being ill, not wicked or lazy. Whether he works or not, he is looked after, cared for and receives attention. He is liked and esteemed, his family is given support. Material incentives are largely removed.

Although there is no need to work in order to earn a living, the patient may be expected to work as part of his treatment. The only reward offered is the intrinsic value of the work itself, the increasing self-esteem and the pleasure his family derives from seeing him recover.

WORK AS AN AID TO TREATMENT

It is essential that the work should be most carefully planned by all those who are trying to help the patient and by the patient himself. Every success on the patient's part must be acknowledged. He must be offered every opportunity to increase his scope. Realistic, lifelike work situations of increasing difficulty are provided and he is encouraged to tackle them. Yet, if he fails, he is protected from the consequences of failure. Even for the patient who remains in hospital, occupation to the best of his ability should be the aim, because without satisfying occupation the patient gets bored and loses his sense of independence.

The first consideration when finding suitable work for a patient is the usefulness of what he is doing. Some patients produce articles for themselves or as presents for their families. This provides a means of retaining contact and a certain degree of responsibility. The nurse should always know for whom the article is designed, and should encourage the patient's endeavours by referring to the pleasure it will give his wife or child to receive the gift. It may be necessary to discuss with the wife how helpful it is for the patient that she should register pleasure when she receives it. If the patient is despondent and feels rejected by his family, the nurse may encourage him to work for her. He may sweep or dust to please the nurse, do odd jobs, or make a cushion if he knows one is needed in his ward. As the patient improves, he may be encouraged to work for the hospital or for others who are not as well as he is. His work should be appreciated and at every step he should be aware of its usefulness.

The patient should be successful in his work. His previous occupation, abilities and ambitions are taken into consideration and work which he can do is provided. Sometimes it would be unwise to allow him to work in line with his usual employment because he might then set himself standards which are too high. However well he does the work while he is ill, it is likely to compare unfavourably with his real work at its best. This comparison would serve only to confirm in his mind the fact that he is a failure.

Normally people set a certain aim and hope to achieve something which is just a little bit difficult. Success leads to rejoicing and the level of aspiration is raised a little higher. Sometimes failure acts as a spur to greater effort. Mentally ill patients sometimes have quite unrealistic aims. Many set themselves such high standards that they are bound to suffer failure. Others are so despondent that they do not try anything which is not well below their known standard of ability. In encouraging the patient to work, he needs help to adjust his standards. The nurse can help him with troublesome details in order to ensure success. Only very gradually should the patient be made responsible for dealing with his own mistakes and encouraged to tackle difficulties. Work should be found for him which he can finish by himself. If the task takes too long, he will become discouraged and perhaps cease trying. The nurse should be entirely clear as to whether to expect perfection from a particular patient or whether to accept inferior workmanship for the sake of seeing an endeavour brought to its proper conclusion.

THE TIME FACTOR IN WORK

For certain patients the hours of working may be an important factor to be considered rather than the work itself. Some who are obsessional may find it almost impossible to arrive anywhere in time and may have to concentrate on time rather than on the work to be done in the occupational therapy department. To psychopaths, regular attendance may provide the main problem, while schizophrenic or hypomanic patients may find it difficult to concentrate for long on one job. The occupation time should be planned for each patient individually. Some patients are responsible for arriving at work unaccompanied and doing so regularly and punctually. Others are accompanied to the occupation department. The number of hours of work varies according to the patient's age and the degree of his illness. In each case it must be decided whether to overlook frequent interruptions and rest pauses, or whether it is important that the patient should keep busy.

GROUP WORKING

Work may contribute considerably towards the socialization of the patient. He may work alone, alongside others or on a project with other patients; he may have to take instructions from others or be made responsible for the work of a group. The domestic work in the ward, for instance, can be so arranged that each patient does his job with a minimum of communication with others, or it may be arranged in such a way that real team spirit prevails. Under such conditions, the patients interact with each other and a leader usually emerges or may be appointed. Valuable observations can be made about the patients' relationships to one another and each has an opportunity, in the shelter of a hospital environment, to try out techniques of interpersonal relationships.

The location of occupational activities will vary with the particular needs of patients and with what accommodation is available in the hospital. Occupational therapy can be effective in the ward setting or in a special building set aside for the purpose. Craft work can give the patient a sense of achievement and satisfaction and can still be used to advantage for certain individuals, but in order to help the patient in his interpersonal relationships, the trend towards patients working in group situations has now become established.

Long-stay patients who are being rehabilitated may require re-education in housework, cooking and shopping. The first two activities may be carried out in groups on the ward, and shopping expeditions may be undertaken in twos and threes at first with a nurse or therapist and, as confidence returns, alone.

Explanations of changes in the monetary and weights and measures systems will require patience and effort on the part of the nurse before patients can be expected to tackle even small purchases alone.

Where patients are expected to be discharged to a group home or hostel, it is much to their benefit to be able to use a telephone and to be able to accomplish minor repairs, all of which could be incorporated into their occupational programme.

It is usually most difficult to find suitable employment for patients who dislike or resent manual work. These may be encouraged to help with typing or in the library. They may help with educational classes for other patients. Sometimes, however, patients from professional fields of work settle down remarkably well to almost any job they are asked to do, provided they can see its usefulness or creativity.

Occupational retraining may be necessary after prolonged stay in a psychiatric hospital or if the patient's illness has left him partially disabled. (Work in rehabilitation programmes is discussed in Chapter 11.)

Whether or not a patient will find suitable employment after discharge depends not only on his mental state but also on the labour market. In times of high unemployment the disabled are particularly vulnerable. The type of occupation which is available to patients while in hospital is also partly determined by the economic state of the country. At one time patients were encouraged to work on the hospital land, as farming was seen as a form of employment most likely to be available to former patients. Later, repetitive industrial work seemed more promising. At present there is a return to horticultural work or work with animals.

RECREATION AND LEISURE

Apart from making sure that all patients spend some time of the day out of doors, leisure time should be so arranged that the patient's background, interests and ability are taken into account. Every effort should be made to encourage the taking up of new interests and hobbies and the trying out, while in hospital, of activities which may be useful after discharge.

It is characteristic of many forms of mental ill-health that the person is unable to plan or enjoy his leisure, and unable also to obtain from it the relaxation he needs. Sometimes he complains that overwork makes it impossible for him to devote any time to leisure activities, and he explains his gradual social isolation to himself and others as being the result of his work. But in reality he may drive himself to work, in order to avoid his social obligations. He may deprive himself of free time, which would expose his inability profitably to occupy his leisure.

Many patients have experienced repeated failure in their attempts to establish social contacts and they have failed miserably to feel at ease in company. They desperately want to be liked, to make friends, to relax and feel happy with others. They envy those who are admired, popular and surrounded by friends. They may often have steeled themselves to attend dances or parties, always hoping to enjoy them, always pretending to have done so, but becoming increasingly discouraged, self-conscious and shy, until finally they feel quite unable ever again to make the effort and shudder at the very thought of attending social gatherings.

Some hospitals have volunteers to help organize the social side of life in hospital, with perhaps the help of a committee of patients. A wide range of recreational activity can be offered, including amateur theatricals, musical appreciation groups, inter-ward or unit debates and keep fit classes.

It is becoming increasingly common for long-stay patients to go on holiday in small groups, usually either early or late in the season when advantageous prices can be arranged for boarding house accommodation. It is usual for a nurse or nurses to accompany these groups, and every opportunity should be taken by the nurse in this situation to take advantage of the more lengthy contact and greater intimacy afforded by the holiday to extend the activities of the patient to the limit of which he is capable.

Social activities

Social activities are well suited to help the patient to gain courage and to be successful where previously he has failed. It is, however, no easy matter to persuade such a patient to make the first attempt, and in no circumstances must a failure be risked. Discos and bingo sessions can be arranged to help to increase patients' confidence. Old-time and country dancing may appeal to some patients.

Activities should be well prepared in advance. The patients need adequate time to get ready. If possible, special clothes should be available and every encouragement given to patients to make themselves as attractive as possible. After the event, the patients will wish to discuss their experiences, and nurses can use the opportunity to emphasize success and to prepare the way for even greater success the next time.

Some patients relax best during informal social activities. They may enjoy party games and may seek new ideas with which to entertain their friends, later gaining prestige and becoming active rather than passive members at a social occasion.

Not all entertainments should allow patients to remain passive. Socials should be organized by the patients in turn. Many patients derive satisfaction from arranging a party, acting as hosts to others, preparing refreshments. Patients may learn to co-operate with each other to make the party a success. Some have the opportunity of taking up leadership, emerging as efficient, capable organizers. Provided the nurses join in, most patients are able to contribute in some way towards the enjoyment of the occasion. Experience of working for a common goal provides a tie among the members of the ward, gives a feeling of unity and solidarity, and helps to raise the morale of the ward.

Radio and television games can be imitated as ward entertainments. These give patients an opportunity for active participation. At all these forms of entertainment the patients mix with those from other wards, make friends, develop social graces and at the same time acquire social skills which may be of considerable use after discharge. However, many patients are left unsatisfied by such forms of entertainment and there should be as many varied kinds of social activities and entertainments as possible in order to give all patients something of interest. No talent should be wasted and every nurse should make it her aim to find something for all of her patients. The slightest hint on the part of a nurse, a word of encouragement, or a creative idea, may encourage some patient to find a new purpose in life. The more unusual the patient's interest, the more he needs a nurse who shares and appreciates it.

Patients value a proper balance between 'going out' and 'staying at home'. Records, radio and television give much pleasure to some patients, but the choice of programme needs careful thought. The young, energetic members of the community need opportunities for developing their interest in 'pop' songs and rhythmic noise, without disturbing the older members or those whose tastes differ. Patients who appreciate serious music or who wish to listen to plays or follow educational programmes should have facilities for doing so.

Where space permits it is helpful to reserve a room, or part of a room, for those who watch television, leaving the rest of the ward free for other activities, or alternatively to reserve one room for those who wish to have peace and quiet while noisy activities go on elsewhere. In some wards patients in their meetings can scrutinize the radio and television programmes for the week and arrive at some agreement about the times when the set shall be switched on. It is always helpful if nurses take an interest in radio, television and record programmes and join the patients in discussions before and after; for very often talking about the previous night's viewing can be the most valuable aspect of television. Often it is possible to develop interests which have been stimulated by television.

Among the activities which take place within the wards are games of cards, chess, draughts, jigsaw puzzles, solving of crossword puzzles or quizzes, singing and the playing of musical instruments. These activities can be particularly valuable in helping to establish personal relationships between nurse and patient or between patients. They offer patients the opportunity of gradual approach to other people. A game of cards can just be watched, the patient tentatively approaching an existing group without too many demands being made on him. He can at first play a silent game with a nurse and very gradually allow himself to get close. Skilled nurses can introduce other patients into the group and gradually withdraw when the patient is able to feel comfortable in a group of patients.

Parties organized by patients in the ward are often greatly enjoyed. Patients' birthdays can be celebrated in some special way, without necessarily having parties for all. It is quite important that the patient whose birthday is celebrated should feel that he is the centre of attention and the cause of the celebration. Birthday cards admired by all, especially chosen food for lunch, first choice in deciding what should be done in the evening, a birthday cake, can be of more value than elaborate parties.

Among activities which can be arranged outside the ward are sports such as swimming and team games, and concert and theatre performances.

Because patients who are mentally disturbed find it difficult to organize their own leisure, much thought should be given to the use of leisure by the nursing staff. However, arrangements should never be made for the patient, without involving him at every stage in planning and in making decisions. Many entertainments are enjoyed much more if one has time to think about them ahead. As soon as possible the patient should have an opportunity of planning, for himself, how he wishes to spend his spare time.

Various types of group activity can be planned within a psychiatric hospital to aid the establishment of contact with others. These can be graded so that, first, there is a spectator level in which the individual contributes little or nothing beyond his physical presence, but is still a participant in that he is sharing an experience, however passively, with others. He is not made to feel socially inadequate or uncomfortable because nothing besides his presence is demanded of him. Beyond this there is a form of group activity in which each individual can perform independently. A contribution is expected from each patient present but no teamwork is necessary; certain forms of occupational therapy fall into this category, as do swimming and painting. On a more demanding level is participation in a group craft project or community singing where non-involvement for a short time will not damage the end-product and reintroduction of the individual's contribution can happen without its being obvious to everyone.

The highest levels of social interaction on a group basis are those which demand continuous co-operation over a shorter or longer period of time. Examples of the former are participation in a team sport such as football, an evening of whist or bridge, or a team activity like formation or country dancing. In the longer term, the presentation of a drama production demands co-operation and involvement over a period of several weeks or months.

Furthermore, there is a variety of people available, some older and some younger, some more dependent than the patient and some more independent, some who can lead and some who wish to be led. The patient can experiment and often changes his friendships as he improves in health and is able to take responsibilities.

The patient is greatly helped in gaining confidence by the fact that he finds himself accepted in spite of his imagined or real shortcomings and in spite of his illness. Even if other patients at first reject him, the staff accept him whole-heartedly and befriend him. Sooner or later, he finds that he is accepted also by other patients. Generally speaking, knowledge of each other's illness and previous life brings patients closer together rather than causing them to reject each other. At first, tentatively, the patient confides in somebody expecting to be ridiculed and despised. If, instead, he finds that an interest is taken in him as a person, he gradually learns to trust others and to respect, in his turn, any confidence reposed in him. The patient's progress may be very slow and he may meet with many setbacks as the social structure of the ward changes.

As patients recover, more unorganized time is needed for private and personal pursuits. Reading newspapers, writing letters, reading books, or quiet chats with other patients may become more important and more valuable than organized activities. There is in some hospitals a serious problem of shortage of space and patients may complain that it is difficult to find a quiet spot and privacy.

Provision of libraries or reading rooms in hospital may be of value, and sometimes patients can find peace in the ward while others are at work or away from the ward at organized entertainments.

Further reading

Morgan, R. & Cheadle, J. (1981) *Psychiatric Rehabilitation*. Surbiton: National Schizophrenia Fellowship.

Willson, M. (1983) *Occupational Therapy in Long Term Care*. Edinburgh: Churchill Livingstone.

21
Psychotherapy

THE PURPOSE OF PSYCHOTHERAPY

Psychotherapy is considered to be the appropriate treatment when the patient's difficulties are thought to be caused by environmental influences of the past and his attitudes determined by factors in his early upbringing and childhood experiences.

Successful psychotherapy helps the patient to develop insight into his difficulties, to become aware of the chain of events which have led to his present condition and to gain some understanding of the motives of his behaviour.

Several forms of psychotherapy can be practised. The choice of specific methods depends on the patient's age, intelligence and degree of illness, and also on the psychiatrist's own training and attitude.

All psychotherapy is based on similar fundamental principles. In psychotherapy a relationship develops between therapist and patient, a relationship which helps the patient to resolve previously unrecognized conflicts and to achieve a better adaptation to stresses in life.

The process of psychotherapy is one in which the therapist listens with interest and attention to all the patient says and also notices the things the patient omits to say. The therapist's attitude, and his words, convey that it is safe for the patient, not only to talk, but also to allow his feelings free rein.

The patient needs to understand and accept that psychological difficulties are as real as physical ones. He must recognize them to be just as serious and must feel able to accept that, just like physical disorders, they require medical assistance to resolve them.

The patient, having gained confidence in the psychiatrist and established rapport in a preliminary interview, feels able to speak freely of anything that comes into his mind without fear of criticism or ridicule.

All psychotherapy consists of communication between the therapist and the patient. In the first few interviews the psychiatrist tends to be active in encouraging the patient to speak. He needs a detailed history, if necessary, and with the patient's permission, supplemented by information from relatives. During these early interviews the psychiatrist can gain a certain amount of understanding of the patient's problems. He cannot, at this stage, expect the patient to have developed much understanding, but on the basis of his own understanding, the further course of action is planned.

The psychiatrist may decide on a course of individual long-term psychotherapy or he may decide to offer the patient supportive psychotherapy or behavioural psychotherapy.

Individual long-term psychotherapy consists of many regular interviews—possibly once weekly lasting 50 minutes for several months or perhaps even years. The broad aims of such therapy are a fundamental restructuring of the patient's personality and symptom relief. The more disabling the patient's internal pressures, the more he may feel in need of such complete reappraisal of his life. Individual long-term psychotherapy is anxiety producing and very slow to show obvious results. It is more likely to be successful if the patient's intelligence is relatively high. Because it is very time consuming, for both the psychiatrist and the patient, it is a very expensive form of treatment. Irrespective of whether the patient bears the cost himself or whether the treatment is carried out under the National Health Service, the decision to embark on such a long-term commitment has to be reached after very careful consideration of all the factors involved.

Individual long-term psychotherapy may adhere to psychoanalytic principles or follow the 'newer psychotherapies', of which there has been a dramatic development in recent years; they make use of concepts from social learning and humanist theories.

Supportive psychotherapy is a form of treatment in which the aim is the relief of symptoms and the reduction of stress. It is assumed that the healthy part of the patient's personality can reassert itself when the current crisis is resolved. Supportive psychotherapy does not aim at uncovering the patient's unconscious conflicts. On the contrary, it aims at achieving better developed defence mechanisms and greater self-confidence.

Supportive psychotherapy focuses on the symptoms of which the patient complains and on the problems which beset him at the time of treatment. It does not necessarily require that the patient should gain insight into the causal connection between past experiences and present difficulties. *Behavioural psychotherapy*, like supportive psychotherapy, is specifically concerned with the removal of disabling symptoms, but uses a behavioural approach to help the patient to learn more accept-able responses to a variety of situations.

The decision about the form which psychotherapy is to take depends to a certain extent on the patient's own hopes and aims. It is only possible to treat a patient by psychotherapy if the patient himself makes that decision. Psychotherapy is not a form of treatment which the doctor actively administers and to which the patient passively submits. The patient in fact does all the active work of talking, thinking, reformulating and reapp-raising. The extent to which he is prepared to do so must determine the treatment objectives. Ultimately the patient must find his own solution and make his own decisions, though he does so with the help of the psychiatrist. It is important to know what kind of life the patient imagines for himself, with what kind of adaptation he would be satisfied, what kind of person he wants to be.

TECHNIQUES OF PSYCHOTHERAPY

The techniques of psychotherapy are based on the methods first developed by Freud, but a number of modifications have taken place.

Psychoanalysis, the technique used by Freud himself, was based on free association. The sessions may take place several times per week, each lasting approximately 50 minutes. It is an individual therapy and relatives are not used, even initially to supplement data obtained. Psychoanalysis may last several years and is too costly to be available under the National Health Service as a rule. The analyst gives no instructions whatever beyond the encouragement to say whatever comes to mind, however trivial or silly it may appear to the patient. As the latter continues to talk to the doctor he remembers more and more details of his past life, details of which he himself has been totally unaware. Each story brings to mind another one. Sometimes the patient finds it difficult to understand why a particular event has been recalled and how various ideas are connected.

Some events are recalled with considerable show of emotion which is often surprising to the patient. This emotional release, termed 'catharsis', is often experienced as a therapeutic event. As the story unfolds the doctor becomes aware of some of the mechanisms which were at work in making the patient the sort of person he is. He can observe what kind of statements are accompanied by deep emotion, such as grief or anger. He recognizes the patient's hostility to some of the people about whom he speaks, and his love for others. He picks out from the mass of recollections those facts which appear to have had a profound effect on the patient's subsequent development and begins to understand the patient's illness. It is not enough, though, that the doctor should understand the patient's illness, the patient himself must understand it.

Psychoanalysts will do nothing to speed up the process of developing insight. They wait patiently until the patient sees the connections between his present attitudes and his past experiences. Other psychiatrists make tentative interpretations to the patient which the latter may be able to accept as true. He may reject most vigorously interpretations which are nevertheless correct, only later to recognize their truth. He may accept the doctor's explanation but not really feel that he understands. Sometimes the patient's reactions show quite clearly that the doctor has been on the wrong track. Once the patient has begun to understand the reasons for his attitudes and his behaviour he may be able to attempt to modify them, and improvement may begin.

Psychiatrists who are not Freudian analysts tend to be more active in offering interpretations and in guiding patients towards discussion of topics which seem significant.

Hypnosis is used by some psychiatrists to assist the patient's recall of dramatic events or to make suggestions to the patient. It is also of value for a patient with aphonia as a conversion symptom. It may only be under hypnosis that the patient can converse with the therapist.

If the patient feels he would like to be able to talk but finds it hard to overcome his own resistance, drugs are at times used.

Intravenous administration of drugs such as diazepam may often facilitate communication by the patient. Recall of painful events is often accompanied by extremely violent emotional experiences which the patient might find hard to tolerate without the help of drugs. This method of bringing into consciousness emotional difficulties which have been repressed is called 'drug-assisted abreaction'.

The root of the patient's trouble may be looked for in the very earliest childhood experiences, in the circumstances of birth, methods of feeding, weaning in babyhood, toilet training, in parental attitudes to the patient as an infant, and the small child's attitude to his siblings.

During individual long-term psychotherapy the patient may be able to recall feelings of these earliest periods of life. There are times when the patient not only remembers, but effectively re-lives these early experiences. His behaviour 'regresses' to a very early stage of development.

The psychiatrist's passive role in psychotherapy is often imperfectly understood. In the early stages of treatment patients may feel disappointed because the psychiatrist does not make positive suggestions or give positive advice. Most psychiatrists refrain from giving any advice, because such action would take away from the patient responsibility for his behaviour. There are some patients, however, for whom a more positive approach appears indicated. Suggestion and reassurance may then play a part in psychotherapy. The psychiatrist's manner, impressiveness and air of competence may play a part in suggesting that the patient is in good hands and the psychiatrist's utterances can help to suggest that the patient is capable of constructive behaviour and of finding a solution to his problems. Reassurance may deal with specific fears, for example a fear that the patient is becoming insane or that his symptoms are unique and beyond the doctor's understanding.

Occasionally positive, didactic teaching about matters of health, for example about the physiological concomitants of anxiety, may accompany psychotherapy.

During psychotherapy, whatever form it may take, there are periods of intense anxiety, when the patient finds it difficult to persevere with treatment. He is helped, during such phases, by the relationship he has formed with the psychiatrist. This relationship is partly determined by the psychiatrist's personality. Partly it is the kind of relationship which the patient, in the past, had with his parents, or with other significant people. The patient is said to have a 'transference' relationship with his psychiatrist. All the elements of love and hate of earlier relationships are repeated as 'positive or negative transference' for the psychiatrist. In his turn the psychiatrist often responds with feelings of resentment to hostility or with feelings of pleasure when the patient seems to be progressing. The psychiatrist's response to the patient is described as 'counter transference'.

Transference relationships are an important aid to the understanding of the patient's feelings and an important prop for the patient in turbulent periods of treatment.

Transference situations have to be resolved, however, before the patient can give up his dependence on the psychiatrist and decide to terminate treatment.

Most commonly, patients receive psychotherapy either in out-patient clinics or privately. As psychotherapy progresses the patient's attitudes gradually change. New relationships develop, old ones undergo considerable modifications. New problems arise as the patient attempts to deal with situations which he has previously found difficult. As new problems arise the patient brings these to the psychiatrist and they form the starting point in the treatment session.

Only rarely does the patient require in-patient treatment during psychotherapy. The reason for admission to hospital may be severe disturbances caused by the treatment, and the patient's relatives may find it impossible to give him the support he requires. Consequently patients who receive psychotherapy in hospital may be among those who are most difficult to nurse.

THE NURSE'S ROLE IN PSYCHOTHERAPY

Supportive psychotherapy

The nurse fulfils various functions depending on the technique employed and on her understanding of the fundamental principles involved. Some psychiatrists are more willing than others to use nursing staff in psychotherapy. If the patient is receiving supportive psychotherapy, the nurse's function is to manipulate the environment in such a way that the patient meets with fewer difficulties than he would outside the hospital. She can reduce the demands made upon him and exert her influence in such a manner that he experiences his surroundings as being friendly, accepting and non-critical. In some instances, without modifying her behaviour in any way and without even a clear understanding of what is taking place, the nurse may be used by the patient to fulfil some of his needs. A patient who is insecure and dependent may lean on a forceful, confident nurse, deriving support and security. A patient who requires someone who is dependent on him may satisfy his need to be protective by trying to help a new nurse.

During the course of behavioural psychotherapy the nurse acts as a suitable person on whom to practice newly acquired social skills. She can serve as a target for the patient's emotions and, because she remains unaffected and detached, can help him to learn control over the expression of his feelings. With more understanding and greater skill the nurse can exploit her special relationship with the patient. She can do this either by her endeavour to minimize tension between therapeutic sessions, thus enabling the patient to use the interviews with the psychiatrist to better advantage, or in some instances she can help to extend the therapeutic sessions. The patient can talk to the nurse, using her to sort out some of his complicated thoughts, ideas and feelings, so making it easier for him to select the most important facts for the therapeutic interview with the doctor.

In some forms of psychotherapy the nurse assumes the role of a significant figure in the patient's life, and enables him to act out in the hospital setting the emotional responses usually triggered off by his own environment.

Psychotherapy always produces changes in the patient's attitude to other people. Different patients' reactions to each other, the way in which groups form and break up, the emergence of friendships and the development of love and hate reactions among patients are always significant as an indication of progress and as a stimulus to therapy. The nurse is in the best position to observe the ward as a whole, to assess the forces of which the ward group is composed, and to exert some influence on the climate of the ward in order to create a therapeutic community.

Role therapy

Interpersonal relationships are of the utmost importance in all forms of psychotherapy. In supportive psychotherapy the patient casts the nurse into various roles, depending on his own previous relationships to other people. Role therapy is a form of treatment in which the nurses, under the guidance of the psychiatrist, deliberately try to assume a particular role relationship towards the patient.

One of the nurses, for example, may deliberately behave towards the patient in the manner in which his father may have behaved and a re-enactment of the patient's attitude and behaviour towards the father is thus deliberately provoked. In this form of treatment it may be necessary to pool a great deal of information about the patient in order to plan the part which the doctor wishes one of the nurses to play. From time to time, discussion between the members of the staff must take place.

If the patient finds it difficult to explain to the psychiatrist where his problems lie, if he lacks the intelligence or fluency to verbalize his difficulties, this method of treatment is often successful in recreating the problems before the doctor's very eyes. The psychiatrist need not rely on the patient's memory of past events, he can use current troubles as they arise to help the patient. As a result of the emotionally charged relationship which the patient develops towards the nurse concerned, the ward routine and hospital life produce the kind of reaction which may have led to the patient's admission. While, normally, psychiatric hospital treatment owes its success to the avoidance of such scenes, in this form of therapy the repetition is deliberately created.

The patient can be helped in one of two ways. Attitudes and the approach of the nurses can help the patient to develop more adequate methods of solving his difficulties or, alternatively, the psychiatrist, who is not in any way involved, utilizes the patient's trust in him to support him during each difficult phase. The doctor himself may adopt a role which is opposite to that adopted by the nurse and as a result of this he is felt to be on the patient's side. The patient feels able to give free rein to his feelings, to discuss and modify his attitudes, and develop new ways of dealing with old problems, because he has the support of the doctor. The nurse, in a similar way to the patient's relatives before, partly causes the patient's disturbed behaviour and at the same time must find some method of dealing with each disturbance as it arises. The nurse has the advantage of previous experience and of relative emotional detachment. In spite of this she may find it difficult to maintain the one-sided relationship which is required in the situation, the patient being deeply attached or violently antagonistic to her, while she remains emotionally detached. She must show that she is affected by the patient's emotional attitude without, in fact, becoming emotionally so involved that she loses the ability to make sound judgements.

In order to maintain this relationship the nurse must have the help of her colleagues with whom she must frequently discuss the patient and her own attitude to him. Her colleagues may be able to point out any gestures or actions which may have indicated impatience or anger without her being aware of it. Discussion with her colleagues may also prevent undue friction among the nurses over the treatment of the patient. Quite frequently a patient who feels angry with one of the nurses ingratiates himself with another and tries to engage one nurse as an ally against another.

It may be most valuable to create the special role of an ally. Often the psychiatrist assumes this role in order to help the patient in his relationship with the nurse. It should be clearly understood by all concerned that somebody must accept the part of always being on the patient's side. But the situation should be planned by the nurse and the psychiatrist, not created and exploited by the patient. If the latter succeeds in creating mistrust and mutual hostility among the nurses, he will become frightened, and lose confidence in the hospital's power to help.

Individual long-term psychotherapy

The nurse's function if the patient is undergoing individual long-term psychotherapy is similar in many ways. There is no need to adopt any particular role, and no need to fear that a wrong approach could harm the patient. It is part of any form of individual long-term psychotherapy that the patient is prepared to tell the therapist all his thoughts, which of course include any thoughts he may have about the nurses. It follows that the therapist is very well informed about the nurses' attitudes, their behaviour and the effect they have on the patient.

The therapist in turn has agreed to listen to the patient's comments, and to regard as confidential anything he may hear. He cannot divulge very much information to the nurses and may only very indirectly influence their attitudes to the patient.

This situation could be exceptionally difficult for nurses, who may feel that the patient is carrying tales to the doctor and that they are being criticized. Sometimes the patient's version of any incident which may have occurred in the ward may appear exaggerated to the nurse and she may feel hurt and insulted if she thinks that the patient's story is believed and that she is not even given a chance to explain.

Nurses should try to understand that this one-sided relationship is fundamental to psychotherapy.

If the patient is treated as an out-patient, he may, for instance, complain that his wife rejects him. This may not be a true statement of fact. The wife may not really reject him at all and may tell about the husband's coldness to her with as much conviction as the husband showed in his version. It does not really matter who is right. If the husband is the patient, his way of experiencing the situation is all-important. The wife, too, may need help and usually the social worker will offer it to her.

If the patient is an in-patient, the relationship to the nurse is parallel to the one described. It does not matter in the least whether the patient's story is true, all that matters is how it appears to the patient. Nurses may require some help in the same way as the patient's relatives, but usually they can give each other the necessary support.

During long-term psychotherapy the patient may pass through a series of extremely difficult phases. He may become acutely depressed, and require careful supervision if there is any risk of suicide. In this case the psychiatrist usually warns the nurses, although this is contrary to the usual practice in psychotherapy.

Periods of excitement, of aggressive behaviour, of violent emotional outbursts, are more difficult to predict and the nurses must manage to the best of their ability to help the patient through the difficult phase. Often these disturbances follow significant interviews, or take place when a particularly painful interview is approaching.

The patient dreams more vividly as he acquires practice in relating his dreams, and often a disturbed night is followed by a day of irritability and moodiness. Sometimes it appears as if treatment is making the patient worse. This is deceptive. Often real improvement follows when the patient has successfully worked through a particularly painful period of his life. At times the patient himself feels despondent about his treatment and this may reinforce the nurses' belief that psychotherapy is not helping very much.

At certain phases of treatment the patient shows a marked resistance to therapy. He forgets his appointments, finds excuses for not attending and is apt to belittle the effect of treatment in his conversation with the nurses. The latter should not fail to understand that the patient's resistance is an indication that a crucial point in treatment is being reached. Discontinuation of treatment may well occur if they reinforce the patient's sceptical attitude.

GROUP THERAPY

Group therapy is a form of psychotherapy which is time saving, because many problems common to several patients can be cleared up jointly. The therapist is able to give more time to the group of patients than he could separately to each individual.

Many patients are helped by group therapy in a more specific way. Diffidence is gradually overcome by listening to other patients discussing their difficulties, and it is possible slowly to gain the courage necessary to speak about personal problems. Listening to others makes the patient realize that he is not alone in his troubles, and that his difficulties are not unique. Often the patient believes that he would be rejected if more were known about his personality. To hear others relate similar facts about themselves without losing sympathy or acceptance may be beneficial.

It is often easier for an individual to understand the mechanism underlying other people's neurotic symptoms than to gain insight into the causation of his own behaviour. A growing awareness of his own motivation may be possible for him as a member of a group.

Group therapy may take place in a day unit, or may form part of the treatment programme during in-patient therapy.

Group psychotherapy has many of the characteristic features of individual psychotherapy. As a form of intensive psychotherapy, a group of 6 to 8 members usually meets regularly with the therapist whose attitude to the group as a whole corresponds to that of the therapist in individual treatment. Therapeutic groups of this nature are usually 'closed' groups, i.e. all patients start and terminate treatment simultaneously. No new members are admitted. It is difficult for such groups to deal with observers, and consequently nurses are not usually present during therapeutic sessions.

Conflicts with which the group deals are related to group membership as well as to the specific problems of individual members. Patients spend only a short period of their day in group sessions. Any anxiety which remains unresolved is taken back to the ward group as a whole and affects the total management of the ward.

Group therapy can also follow the pattern of supportive psychotherapy. Groups of patients meet regularly, discussing, in the first instance, any topic of current interest to the ward. Such groups are usually 'open' groups. New patients can be invited to join and as patients recover they leave the group. In group therapy of this kind one staff member assumes the role of convener of the group. Often this is a psychiatrist but, increasingly, nurses are developing skills in the management of such therapeutic groups.

In group therapy of this kind it is possible and desirable to have observers, who are able to note and report the various forces which act in the group. The presence of an observer is of course one of the factors which influence what happens.

In therapeutic groups of this kind the events of the ward often form the official part of the agenda. The way patients organize their time, the manner in which they carry out their responsibility, the frustrations they experience in relation to the hospital staff are profitable topics for discussion. They constitute common business and, therefore, offer an opportunity to all to contribute to the discussion. The way patients use this opportunity reflects their personal problems and attitudes.

Some patients find it very difficult to speak, and it is the business of the other members of the group to explore the reasons for the difficulty and to help the patient to deal with it. Patients who monopolize the floor during a meeting similarly give others the opportunity to understand their need to dominate and to deal with the situation.

There are often long silences during group meetings, when the leader waits for tensions to become manifest or for topics of high priority to emerge. Facile chatter about trivialities often occurs when some important business threatens to be too painful to discuss. Chatter is pleasant for the group members. Silence is difficult to tolerate; yet silence can be a very important part of treatment. During a period of silence members can examine their feelings towards each other and towards the therapist. They become aware of hostility and tensions or of depressive moods or thoughtful reflection. During a period of silence people often watch each other and detect signs of anxiety by the way people fidget or pass around cigarettes, or tap their feet, or hide their faces. During a period of silence they can also sometimes detect genuine interest or concern or sympathy in the faces of other patients or of staff members. Knowing when and how to break a silence is very difficult. If it has gone on too long it becomes very difficult to break but if the leader is anxious about silence he may deprive some members of the group of valuable experience.

In many group meetings patients express criticism of the staff.

This is to be encouraged for a number of reasons. Patients need a safe outlet for their hostile feelings. At some stage staff are certain to become targets of such feelings. Group meetings should provide a safe forum for discussion and in this way help the patient to cope. The patient's feelings may in the course of such discussion become more obvious to the staff and to other patients, who as a result of this may understand the problem better and become more able to help.

The patients may gain insight into their own problems as a result of the response they obtain from members of the group.

Of course it is always possible that good grounds exist for patients' complaints about the staff. Their complaints should not automatically be regarded as evidence of displaced feeling.

There is a danger that a split may occur between patients and staff if the staff react defensively to the patients' complaints. To be effective, groups need to develop a certain cohesion and identity. If staff members predominate in number or in articulateness, two groups tend to form instead of one, a staff and a patient group, with rivalry and competition instead of co-operative effort.

During group meetings a certain amount of clarification takes place of the patients' problems. By making observations about the patients' behaviour, rewording certain statements, explaining how the problem appears to the onlooker and tentatively interpreting what it might mean, patients begin to gain a new level of understanding of their own and other patients' difficulties. One of the advantages of group therapy lies in the fact that patients can exert therapeutic influences on each other. This will be discussed more fully in Chapter 25.

FAMILY THERAPY

Family therapy is a form of group therapy in which not only patients and staff, but also the patient's family, participate. Sometimes, in hospital, multiple family therapy is practised, i.e. several patients and their families meet and discuss problems which they have in common. This form of treatment has been found especially beneficial in work with children and young people. Sometimes, particularly in the treatment of patients with marital problems, family therapy is carried out in a group comprising the patient, many of the relatives who play a significant role in the patient's life, the doctor, nurses, social worker and any other professional person concerned with helping the patient. This approach is particularly useful in a day unit, or, occasionally, in the treatment of the patient in his own home. The treatment team may find it useful, initially, to see the patient in his own surroundings, in the company of the people most concerned with his illness and with his treatment, if he is not admitted to hospital. To see the patient and his family together allows the staff to observe the interactions between the patient and others, and often makes it easier to understand the psychodynamics of the illness.

The value of family therapy lies in the fact that interactions are collectively explored, that all the significant people are actively involved in the treatment process, and that not only the patient's difficulties, but also those of the people who have to cope with the patient, receive attention.

The fact that several staff members may participate means, very often, that each identifies with a different family member and that the complexity of the problems is more clearly appreciated. Relatives may feel better able to give constructive assistance when they sense that they have the sympathy of at least one member of staff. When the whole family participates in group therapy it is sometimes difficult to think specifically of the patient as the one who receives treatment. The whole family may become the client or different family members may take on the patient role in turn.

All psychotherapy creates tensions and strains relationships. In family therapy the patient cannot escape confrontation with his relatives by talking privately about them to a sympathetic listener. The intense feeling with which family problems are publicly discussed can lead to much greater understanding within the family. It would be difficult for any one therapist to be continuously aware of the complicated communication patterns which emerge during family therapy. To have several observers, able, after the group meeting, to compare impressions and discuss interpretations may be a great advantage in this form of treatment.

Further reading

Bloch, S. (1979) *An Introduction to the Psychotherapies*. Oxford: Oxford University Press.

22
Behaviour Therapy

Maladaptive behaviour is generally recognized to have its origin earlier in life. Psychotherapy is based on the assumption that *insight* into connections between earlier experience and current difficulties is therapeutic. It is sometimes possible to bring about changes in behaviour more easily by assuming that the maladaptive behaviour is learned and that new and better adaptive behaviour can also be *learned*. The aim is to change the presenting behaviour without delving into the patient's past.

Those who are mentally ill have an unacceptable amount of awkward behaviour in their dealings with others and with their environment. Since the awkward behaviour generates further anxiety for the emotionally disturbed person, it may well bring about further non-acceptance, creating a vicious circle. Under the broad heading of behaviour therapy (also known as behavioural psychotherapy or the behavioural approach), a variety of techniques has been developed to extinguish the troublesome behaviour and establish new and acceptable modes of interaction with others. All behaviour therapy methods are based on knowledge derived from the psychology of learning, one central feature being 'reinforcement'. Behaviour is influenced by the changes that the behaviour produces in the environment: the consequence. When a favourable consequence arises as a result of a specific behaviour, this is positive reinforcement, which increases the chance of this behaviour being repeated. We use this aspect of learning theory in the socialization processes applied to bringing up children, in that they learn how to behave either because they receive some tangible rewards, e.g. sweets when successful, or because mother's approval and love act as a reward for certain forms of behaviour, but are withheld for other forms of behaviour.

Some of the terms used in behaviour therapy require explanation. It might be said that behavioural methods of treatment originate with the classical form of conditioning used by Pavlov when he noted that dogs salivated when food was

273

presented to them—unconditioned response. He found that when a bell was rung at the same moment as the presentation of food, only one response, salivation, was elicited. It was then discovered that if the stimuli were paired often enough, eventually only one (the weaker, or conditioned stimulus) would produce salivation in his dogs. This he called the conditioned response. Another term used for this pattern of behaviour is 'classical conditioning', as distinct from operant conditioning, the kind most commonly used in behaviour therapy. When the word operant is used in this context, it implies that every response to a stimulus, or every unit of behaviour, will operate on the environment in some way, producing a consequence. Operant responses can be defined and measured perhaps by frequency, intensity or duration. Operant conditioning uses positive reinforcement (favourable consequence) to increase desirable behaviour or decrease unwanted behaviour.

BEHAVIOURAL ASSESSMENT

Before any behaviour therapy technique is considered, a comprehensive assessment of the patient's problem(s) is carried out. Part of the assessment process includes an initial interview aimed at uncovering details of the problem behaviour, with special attention focused on how the patient feels about it. For example, if the patient has a fear of crowds, the circumstances in which anxiety is experienced are elicited. Does the patient feel anxious once he has entered the crowded supermarket or (as is more usual) do symptoms arise at the prospect of going into the shop? (At this point a hierarchical list may be drawn up for the patient, grading anxiety-arousing situations from the least to the most stressful.) Emotions and thoughts associated with the feared situations are also noted; fear of fainting and autonomic symptoms such as palpitations are commonly reported. The person's response to the stressful situation is determined. For example, does he leave before symptoms subside?

The patient's motivation to change his behaviour is also assessed. Social and material rewards (reinforcers) are discussed. They are important if behaviour is to be modified or new patterns are to be established and improvement maintained.

Goals of a realistic nature are jointly negotiated, followed by consideration of the possible methods of treatment best suited to the patient's particular problem. When a particular technique is decided upon, a full explanation of the aims of the programme and methods to be used must be given to the patient. A written contract outlining what the patient has to do for himself, such as regular practice (homework), may be signed. If the patient cannot give valid consent to the programme, his relatives should be contacted. This is in accordance with the recommendations of a working party's recently published ethical guidelines on behaviour modification. Assessment may also be carried out by the use of rating scales and questionnaires.

In order to be able to evaluate progress, certain observations and measurements (baselines) are usually recorded before the agreed programme is introduced; they give an indication of the extent of the problem. Using the example of a long-stay patient with frequent episodes of screaming loudly while rushing up and down the corridor, baselines would include a recording of the number of times the screaming occurs, the time of day and the number of staff on duty when it happens. Also included in the assessment process for this patient might be the behaviour of the staff towards the patient's screaming, because the staff's response may be reinforcing his behaviour.

As preparation before the programme begins, it may be necessary for the patient with a phobia to learn techniques of self-relaxation. The ability to relax is part of the behavioural technique of systematic desensitization.

There is now a wide variety of techniques available to the behaviour therapist. Only a few of the more commonly used will be briefly described.

OPERANT CONDITIONING

This form of treatment can be used to decrease behaviour which the patient himself complains of, such as stammering or nervous tics. For example, in the case of a tic where it has been established that there is no disease of the brain which might cause this difficulty, baselines would be required to establish the frequency and the circumstances under which the behaviour occurs. In the case of gross blinking, which is a common manifestation of nervous tic, the observer could use a mechanical counter to record the number of responses per minute under different circumstances. An alarm clock could then be set for as short a time as the tic is not normally emitted, and when the bell rings, the patient is immediately reinforced for not exhibiting undesired behaviour. The time intervals are progressively increased in treatment sessions, and gradually extinction of the unwanted behaviour should occur.

Systematic desensitization

The basis of this exposure technique is the deduction that anxiety aroused by a specific situation can be suppressed by the simultaneous evocation of the antagonistic response. Wolpe called this reciprocal inhibition, and used relaxation techniques to bring about this response. It is also known as counter-conditioning; the relaxation counters (inhibits) the anxiety. The patient is subjected to a graduated brief exposure to the feared object or situation, e.g. spiders or birds, while in a relaxed state. Progress up the hierarchical ladder can be in imagination, supplemented by audiovisual aids, or in real life (*in vivo*) if practicable. The procedure used in the case of a patient with a spider phobia is gradual exposure from tiny hairless to large-bodied spiders with long legs. The setting for the treatment session would be carefully arranged to be as relaxing as possible, with a comfortable chair and perhaps a favourite piece of music being placed. The anxiety-provoking stimulus (mildest first) would then be introduced into conversation and the level of anxiety produced in the patient noted. The patient may be asked to imagine the feared or avoided situation. When the patient can talk comfortably about the first item in this particular hierarchy of tension-producing situations, the next would be introduced. The therapist may handle the feared object and encourage the patient to do the same. This is referred to as passive and participant modelling. At each session it might be necessary to regress one or two steps initially, but eventually the patient, because of the relaxed and rewarding atmosphere, will be able to withstand the idea, and perhaps the sight, of even the most frightening article on the pre-arranged list.

Another technique in the spectrum involving exposure is known as *flooding*, i.e. prolonged exposure to the situation causing anxiety. For example, the agoraphobic patient, accompanied by the therapist, must remain in a crowded supermarket for an hour or so until the anxiety lessens—the longer the exposure the better. Recent research has shown that for flooding to be maximally effective the patient must practise the required behaviour regularly. Family co-operation may be required to help the patient during practice sessions.

Patients suffering from obsessive–compulsive rituals may also be helped by sustained contact *in vivo* with the anxiety-arousing situations. The aim is for the patient to remain 'contaminated' with the object until he becomes less anxious. The nurse must gently but firmly dissuade him from performing his usual elaborate ritual, involving perhaps the use of disinfectant and the rinsing of his hands innumerable times (i.e. 'response prevention'). If the patient were allowed to do so, it would mean termination of the exposure. Extensive supervision is not always required; to tell the patient he must desist from performing his ritual is often enough. Exposure to the cue (e.g. a soiled towel) and prevention of the ritual must continue for at least an hour. Supplementary modelling by the therapist may be useful. He touches the soiled towel and eats something with his hands immediately afterwards; the patient is then expected to do likewise. If sessions are held on an out-patient basis, practice sessions at home are recommended.

Less successful is the technique of *thought-stopping*, used for patients with obsessional thoughts. The patient is taught to interrupt an obsessional thought, at first by the therapist shouting **stop**, and making a loud noise. Later the patient interrupts his own thought by saying **stop** to himself.

Self-instructional training—a form of cognitive behaviour therapy—also focuses on the patient's thoughts, particularly on the way faulty or negative thinking can influence feelings and behaviour. For example, the cognitive therapist may teach the patient who is facing up to a stressful situation to give himself positive instructions designed to displace self-defeating negative thoughts ('I may feel like fainting but I know I won't').

Another cognitive approach assumes it is the patient's irrational beliefs which cause him to misinterpret events around him. The cognitive therapist tries to persuade the patient to alter his pessimistic way of looking at the world and to adopt more productive, less self-denigratory beliefs and attitudes. A simple example may be to encourage the patient to concentrate less on how dull and boring a conversationalist he thinks he is and to believe he will improve; in social situations, to pay more attention to what his companion is saying and less to his own 'performance'.

A recent controlled trial in the community found cognitive therapy to be an effective treatment for depression when used in combination with conventional drug therapy. When used for this disorder, one of the treatment goals is to help the patient to learn to interpret his experiences in a more positive, less pessimistic way than he is in the habit of doing.

Social skills training

A number of recent studies testify to the effectiveness of this form of behaviour therapy, and a number of manuals are available to guide the novice through the various approaches used.

Social skills training is based on the principle that social (like psychomotor), skills are learned and can be taught *de novo*, for example to the mentally handicapped person, or re-taught when lost as a result, for example, of social withdrawal on the part of the long-stay patient.

A social skills programme may be used in conjunction with other conditioning techniques for the agoraphobic patient who has become uncertain about how to behave in social situations that have been avoided for so long.

The long-stay patient may, in tandem with or after a token economy programme, require to relearn social skills as part of a rehabilitation programme before discharge. A careful assessment of the patient's present level of social behaviour is made. Rating scales compiled over a period may reveal certain social skills deficits, including failure to initiate, sustain, or end a conversation, or show the lack of effective use of non-verbal communication skills during social interactions.

Most social skills treatment packages include assertion training. This concentrates on encouraging the patient to assert himself politely but firmly in situations which provoke maladaptive anxiety responses. The classical interaction commonly practised in social skills training programmes is the assertiveness required when returning faulty goods to a shop; saying no, without necessarily apologizing, rather than meekly acquiescing to an unreasonable request is another example of an area of difficulty for many unassertive patients. Social skills training may be carried out on a one-to-one basis for very specific individual problems, but more commonly it takes place in groups—they provide a ready-made social situation. Goals, set after discussion with the patient, are graded. For example, the first few sessions may deal simply with greetings and introductions; later ones may progress to the more complex goal of knowing how to conduct oneself at a job interview.

A variety of techniques is used during social skills training sessions. These include, for example, modelling: a topic is selected, such as the use of eye contact during a conversation, and the therapist and co-therapist begin by role playing a situation. It is then the turn of the group participants, split up into pairs in order to practise this exercise. Video recording apparatus may be used in these sessions to demonstrate faults in performance. Feedback by the therapist is an important ingredient of the programme and it should include praise whenever possible, and constructive, rather than critical, comments. The corrected behaviour is then practised. To promote generalization, the nurse should ensure that the patient is given every opportunity to try out his newly acquired social skills and also to discuss the degree of anxiety experienced when doing so.

Token economy

Operant conditioning theories are sometimes used for a patient in the long-stay ward to help improve his quality of life and rehabilitate him, if possible, for life outside hospital, but at least towards more independence from the nursing staff. A token economy is an example of a system which provides a motivating environment for the long-stay patient, based on operant reinforcement theory.

The token programme may be applied on a ward-wide basis, or only a small group of patients may take part. Patients showing the typically negative symptoms of chronic schizophrenia, such as lack of initiative, social withdrawal and lack of social skills, and also dependence on the nursing staff for carrying out everyday living skills, have been shown to benefit from this form of behaviour therapy. It aims to foster spontaneity and independence. 'Tokens' are given contingent on the occurrence of specified desirable behaviour; they may also be used to decrease undesirable behaviour. A full explanation of the programme is given to the patient, and his consent is obtained. Tokens must be given immediately, or as soon as possible, after the task is completed; later the patient may exchange the tokens for so-called 'back-up reinforcers', such as luxuries from the ward or hospital shop, or for the pleasure of staying in bed on a Sunday morning instead of having to get up for breakfast. Relatives may have to be asked not to give the patient reinforcers on a non-contingent basis—staff must also agree to this condition otherwise the programme will fail.

In the area of self-care, for example, the patient may receive tokens for carrying out everyday activities like getting up in good time for breakfast, making his own bed, selecting his clothes, dressing and attending to his personal hygiene. Whenever an occasion warrants tokens, the nurse must pair them with verbal praise; eventually tokens will be phased out, first by offering intermittent reinforcers, later by leaving only social reinforcement, a more natural reward for desirable behaviour. Token economy programmes have been abandoned in many hospitals (some countries have declared their use illegal). Their replacement by methods which include systematic instruction by the nurse, e.g. making use of verbal and non-verbal prompts which help to initiate behaviour, and social reinforcement, have in themselves been found to be enough to bring about desirable behaviour patterns. The 'adoption' by a nurse of a long-stay patient with whom she is particularly concerned may, where staffing levels permit, prove successful in changing a patient's behaviour.

Token economies may still be favoured in hospitals where staffing levels are low. However, it has been found that unless nursing staff are adequately prepared for the token economy programme, they may be liable to experience considerable difficulty in adjusting to their new role as a passive observer, i.e. standing aside while the patient attends to his own needs. The nurse is expected to provide encouragement, support and feedback, and also to discuss goals, but not to assist the patient physically with his self-care activities. Ward routine may have to be altered to accommodate the patients whose progress is very slow initially. The nurse must also resist the temptation to ensure the patient exchanges his tokens, and also, if and when he does so, desist from monitoring his purchases.

If token economies are used, it is important for the patient whose original target behaviour has been met, to have the opportunity to graduate to a unit or perhaps to a hostel-type ward where he can use, and improve on, his recently acquired skills with the minimum of supervision from staff.

AVERSION THERAPY

A form of behaviour therapy, first introduced some 50 years ago, in which the process of 'deconditioning' is used. Patients suffering from alcoholism are occasionally treated by aversion therapy. The aim is to destroy the association between drinking and pleasure, by substituting for it a conditioned response of aversion to alcohol.

The patient, on several occasions, is given an emetic, for example apomorphine by injection, with his drink. The feeling of nausea which results from the emetic will gradually become a conditioned response to drinking alcohol, to the smell of alcohol or even the thought of drinking alcohol.

Although this method of establishing a conditioned response of nausea to alcohol may be effective, the results are not lasting unless the connection between vomiting and alcohol is periodically repeated by the use of an emetic. The use of chemical aversion therapy has been largely abandoned.

Another form of aversion therapy is the giving of an electric shock to the patient while he is drinking alcohol. The shock is delivered through electrodes attached to the patient's wrists. The main advantage of this method over chemical aversion is the precise timing achieved by giving the aversive stimulus (the shock) simultaneously with the drinking of alcohol. It has been suggested that the aversion established is to the taste of alcohol.

Aversion therapy has also been used for patients suffering from sexual perversions.

Patients undergoing aversion therapy require the support of a sympathetic and optimistic person. It is often difficult for the patient to feel in any way positive about the treatment. The unpleasantness is so great that there are many occasions when the patient does not feel it worthwhile to continue. His despondency may take on suicidal proportions.

The symptoms which are removed by behaviour therapy may at first sight appear to be isolated, and the patient may otherwise have appeared healthy and well adjusted. When the symptoms disappear the full impact of the patient's underlying disorder may become evident, and more intensive therapy may become necessary. This is particularly the case with patients suffering from alcoholism or from sexual perversion whose whole social life may have been determined by their disorder. When such patients sever their association with fellow sufferers their underlying personality problems may become evident.

Treatment programmes

Considerable professional expertise is required to devise a treatment programme for an individual patient or group of patients. It is often a complex procedure planned by a psychologist or a nurse behaviour therapist. As well as assessing the patient and planning the treatment programme, the nurse-therapist may also act as a clinician in the hospital and in the community. Other roles of the nurse-therapist include that of adviser and teacher to non-specialist colleagues. The nurse behaviour therapist receives a highly specialized training; his/her work represents an important growth area in the field of the extended role of the psychiatric nurse.

Further reading

Barker, P. (1982) *Behaviour Therapy Nursing*. London: Croom Helm.

Greenberg, D. (1981) *Behaviour Therapy*. SK & F Publications. Vol. 4, No. 3.

Joint Working Party of Royal College of Psychiatrists, Royal College of Nursing, British Psychological Society (1980) *Report of Joint Working Party to Formulate Ethical Guidelines for the Conduct of Behaviour Modification*. London: HMSO.

Meichenbaum, D. & Genest, M. (1980) Cognitive behaviour modification. In: *Helping People Change*, ed. F.H. Kanfer and A.P. Goldstein, 2nd edn. Oxford: Pergamon.

Teasdale, J.D. et al. (1984) Cognitive therapy for major depressive disorder in primary care. *British Journal of Psychiatry 144*, 400.

Trower, P., Bryant, B. & Argyle, M. (1978) *Social Skills and Mental Health*. London: Methuen.

Watts, F.N. & Bennett, D., eds. (1983) *Theory and Practice of Psychiatric Rehabilitation*. Chichester: J. Wiley.

Wolpe, J. (1982) *The Practice of Behaviour Therapy*, 3rd edn. Oxford: Pergamon.

23
Nurse–Patient Relationships

It was said earlier that the progress of psychotherapy depends on the relationship which develops between the therapist and the patient.

The relationship between the doctor and the patient in individual psychotherapy is unique, and it is based on the understanding that communications between the patient and his doctor are absolutely confidential. Nurses are therefore often ignorant of what goes on in psychotherapy sessions.

The patient may feel somewhat suspicious of the staff, wondering if the promise of confidentiality is being kept. His conversation with the nurses may be designed to test whether the trust in the doctor is well founded. It is in such a case helpful to the patient to find that nurses do not have access to case notes and only know as much about him as he himself chooses to disclose to them. The patient may also derive comfort from observing the fact that case notes are carefully locked away.

To the nursing staff, communication about the patient is important if they are to act intelligently and as a team. In the case of patients undergoing psychotherapy such communication is, however, best carried out in verbal reporting and in staff meetings rather than by reading case notes which contain confidential information. In the first instance, at any rate, it is easier for the nurse to approach the patient if she is unbiased and uninfluenced by advance information.

In some hospitals it is the practice to keep full psychotherapy notes locked away, but to make available to the staff notes in the form of a summary, so that some degree of planning is possible.

Often the relationship between doctor and patient is not the only significant relationship to occur during the patient's stay in hospital. Other members of staff may develop relationships with the patient, which have therapeutic or anti-therapeutic results. By design or by accident, members of staff other than the patient's doctor may even take on the main therapeutic role.

Their therapeutic role depends on the type of relationship formed with the patient. Nurses sometimes use adjectives like 'good' or 'bad' to qualify the word relationship, when they discuss what happens between the patient and themselves. Such judgements are often invalid, as it is extremely difficult to describe what kind of relationship is good or bad for the patient. It may be good for the patient to have a negative relationship, for example one of hostility towards a nurse, if this enables him to discuss his feelings, not only about the nurse but about other significant people in his life. It may be bad for the patient to have a positive relationship with a nurse, if such a relationship allows him to remain excessively dependent, or if it prevents exploration of aggressive feelings.

The pattern of relationships into which any person enters changes throughout life. Every contact a person makes contributes something towards the formation of relationships and the quality of every human contact depends to some extent on the relationships which already exist. Without contact with people one cannot learn to relate to them. A child who has very little contact with his mother, for example, cannot learn to enter into a relationship with her. Only repeated contact with the mother enables the child to develop trust and love, and only repeated contact with the child enables the mother to develop the concern and tenderness for the child which are characteristic of a mother–child relationship. When a mother–child relationship has been established, its existence affects every contact the mother and child have with each other. The mother's correction is acceptable to the child or the child's temper is acceptable to the mother because of the relationship which already exists between them. The child allows and expects the mother to bath him, tuck him up in bed and kiss him, activities which he would resent from a stranger with whom he has no loving relationship.

Relationships between people are always characterized by their emotional content. Loving, caring for, prizing, being concerned, are the positive emotional characteristics; hating, feeling angry, disappointed or frustrated, the negative emotional characteristics of relationships between people. Loving and hating often occur together; being pleased and disappointed are the opposite sides of the same coin in a relationship. One cannot feel angry with a person about whom one does not care; one cannot hate a person whom one does not also, at other times, love.

In the course of life one establishes relationships with people differing in quality, in intensity and in the extent to which they are reciprocated.

The relationships between mother and child or between father and child or between siblings often develop into the prototypes of the kind of relationships one enters into later in life. Mother–child relationships and father–child relationships are different in quality but may be similar in intensity.

In any relationship between two people, the participants may have similar or dissimilar status, and their roles in relation to each other may be alike or different. The parents' role differs from that of the children. Parents are expected to give care, children to receive care; parents are expected to be protective, children are expected to be dependent. The parents' status is different from that of their children. Status determines the rights and obligations of each participant in a relationship. The parents' status entitles them to give commands and administer punishment. The children's status obliges them to obey and to submit but gives them the right to behave in childish irresponsible ways. As children grow up, role and status change in the parent–child relationship, often accompanied by a considerable amount of conflict.

Sibling relationships and friendships are relationships in which the participants' roles are similar and status is equal.

The way in which people address each other is often an indication of the extent to which reciprocity exists in the relationship. Children address their parents as 'mother', or 'dad', parents call their children by Christian names, or sometimes nicknames. Friends, or brother and sister, call each other by Christian names.

Many patients have experienced, in childhood, difficulties in some of their basic relationships. These difficulties have resulted in disturbed relationships with people in adult life. Marital problems, difficulties in coping with employers, problems in dealing with subordinates are often indications that the patient has failed to come to terms with his own changing role and status in society. Experience of life in hospital should enable the patient to learn how to deal more effectively with the changing relationships into which he enters.

The very fact that a person has decided to become a patient allocates to him a special role and a new status. It becomes the role of a patient to be dependent, trusting, submissive, and rather like a child. A patient has a special status in being the most important person in the hospital, the person whose existence justifies the existence of the whole organization. On the other hand, the patient's status is low. He cannot exercise his right to make decisions and has abdicated from responsibility.

The role and status of a patient are in fact very similar to those of a child. The patient's need for protection causes him to cast members of staff into parental roles. He assigns to the staff superior status, and expects from them behaviour appropriate to that of father or mother.

The parental role is one which the nurse often assumes; often with beneficial results, but accompanied by certain disadvantages. It may be appropriate to examine in detail what is involved when a nurse takes on a mothering role. It entails authority on the part of the nurse and submission on the part of the patient. The nurse takes on certain commitments to the patient. It is a one-sided relationship. The nurse is concerned with the patient's welfare, not her own, with the patient's thoughts, feelings, interests and problems, not with her own. In her mothering role she has to be accepting of the patient, no matter what his behaviour may be. Her acceptance is unconditional. Yet it is also her duty in her mothering role to indicate disapproval and disappointment. As a mother, she gives encouragement and support, always expecting the capacity to improve and to excel, yet knowing and making allowances for shortcomings.

In her mothering role the nurse is not only concerned with the patient while he is in her physical presence. She is concerned with all he does. She knows his friends and their influence on him. She is interested in what he learns and how he spends his leisure. She arranges for him to be looked after by others when she is not available herself, or when she cannot help. When the patient is in need of a dentist, for example, she arranges it, accompanies the patient and afterwards is concerned with comforting him if he is in pain. She is concerned also with his aspirations and plans for the future.

The mothering role can provide considerable satisfaction to

the nurse and to the patient, so much so that the patient may be prevented from outgrowing his dependency. Good mothering makes provision for growing independence, but the authoritarian attitude of some nurses makes it difficult for them to recognize this.

The mothering role of the nurse and the function of a real mother are dissimilar in many ways. In real life the role of the mother is complementary to that of the father. Conflicts between father and mother about the child, and jealousies between children about their parents are normal events in family relationships. Father and mother have an important relationship with each other, which is significant to the children.

In hospital it is almost impossible for such triangular relationships to be reproduced. Often the nurse may have to assume the role of father and mother—of authority and protection simultaneously, making it difficult for her to be as accepting as she might like to be.

When a doctor or another nurse takes on the father role, difficulties may arise in the sharing of parental functions. Relationships between the nurse and the doctor can never be as close as is expected of father and mother.

Relationships between doctor and nurse are seldom close enough to withstand serious disagreement about a patient, and the resulting anxiety tends to spread rapidly from the nursing staff to the patients. Because the patient's anxiety appears to aggravate rather than improve his condition, the beneficial effects of the relationship with the nurse are often obscured.

Relationships often get strained when they are exposed to public scrutiny and criticism. Nurses' relationships with their patients are often scrutinized by others, higher in the nursing hierarchy. Any indication that the patient's behaviour meets with disapproval may make the nurse feel defensive and inadequate in her role performance.

The greatest difficulties in fulfilling a mothering role towards a patient are related to the staffing pattern of the wards and the nurse's responsibility to a number of patients. In real life only one person has the role of mother. Even if mother is asleep, or ill, or away, her place cannot be filled by anyone else; attempts by paid helpers or by grandparents to substitute can never be wholly successful while a real mother exists. In hospital the nurse's mothering role is confined to her hours of duty. When she is on holiday or ill or off duty, someone else automatically steps in. Real mothering only comes to an abrupt end through death. The hospital relationship between the nurse and the patient comes to an end when the nurse decides to leave, or when she is moved to another ward. Even when a patient is very well prepared for the separation, resentment and grief are inevitable if the relationship had any emotional significance for the patient. The more the relationship between the patient and nurse resembled a mother–child relationship, the more damaging sudden termination of the relationship will be.

If a patient whose relationship with his own mother was unsatisfactory is to gain any benefit from experiencing a mothering relationship with a nurse, his new experience should be a corrective one, not one that reinforces his expectation of disappointment and frustration.

Because the hospital organization is such that the patient is almost certain to be disappointed, it would seem that something other than spontaneous mothering activity is required from the nurse.

Nurses and patients sometimes enter into relationships which resemble sibling relationships or friendships more than mother–child relationships. If the nurse can fulfil the role of friend or older brother or sister, the patient may benefit by using her as a model on which to pattern his own behaviour, or by identifying with her and consequently becoming aware of his own positive attributes.

Many patients need friends. Their isolation from people and inability to make and keep friends may be the cause or the result of their illness. The opportunity to find a friend in hospital may be of great therapeutic significance. The relationship between the nurse and the patient cannot, however, develop into real friendship. What characterizes friendship or sibling relationships is mutual trust and mutual exchange of confidence. Friends make demands on each other and take it for granted that their demands will be met. Friends treat each other as equals, share each other's troubles and difficulties. It is not possible for the nurse to burden the patient with her problems or with her personal affairs, and consequently, the relationship becomes one sided. The choice of meeting places and the duration of contacts is often one-sidedly determined to suit the convenience of the nurse not the patient. In conversation between the nurse and the patient the focus is on the need of the patient, not the need of the nurse. The relationship between nurse and patient is often of greater importance to the patient than it is to the nurse. To the patient it may seem a unique relationship—the nurse may be the only or the best friend the patient ever had. But to the nurse the patient is only one of many with whom she relates. Her personal family or friends provide the satisfaction of closer bonds. She does not regard her relationship with the patient as a significant event in her own life and she does not plan that the relationship should continue indefinitely. If the patient regards the relationship with the nurse as a personal, rather than a professional one, he may become disappointed and his previous antisocial attitudes may be reinforced.

There are occasions when the nurse does put herself in the role of friend to the patient, and the actions of a friend come to be expected by the patient. This may occur because of an intuitive affinity between the two people concerned. More often it occurs because the patient's suffering is particularly obvious and his appeals for help particularly urgent. The patient may succeed in making the nurse feel sure that she understands him much better than anyone else, and that only she can be relied on to provide the right approach and the right support. This kind of relationship is rarely beneficial to the patient. It leads to increasing demands, and as the nurse begins to feel resentful of these demands, she tends to withdraw her support. The fact that the patient is not responding causes the nurse to feel guilty and disappointed and eventually angry with the patient.

The nurse who feels that she has some special ability to help the patient, which others lack, tends to be criticized and resented by her colleagues.

The term 'involvement' is sometimes used to describe this relationship in which the nurse's own emotions render her unable to view the patient's problems objectively, and in which the patient's lack of progress becomes a personal challenge to the nurse. Nurses tend to become secretive about such relationships. The patient in the long run tends to be let down and the nurse to become profoundly unhappy.

It is possible to prevent relationships between the nurse and the patient from reaching an untherapeutic level, by ensuring that free discussion takes place among nurses in staff meetings about their feelings for the patients, and their feelings about each other. To expose one's work to the critical evaluation of one's colleagues is not easy, but it is a necessary corrective and support.

To become emotionally involved may not be helpful to the patient, but it cannot be prevented by prohibitions or warnings of danger. The secrecy often surrounding involvement may be the result of expected disapproval. Instead of pretending that involvement does not occur, it is better to acknowledge its existence and co-operate with colleagues in finding a solution to the problem.

A solution may be found by trying to establish a transference relationship rather than one of personal friendship. In a transference relationship the patient uses the nurse in place of his own friends or relations to become the target for love and hate, and the object of admiration and criticism. The termination of such a relationship is carefully planned as a part of the treatment.

A transference relationship is similar to the relationship which the patient forms with a psychotherapist. Such relationships enable the patient to experience close human contact, to enjoy approval and encouragement without the danger of being disappointed. They help the patient to face his feelings and to cope with them.

It is essential that the nurse should be capable of deep feeling for and emotional understanding of the patient, and that she should have insight into her own emotional response to him. One way to achieve such insight would be for each nurse to undergo a personal analysis; but few people would consider this practicable or desirable. Some people advocate instead a systematic review of what goes on between the nurse and a patient, by a process of regular supervision from a trained person. This method is adopted in the training for social case work. Regular group discussion with the members of the ward team in an atmosphere of acceptance and co-operation may be the most effective way of alerting nurses to the significance of their own attitudes and behaviour.

24
Nurse–Patient Interactions

During his stay in hospital the patient establishes contact with many people. His contacts with other patients may be the most helpful and significant ones. These will be discussed in the next chapter. Here the contacts with nurses are discussed.

During the first few days in hospital the patient is among strangers. He naturally feels insecure and diffident. His attitude to the people who are concerned with his treatment is affected by this. Some people show their anxiety, others appear full of self-confidence or even a little brash or aggressive. When the patient settles, his behaviour may be very different from the initial impression he created. It is important to take his first approach seriously, as his attitude on admission may be characteristic of the way in which he behaves towards strangers. His shyness and diffidence or his apparent aggressiveness may be part of his difficulty in meeting people.

The preliminary period of getting to know one another is a very important phase in establishing confidence. No patient is quite free from preconceived ideas. 'Hospital', 'psychiatric hospital', 'nurse', 'psychiatric patient', are all words which conjure up mental pictures for everybody, pictures which often correspond very little to reality and are determined by past experience and by some ideal which is popularly accepted.

The patient's ready-made attitude to nurses may be important in helping him to accept hospitalization. To many people the title 'nurse' and the nurse's uniform stand for all that is good, kind and competent. This stereotype is, of course, quite unrealistic; nurses are people, each nurse is different and no nurse embodies all the good qualities which patients expect in the ideal nurse. Nevertheless, the fact that patients tend to be well disposed to nurses and to trust them may reduce their anxiety on admission.

The presence of nurses may also help to convince the suspicious patient that he really is in hospital and to accept that he is ill. This first, reassuring effect of the nurse's uniform may possibly be the only justification for wearing a uniform at all. The wearing of uniform becomes harmful if it gives the nurse a false sense of security and leads her to adopt an attitude of authority and superiority over the patients, which is incompatible with a therapeutic attitude. Uniform has the effect of giving to all who wear it similar roles and status. When a patient needs a nurse, any one of the people in a nurse's uniform will satisfy his needs, but by the end of the first few days a patient in a psychiatric ward knows each nurse as an individual and has formed an opinion of each.

If nurses do not wear uniform they find it easier to accept the fact that they must establish 'their position' in the ward personally and cannot expect to be treated with respect as of right.

Introductions are important in stressing the nurse's personality rather than her role. The patient is often more interested in her name than in her rank in the nursing hierarchy. Many patients appreciate it if nurses are willing to be called by Christian names.

The process of becoming acquainted is a mutual one. While the nurse tries to find out as much as she can about the patient in order to help him, the patient tries to find out as much as he can about the nurses in order to establish which ones can be trusted. Some patients try to ask questions about personal matters and attempt to interview the nurse about her family, her social life, her views and interests. There is no need to answer such questions. They can be deflected by indicating that the nurse is more interested in talking about the patient than about herself.

The nurse gets to know the patient in conversation and in joint activities. Some nurses find it easier to contact the patient while some activity is in progress. The personal attention which the nurse gives to the patient gives the opportunity for communication. The nurse who admits the patient, who deals with his property and clothing, who shows the patient around the ward and who has met and spoken to the relatives on the first day is often the one in whom the patient feels particularly confident.

Everything the patient does in the hospital should be fully shared by nurses. The patient's work in the occupation department, his activities at social events, his use of leisure in the ward, should be of interest to the nurse both at the time when she is present and participates, and later as topics of conversation. The more common experience the nurse has with the patient, the easier she will find it to talk to him. The fact that the nurse shows interest in the patient's daily life encourages him to believe that she has his interest at heart.

Conversation with the patient rarely touches on personal problems in the early stages. At no time should the nurse ask direct questions or appear to be prying. The aim of talking with the patient is not to find out about his illness, but to get to know him as a person. Anything that interests the patient is a good starting point—clothes, sports, his occupation, the radio or television programme, the contents of the newspaper. Gradually it becomes possible to build up a picture of the way the patient spent his life prior to admission and of the way in which he plans to live when he is discharged. It is possible to plan nursing intelligently only if it is known how, from his point of view, it is desirable to live.

Most patients, if their illness permits, are willing to talk quite freely about the kind of house or flat they live in, the amenities or inconveniences of their place of residence, the neighbours, the shops, the other people in the household. Such conversation can remain completely neutral and yet allow the nurse to become aware of the patient's social standing, his attitude to neighbours of higher or lower social class, his views about the importance of pubs, cinemas and clubs in the neighbourhood, about schools, about the behaviour of children. The patient readily reveals his political outlook when he discusses the shortcomings of his local authority, for example in the matter of refuse collection or the provision of housing.

Without having asked any personal question at all, a conversation which starts with such a topic as the patient's home can give a fairly good understanding of the patient's basic attitudes to a very wide range of experiences. A television programme, for example, can begin a conversation which explores the range and depth of the patient's education, of his interests in art, music, literature or theatre. Discussion of the newspapers not only has the value of keeping the patient informed and up to date but also touches on many opinions.

Politics and religion are topics which cannot really be avoided, though some nurses endeavour to do so. These subjects are so important in most people's lives that any conversation attempting to circumvent them becomes artificial. There is no harm in hearing the patient's views or in stimulating him to further thought. These subjects only become difficult if the nurse's own views are so dogmatic, or if she is so emotional about them, that she cannot listen calmly to the patient. It is also important that the patient should feel completely free from pressure and that he should never come to think that his treatment might be jeopardized by the fact that his political or religious convictions are not those of a particular member of staff.

Most conversations, however apparently neutral the topic, tend to reveal some of the patient's specific difficulties. Although the nurse may not have asked a question, she may soon become aware that the patient's political opinions have a delusional quality or that the topic of the educational system of the country is one about which husband and wife disagree, or that, although the patient's mother lives next door, she never visits. It is much better for information to be pieced together gradually than to press the patient for personal details.

While the nurse gets to know the patient, the patient learns a great deal about the nurse. Every occasion when nurse and patient are together offers as much opportunity to the patient as it does to the nurse. The nurse's tact, the genuineness of her interest, are among the personal characteristics the patient notices. Gestures, facial expression, tone of voice sometimes convey much more than actual words. A patient can usually judge if the nurse enjoys spending time with him or is merely doing so from a sense of duty. Any sign of impatience, of looking at the watch, is easily detected. Patients remember, often more readily than the nurse, what was talked about on the last occasion. If the nurse forgets, it is interpreted as a clear sign that she could not have been very interested, and this may be disappointing or even insulting to the patient. By contrast, to refer back to something the patient mentioned last time or to ask him about his activities on the day the nurse was off duty indicates interest.

A patient not only judges the nurse's behaviour to him personally but also takes into account her behaviour to others. It is comforting to see another seriously disturbed patient competently and kindly dealt with and extremely worrying to see a nurse ignore someone in need of help or deal hastily with another patient. Each patient feels that the treatment meted out to another might easily happen to him and that any nurse who is inconsistent in her behaviour is not to be trusted.

Each patient's personal needs also determine the way in which he sees and uses the staff. A patient may find among the nurses one whose interest and concern he values and whom he hates at the same time for making him dependent on her. Another patient, feeling weak and insecure, develops a growing attachment to a nurse whose forceful personality he needs, while yet another treats the same nurse with hostility, rudeness and scorn, because he sees in her a representative of authority and he treats authority with his usual defiance and resentment. The patient's attitude to any one nurse may change during his stay in hospital, sometimes rapidly, sometimes over a period of time. It is usually interesting and worthwhile trying to find out what has caused changes in relationships, but this is not always possible to establish. Something in the nurse's tone of voice, her facial expression or her manner, may have conveyed to the patient disapproval or criticism, even if none was intended. Some reaction may not have been in keeping with the role which for the time being the nurse has fulfilled towards the patient. The patient may have expected protection and found that the nurse expected him to manage without it. He may have hoped for disapproval, but found the nurse non-committal. He may have expected affection and have felt rejected.

The ease with which nurse and patient establish contact depends to a large extent on the personal characteristics of the people concerned. Patients and nurses of similar social class tend to find it easier to talk to each other than those whose social class background is very dissimilar.

The patient's age plays a part in interactions. Some nurses find older patients or very young patients easier to talk to than patients of their own age group.

It is often assumed that the presence of nurses of the opposite sex to the patients has beneficial effects on the atmosphere of the ward, but some patients may find it easier to converse with nurses of their own sex.

Nurse–patient interactions may change according to the function the nurse fulfils in the ward. The ward sister, as the head of the nursing team, more often represents a mother figure to the patients than does the junior nurse. She may be loved by some patients, hated by others, obeyed or defied according to each patient's previous experience. Her presence in the ward may help to reassure one patient, and cause anxiety to another. One patient may cling to her and seek her attention at all times, another avoid her whenever possible.

The nurse who has newly arrived in the ward may have to wait a few days before patients feel sufficiently comfortable with her to establish any contact. Some patients may, however, welcome the opportunity to offer guidance and, in doing so, gain self-confidence and assert authority. Interaction between nurses and patients depends to some extent on the opportunities for frequent informal contact which arise. The architectural layout of the ward may facilitate such contact or render it difficult. Staffing problems and excessively large numbers of patients in the ward may make it more difficult to find occasions for informal chit-chat.

The more often nurses and patients see each other, the easier it becomes for patients to approach a nurse when the need for communication arises.

Not all interactions between nurses and patients exert an influence on the patient's recovery. Many merely serve to make the patient's stay more interesting, to reduce boredom or to convey to the patient a general sense of concern and interest in his welfare. A few interactions, however, lead to important developments in the patient's treatment. These arise from the nurse's sensitive appreciation of the patient's mood, preoccupation, and thought, gained during casual contact with him. Unless frequent interactions occur, the opportunity for extended contact will be missed.

The patient's diagnosis affects the extent to which he chooses to make contact with nurses, and also the extent to which nurses choose to interact with the patient.

It would seem that depressed patients find it particularly difficult to approach nurses, though they experience the need for contact most. Nurses are often aware of the patient's isolation, yet have inhibitions in approaching him. It is sometimes difficult to feel that one has established contact with a patient suffering from schizophrenia, even though interactions may have taken place. Some patients suffering from neurotic disorders make their need for contact known; others, however, are easily left out and ignored. Patients who have been in hospital for a long time may find their contact with nurses diminishing as the nurses whom they knew leave the ward to be replaced by others who devote their attention to newly admitted patients.

It seems important to offer some contact to all patients so that those whose need for interaction is greatest have the opportunity of having their need recognized. Contact with nurses for as prolonged a period as possible may become a vital factor in the progress of some of these patients. Deliberate and prolonged contact with patients makes great emotional demands on the nurse. She tries to help the patient without necessarily succeeding, or knowing whether her efforts are appreciated. Rejection by the patient is often very hurtful and it would be easy to withdraw, yet what the patient may need is acceptance and perseverance in spite of his rejecting attitude. To withdraw from contact may merely serve to reinforce the unhealthy pattern of interaction to which the patient is accustomed.

Even more difficult to tolerate than overt rejection is the silent apathy or the unemotional withdrawal of some psychotic patients. With such patients, the nurse has to learn the art of being with a patient without doing anything at all. Silence can be very uncomfortable. If one tries to make superficial conversation or fidgets or tries to encourage the patient to do things, he may become more and more tense. Quiet, relaxed, silent companionship may help the patient to realize that contact with people is safe.

It is not always easy to know whether touching is found to be helpful to the patient. When one feels sympathy or concern, when one wants to protect or comfort, one tends to touch people gently, hold hands, stroke the forehead. This may be appreciated, but some patients shrink from touch. It should then only be offered when the patient makes the first move. Some patients, on the other hand, seek closeness with the nurse. They try to cling, embrace, kiss or cuddle the nurse. It may then be the nurse who shrinks from such contacts and makes the patient feel rejected.

In conversation or in play the physical distance between nurse and patient may be important. Sometimes patients come very much closer to the person to whom they are speaking than is usually the case among healthy people. Eye contact cannot be maintained when people get too close to each other; they then have to look past each other. It is possible that some patients find close bodily contact more tolerable than looking into the interlocutor's eyes.

The nurse's touch may convey a negative message. If, for example, the nurse touches the patient while he walks through a door, it may almost seem like pushing. It would always seem advisable to observe how often, in the course of a day, a nurse touches a patient and to try to decide whether more or less touching is indicated. When more bodily contact seems desirable, physical care is often a good way of providing it. Bathing the patient, combing hair, massaging his hands, may be ways of offering bodily contact.

During occupational or recreational periods, occasions may arise when bodily contact can occur. Dancing, for example, or certain gymnastic exercises require that people hold each other's hands or help each other to turn or jump, give each other support to maintain equilibrium. In playing games, proximity to a nurse may be more acceptable to the patient if a table is between them than if they are sitting side by side.

The patient's difficulties in tolerating bodily contact, or in making excessive demands for it may have many reasons. One of these may be the arousal of sexual feelings. Another, especially in the case of patients suffering from schizophrenia, may be the patient's inability to create a satisfactory body image of himself. Educational influences and cultural background play an important part in determining the most comfortable way of making contact with people. The patient does not have to become consciously aware of the significance of what he is doing, but at times it may be helpful if he recognizes consciously any problem he may have in relation to physical closeness.

Most interactions between people involve talk. It is the nurse's function to enable the patient to talk as freely as possible. An interested, listening attitude, is a necessary beginning but it may not be enough. It may also be necessary to develop special techniques of communication. If the patient is to speak freely, the place and the time must be right and the atmosphere conducive to talk. One cannot generalize about these factors. Sometimes sitting comfortably in armchairs is right, but sitting down is not always necessary. Some patients can talk best while walking up and down the ward or the garden. Some patients talk when they are lying down in bed and the nurse sits beside them. Some patients can talk in the bath, others find that the best time to talk is over a meal or a cup of tea. Some patients can only talk freely if they are alone with the nurse, others do not mind talking in the presence of other people or may even need their presence to give them courage. Only very few patients feel able to talk seriously to a nurse as soon as the approach is made. A few patients feel under such pressure that they are constantly in search of a nurse who will listen. Most patients, however, need a period of superficial social chit-chat before they can get to any important point they wish to make. Occasionally the patient can only speak about important matters at the very end of a period of interaction. When preparations for leave taking are obvious, the patient says: 'Oh just one more thing ...' and then proceeds to talk about highly significant matters. Because this is known to happen, it is sometimes thought to be a good idea to tell the patient approximately how long the contact is likely to last. For example, it may be possible to say: 'I have half an hour now in which we can talk, then I shall have to attend to the medicine round' or 'I shall have to leave the ward at 5 p.m., we can go somewhere and talk until then'. It is also easier to sit with a patient in silence if both the nurse and the patient know in advance how much time is available. If a time limit is not set, there is a tendency to keep looking at one's watch and give the impression to the patient that one is longing to escape from contact with him.

Encouraging grunts and nods are often enough to keep the patient talking. Sometimes it is necessary to say a little more, 'Go on', 'Yes and then?', 'Tell me more', or 'I should like to hear more about this'. Acceptance of what the patient says as valuable, interesting and important helps the patient to continue. While the patient is talking he is sure to watch the nurse's face for signs of approval or disapproval. Neither approval nor disapproval helps. As soon as the patient senses moral indignation, disapproval or condemnation, or as soon as he feels that he has hurt or embarrassed the nurse, he is likely to stop talking.

If the nurse approves, there is always the danger that sooner or later she will disapprove. For this reason the patient may be constantly on the alert to detect whether any disapproval might be forthcoming, and may in fact challenge or provoke the nurse to reject him, to disagree or to indicate her disapproval.

Sometimes nurses find quite spontaneously the right words and gestures, the right openings and responses, to make the patient feel at ease. More often though, nurses who merely act on intuition and commonsense may find that their response has reinforced the reaction with which the patient had, previous to admission, met attempts to help him. The nurses' interaction with patients should develop into a purposive activity and the objectives for the patient should be clear.

Sometimes no more is required than to provide an active listener. One can indicate that one is such a listener by making observations about the patient's state of distress, for example: 'I notice you are twisting your handkerchief ... you appear tense ... you seem to have been crying'. 'Would you like to talk about this?' 'Would it help you to tell me?' might be the kind of remarks which encourage a patient to talk more freely.

It sometimes helps to recognize how painful and distressing things must be for the patient. 'I can see that this makes you feel frightened' or 'This has made you feel lonely' may indicate the nurse's empathy with the patient.

For some patients, the objective is to gain insight; for some to develop emotional control. It may help the patient if the nurse assists him to look at a problem more closely, to examine it from more points of view, and to express his thoughts more clearly.

If, for example, the patient talks about the attitude of his family, it may help to ask him to describe it more fully or to say: 'And how does your sister feel about this?' or to explore a specific incident more fully by asking 'and then what did you say? ... what did your sister say?'

To help the patient to gain emotional control it is sometimes useful to state how the situation is perceived by the nurse, e.g. 'You are angry' or 'You seem angry with me', or 'You are angry with me because I did not give in to you' or even 'I have the impression that you are doing this to make me angry'.

It is almost impossible to continue behaving in an uncontrolled manner once the difficulty has been recognized and openly stated.

Talking is not made easier by asking probing questions about the patient's life history or about his emotional difficulties or about his beliefs. Insight is not gained by asking 'Why?' If the patient knew why his behaviour is disturbed, he would not need the nurse's help. He might discover 'why' if the nurse helps him to explore 'when, where, how, how long, what else, who with'.

Patients sometimes ask for advice. Advice is, however, rarely what the patient needs. Very often the patient who asks for advice merely wants someone to confirm that his own decision was the correct one.

It is hardly ever useful to give advice. If it were taken, the patient would place the responsibility for his action on the adviser, whereas the aim is to help the patient to make his own decision and himself to take responsibility for his own action. Advice given without due consideration of all relevant factors is useless, and conflicting advice undermines the patient's confidence in the staff and increases his difficulties. A nurse who gives advice too readily indicates to the patient that she considers herself competent to solve a problem which has proved to be a difficulty to him. This attitude may discourage him from further discussion of his conflicts, which he may feel are not taken seriously enough.

Of course, a straight refusal to give advice may be resented, as is a refusal to answer direct questions. The nurse can avoid giving advice or answering questions by restating the problem, rephrasing it, trying to get the patient to clarify it. A co-operative effort can be made to understand the full implication of any proposed action and to explore the patient's feelings about it. In the last resort the patient must feel free to make his own decisions, even his own mistakes.

Nurses are sometimes tempted to use their knowledge of psychological mechanisms to offer interpretation to the patient of varying depth and complexity. It is doubtful if such interpretation can be of help to the patient. Premature interpretation, even if correct, tends to be rejected and may render communication more difficult. When the patient is ready to accept interpretation, he has probably also gained sufficient insight to make his own interpretations. The patient may, for example, relate how his wife always pushes him around. The nurse may rightly interpret that the patient is trying to say: 'You are pushing me around in the same way as my wife does'. But it would not help to say to the patient: 'What you really mean is that I am pushing you around'. Insight is an experience which cannot be imposed.

During prolonged contact with a patient, interactions arise in which the nurse is uncertain how to respond. Inevitably there are moments when her reply is tactless and she becomes aware of having offended the patient. Inevitably her response occasionally has the effect of cutting the patient off. Moments of guilt are bound to occur and there are periods of helplessness when nothing one says seems to make any difference, and periods of frustration when the patient seems to be getting worse rather than better.

All nurses need the opportunity to discuss with other colleagues the interactions they have with patients. At times the nurse should recapitulate, if possible, verbatim, what the patient said and did, what she said and did in response, and how the patient reacted.

Where several nurses interact with the same patient, some comparison is necessary to learn from each other the different ways of dealing with similar problems and to gain an idea of the extent to which the patient's behaviour is the response to the way he is treated by different members of the staff. Discussion with other nurses is also needed to gain better understanding of the social factors involved in determining how people react to each other. A greater understanding of the complexity of human contact can be gained by a careful study of one's own contribution and experience.

Because prolonged contact with patients, particularly with those who need it most, causes stress to the nurse, supervision, frequent discussion and personal support are necessary for the nurse to retain her own emotional equilibrium, to gain increasing insight into her own problems, and to develop her therapeutic skills in relation to patients.

Further reading

Altschul, A.T. (1972) *Patient–Nurse Interaction*. Edinburgh: Churchill Livingstone.

Bradley, J.C. and Edinberg, M.A. (1982) *Communication in the Nursing Context*. New York: Appleton-Century-Crofts.

Macilwaine, H. (1978) Communication in the nurse–patient relationship. *Nursing Mirror 146* (7), 32.

25
Social Therapy;
The Therapeutic Community

In previous chapters it was shown that psychotherapy is a form of treatment in which the origins of the patient's problems are explored. With the exception of behavioural psychotherapy, it is concerned largely with the past.

Social therapy, by contrast, is concerned with the present. In daily contact with other people in the ward, the patient's problems are displayed. He may, for example, feel intense resentment regarding the way in which his mother has treated him. He talks, in his psychotherapeutic interview, of his mother's lack of understanding, of her aggressive attitude to him, of her preference for his brother. He may, in the ward, talk in a similar way about the ward sister. She too, he says, lacks understanding and sympathy, she too dislikes him and shows preferences for other patients. It becomes clear to the doctor and the sister that he is 'projecting' on to the sister attitudes she does not really have, at least not at the outset of his stay in hospital.

In the ward it soon becomes obvious, however, that the patient's behaviour is so hostile and provocative towards the ward sister that before long her attitude may well be as he describes. He does not at first realize the part that he himself plays in creating unfavourable attitudes in other people. In the ward the other patients and the staff can confront him with the effect his own behaviour has on others. When he begins to see how he himself creates antagonism in others he may begin to reflect that he might have provoked his mother in a similar way. He may gain a deeper understanding of his past problems from an investigation of his current ones, just as an awareness of his past attitudes may help him to understand his present ones.

THE PATIENT AND THE GROUP

The patient's relationship to the group as a whole is also important. He may feel that he 'belongs' and is accepted by others and may derive benefit from his popularity. Whether he emerges as leader or assumes a subordinate role may depend on his previous personality and experiences and may indicate the kind of social setting most congenial to him.

If he remains an outsider and is not accepted by the group, he may require help from others in the group to restore his self-confidence, raise his opinion of himself and at the same time become aware of his own attitudes to group membership.

When difficult situations arise in the ward the patient's attitude to the staff may give an indication of his progress. Jealousies between patients who have the same doctor, or competition for the attention of the charge nurse, may indicate the patient's dependence on the hospital. His growing sense of security may manifest itself in the manner in which he identifies himself with the group of patients. As a member of the ward group he may for the first time find courage to criticize the hospital or those in authority. He may become less frightened of his feeling of rebellion, able to understand his attitude and to revise it. Gradually his growing social awareness may lead to a sense of belonging to the ward as a whole. Co-operation with others may replace dependence or self-assertion. The patient may understand the emotional interaction which takes place between staff, other patients and himself, and he may be able to use his newly won confidence in order to help other patients who are less well.

In social therapy use is made of the fact that everyone—staff and patients—acts as observer and as participant in the interactions that take place. Jointly, they are often in a much better position to understand what the interactions mean, than are the individual participants of such interactions.

Patients may be able to observe that even the apparently private relationship between one nurse and one patient affects the ward community as a whole. Many of the patients' difficulties affect not only attitudes to staff but also attitudes to each other. Hostilities, friendships, close attachments between patients are important to everybody. The way in which some patients make a bid for prominence and leadership, the way in which rivalries and jealousies develop and are dealt with, the way in which one patient is helped by another, or the way in which someone is rebuffed or hurt, are all crucial to the feelings of every single member of the ward community. Social therapy is an attempt to manipulate the environment in order to produce change in the patient's behaviour and to use to the fullest possible extent the contributions of all staff and all patients in a treatment plan.

Patients can only learn to contribute effectively if the general climate of the ward permits them to use their initiative and their judgement, and if they have freedom to express their opinion. They need the opportunity to make decisions and to deal with the problems which arise as a result of their decisions.

Whether a hospital can provide the patient with such an environment depends to a large extent on the nursing staff. Nurses are sometimes found to be so authoritarian in outlook and action that patients are given very little opportunity to exercise their initiative. Nurses tend to decide what is good for patients and tell them how to behave. Nurses who behave in an authoritarian way often do so because they themselves are members of a hospital organization which is authoritarian in outlook. Nurses in the ward tend to be low in the hierarchical arrangement of the hospitals. Orders from above may reach them without explanation or opportunity for discussion. They gain approval from those in senior positions if they carry out orders smoothly. They, in turn, give instructions to patients and expect them to be carried out smoothly.

If patients are to take responsibility, nurses also need to feel free to make decisions and to accept authority.

Free and open communication is only possible for patients if nurses can communicate freely with other members of the staff. Mutual understanding and respect are essential ingredients of successful staff co-operation. These grow gradually and slowly. There are many obstacles to understanding which must be patiently removed. The tradition of some psychiatric hospitals is against free speech from nurses in the presence of doctors. Where formerly the Medical Superintendent reigned supreme, it is hard for doctors to exchange opinions freely, let alone for nurses to offer theirs. Traditionally nursing is arranged in an hierarchical order which may be a hindrance to free expression of opinions.

STAFF MEETINGS

A programme of re-education of all staff members may be necessary to enable them to use social therapy effectively.

Frequent staff meetings have become an essential part of the organization of most psychiatric hospitals. The mere arrangement of staff meetings, however, is not sufficient to ensure that they are of use to all concerned. Sometimes nurses find it difficult to speak at meetings and they keep information to themselves which might have been of great value had it been shared. Junior nurses, particularly, find it very hard to talk in the presence of their seniors, especially if they feel in some way critical of a senior. Again, nurses may find it hard to speak freely before doctors or social workers. Antagonism between any two members of the staff may make it very difficult for them to discuss any topic objectively and unemotionally. In any discussion about patients, personal feelings tend to become obvious to others and it is understandable that the individual should try to protect himself from exposure. Silence may be one way of achieving protection. Apparently free discussion, but of trivial points, is another device.

In any discussion the opinion of an individual may not be well received by the others; there is, moreover, always the danger that such an opinion may seem silly to others. There is no way of finding out except by risking exposure, but exposure may be uncomfortable and therefore there is a tendency to try to avoid it. Staff meetings inevitably have their painful moments. It is part of the professional growth of each nurse to learn to deal with her own emotions, whether they are aroused by colleagues or by patients. Every difficult experience during a staff meeting can help her to gain more understanding of the interaction which takes place among people and of the way in which attitudes can be modified.

WARD MEETINGS

The chief instrument of social therapy is the meeting of patients for the purpose of solving the problems of communal living. Patients must have the chance to solve genuine problems which resemble those of real life which patients are likely to lead after discharge.

The patients' physical environment needs to be under the patients' control. If the ward resembles a luxury hotel or an airport lounge, life within it takes on an unreal quality and feelings of transience and detachment prevail. Patients feel that no decisions need to be taken because the ward cannot possibly have any personal meaning for them. When there is overcrowding in the ward and squalor in the environment, no decisions can be taken by the patients which can make any difference to their quality of living.

Some identification with the hospital and with the ward in particular is necessary. It is useful to observe how the possessive pronoun is used in the wards. If the charge nurse refers to *my* ward, she is likely to be the person who makes decisions about choice of furniture, arrangement of ornaments, spending of money on equipment. Where social therapy is being used the patients need to feel that the ward is 'theirs'. *They* decide about the character of their personal environment, arrange personal property and make responsible decisions about the maintenance, repair and replacement of furnishings and equipment. Patients show visitors around their ward. They explain the ward to new patients. They take pride in the appearance of the ward, or feel embarrassment if visitors call when the ward is untidy.

Meetings of patients can be used to define the extent to which they feel responsible for their environment. If they do not feel responsible, they will interpret any shortcomings as evidence of insufficient concern for their well-being. 'They' are blamed for not providing all that is needed. 'They' won't give us ashtrays, 'they' are slow in carrying out repairs, 'they' don't seem to care! 'They'—the authorities—are never clearly identified. As long as they can be blamed, patients can remain passive, and avoid looking at their own problems. As soon as patients begin to ask 'How can *we* solve this problem?' or 'What can *I* do to help to solve it?' or '*Whose* problem is this? Is it my own?', some useful exercises in decision-making follow.

Patients in their meetings can deal with decisions about the way their life is arranged. They may decide that something needs to be done to make arrangements better known or more comprehensible. They can impose structure by agreeing on time-tables. Arrangements of events can be made known on notice-boards, in bulletins or through the medium of a news-sheet. Patients can control the amount of contact they have with each other by allocating certain rooms for television viewing, others for silent occupations, others for social gatherings. Arrangements of chairs around the fireplace or around small coffee tables will help to establish contact in small groups.

Patients can be responsible for making and enforcing rules necessary for communal living. They learn very easily to cope with their own deviant members, and they benefit from the experience of having authority.

The distribution of the work of the hospital is the business of patients' meetings. Every task that can be organized or performed by patients should be. Nurses and patients work together, but patients decide what is the nurses' share of the work and what their own. Arrangements for bedmaking, sweeping, dusting, washing up, can be left entirely to patients in some wards. Decisions about times for getting up or for going to bed, for the hours of use of record player, radio and television, can be reached without staff intervention. Preparation for evening entertainments, provision of refreshments, invitations to patients in other wards are examples of the kinds of activities which patients can take over. The purpose of patients' activities should always be clear. It should never be a matter of 'helping the staff', but rather of 'patients' responsibilities' with which staff help only when a patient's illness makes this necessary. Responsibility is usually accompanied by difficulties and frustrations and these should be shouldered by the patients themselves.

If the cleanliness of the ward is the patients' responsibility, they must find ways of dealing with those who do not pull their weight, they must suffer the discomfort of living in a ward which has not been cleaned, they must bear the criticism of the hospital authority if the ward is dirty. Each of these frustrations can become the topic for discussion at a ward meeting, sometimes in a general kind of way, for example by examining what is meant by sense of responsibility and how it is acquired, or in a specific way, for example by discussing a particular patient who will not do his share of the work in spite of all the different approaches tried by the other members of the group.

No decision is permanent. The ward community is complex and constantly changing. The patients are continuously provided with new problems to solve.

There are many possible methods of involving patients in discussions. In some instances the entire ward population meets once a week. In other hospitals meetings are held daily and include as many of the patients and staff as are able to be present at the time. In some instances group meetings take place several times each day, but the composition of the group and the purpose of the meetings differ. Group therapy is discussed in Chapter 21.

When meetings are held infrequently, for example once per week, they tend to deal with administrative routine aspects of ward life. Ward chores may be arranged and entertainments or outings organized. Patients may be able to discuss difficulties encountered in community living, for example the fact that the television set is used too noisily or that some patients feel the need for a quiet place for reading. The value of occupational therapy may come under scrutiny. Quite often the quality of the food is raised for discussion and at times hospital rules are questioned. It is possible to conduct meetings of this kind quite informally, without an agenda and without an official chairman, or alternatively patients may wish to arrange a more formal opening of the meeting, by keeping records of business, reading or circulating minutes and preparing an agenda.

There may be value in both kinds of meeting. If the opening phase is left entirely unstructured, there may be some initial silence which may then lead to tension and consequently to some very significant topic being raised. At the same time this may frighten some patients who may find it difficult to make the effort to attend. Some patients may hesitate in these circumstances to speak or bring up their points of view because they feel sure that all other business is more important and because they themselves feel so insecure and insignificant.

A more formally conducted meeting may have the advantage of making a definite place on the agenda for business raised at other times by the more diffident patients. It also gives the opportunity for practising the holding of office and patients can elect their chairman and secretary. A great deal of what needs to be said will, however, never be raised at all at a formally conducted meeting because there never seems to be a right time and place for it.

When meetings are held infrequently content rarely goes beyond factual business. By the time feelings between patients are overtly aroused there is often insufficient time left to discuss these fully and to help each person to understand and cope with them. The meeting closes at a point of high tension and what happens after the meeting becomes the really important factor. The next meeting is too far away to allow feelings to remain unresolved, so immediately after the meeting nurses may try to help the patient who is disturbed, or patients, over their cup of tea or in various corners in the ward, themselves deal with the feelings of which they have become aware. The meeting may have served the purpose of making everyone more aware of a problem; the solution of the problem takes place elsewhere. The following meeting begins without reference to the previous one though the continuity may become obvious by the way everyone studiously avoids raising another emotionally charged topic.

If meetings are infrequent, it is difficult to discuss problems between patients and staff. Although often patients may wish to criticize staff, they may not venture to do so overtly. Consequently criticism of staff may often only be implied. For example, talk about hospital rules may really imply criticism of those who made them; talk of disturbance caused by a patient may include hints that the nurses ought to have prevented it. If patients are to explore freely their feelings about staff, meetings need to be held fairly frequently.

Not only their frequency, but also their size and composition determine how meetings are used. If very large numbers of patients are present, it is impossible for everyone to speak. The silent members are less conspicuous than they would be in a smaller group. New members can join the group unobtrusively and can gradually gain confidence as they listen to a number of people speak.

On the other hand, in a very large meeting it is impossible for everyone to sit face to face. It is easy to remain outside the group and to be overlooked altogether. Patients in a large meeting always outnumber staff. In some ways this can make it clearly a patients' meeting, but it can also lead to a very conspicuous dominance by any member of staff who assumes leadership.

If the number of patients is small, any person who absents himself from the meeting is at once missed, whether he remains away altogether or whether he is physically there but chooses to remain silent. In a small meeting it is possible to become aware of every person in the group. Not only what people say, but also their facial expression, their way of sitting in the chair, their sidelong glances at other people, their fidgeting, smoking or mannerisms become important. There is no way of disguising their attitudes to each other and consequently every person's awareness of tensions in the ward is heightened and every person feels conspicuous in the group. When there are few patients the staff ratio is often relatively high and it becomes necessary for the staff to join in if they do not wish to create the appearance of a split between patients and staff.

In small groups feelings are frequently discussed because they cannot be covered up so easily, even if speech is avoided. How freely patients can express their own feelings, how safely they can involve the staff and how constructively they can use group meetings, depend largely on the level of understanding reached by the staff.

Meetings can be used to make decisions about the way in which patients spend their time. Because the patients themselves make the decisions and because decisions are reached publicly they have a reasonable chance of being carried out. On the other hand, failure to carry out a decision can become a topic of discussion. Many patients have special difficulties in carrying out their own decisions. They benefit from seeing the effect their behaviour has on others and also from realizing that other people have similar difficulties.

THE THERAPEUTIC COMMUNITY

Life in hospital should offer all possible opportunities for the patients' difficulties to become overt. Living in a relatively confined space with a number of other people, all of whom are difficult, is inevitably frustrating and tension producing. Patients who are inconsiderate to others, for example, inevitably demonstrate this early on and soon other patients comment on the effect this has on them. Any attempt to change, to show more consideration for others, is also noticed and the patient learns by direct experience the pleasure of receiving other people's approval. In meetings patients learn to recognize other people's strongly held values. Other people's comments mirror back varied aspects of the patients' own personality.

In hospital the patient needs the opportunity to shoulder responsibility for a job and if being unreliable is one of his problems, he needs a chance to demonstrate how and why it is difficult for him to perform his allotted task. The annoyance of the other patients at being let down is part of the necessary treatment. Knowing that the difficulties are understood and being given repeated opportunities to try again help to make progress.

There are some events in the ward for which patients can assume partial responsibility but where the staff cannot ultimately divest themselves of their share. It is, for example, useful that all patients should be concerned if one member of the group attacks another. Everyone may feel in some way responsible because they did nothing to prevent the outburst. Someone may have been particularly aware of the rising anxiety but failed to draw the nurse's attention to it. Someone may feel that he has contributed to the incident by his own unfriendly attitude to the patient. It is the business of all others to try to understand the aggressive feeling of the patient, while at the same time becoming more aware of similar feelings in themselves. Fear, anger, irritation, guilt, sympathy, are common ground for patients and staff in the ward. The ultimate responsibility for protecting the patients from the effect of violence remains that of the staff, and patients need to know how far they can rely on staff to carry out their duty. Ward meetings are good opportunities to clarify the feelings between patients and staff with regard to such points.

The term 'therapeutic community' has been used to describe a hospital where every aspect of community life is planned to serve a therapeutic aim. Group discussions are an essential part of a therapeutic community but they serve their purpose only if there is worthwhile community life and if the staff have developed attitudes in which they can accept each patient as a full member of a therapeutic team.

Although the patients in a therapeutic community adopt functions and responsibilities which, in different settings, belong to members of the staff, there are certain specific roles which belong to the staff.

The staff are the more permanent members of the community. Patients leave the hospital as they improve. The staff are responsible for the growth of a specific culture within the hospital. The culture of a therapeutic community is one in which equality is highly valued. Relationships change in such a way that people feel increasingly confident of each other. Every effort is made to blur the role distinction not only between different categories of staff but also between staff and patients. The universal use of Christian names may contribute to the realization of role fusion.

This fusion of roles, however desirable, produces certain stress at times. Staff members may find it difficult to discount entirely the specific skills acquired before they started to work in a therapeutic community.

Doctors, social workers, occupational therapists and nurses may rightly feel that their training enables them to make specific contributions to the community. Their different level of remuneration, their membership of different professional organizations may render it difficult for them to operate realistically in an egalitarian setting.

A therapeutic community which has been in existence for a period of time develops norms of behaviour which may not be relevant to the culture outside the hospital. For this reason, however therapeutic the cultural values of the community may be, criticisms from outside are common. Those who belong to a therapeutic community are often accused of being too 'permissive'. New staff members may for a time share the standards of the outside community, and fail to understand the objectives of the therapeutic community. The established staff may find the new staff members too 'judgemental', too 'authoritarian' or too 'custodial'.

The duty of the staff is to interpret the therapeutic community in an unambiguous way to the outside and to mediate between the demands and interpretations of the outside community and the patients.

People who work and live with each other develop an understanding which makes communication easy, even if a great deal is left unsaid. People's tone of voice is understood, their background is known, shared experience is referred to without it being made explicit, and understanding of each other's difficulties is taken for granted. Psychological insight is achieved in co-operative exploration and as a result of cumulative experience.

Conversation between people who know each other well often becomes unintelligible to outsiders. New patients and new members of staff may find the experience of entering such a community profoundly unsettling because they cannot understand the hints, the jargon and the ambiguous statements which established members use in communication. Making the environment explicit to new patients in a friendly unambiguous way is the function of the staff.

Social therapy is a form of treatment which is of value to patients suffering from a wide variety of disorders. Some psychiatrists see this form of treatment of special value in schizophrenia, to counteract the patient's tendency to become isolated. The patient's problems of identity confusion and disorder of ego boundary can be most effectively attacked by social therapy. Some neurotic patients find the experience of value. Co-operation with others, exercise of authority, and practice in assuming responsibility enhance the patient's self-respect. Participation in group activities and discussion with patients and staff help to develop insight and promote emotional growth.

Social therapy is of particular value to patients suffering from personality disorders. Patients suffering from psychopathic disorder do not respond easily to any other form of treatment. Their distrust of authority and their general antisocial attitudes make it difficult for them to accept treatment of any other kind and to persevere with it. In a therapeutic community these patients are submitted to the control of other patients like themselves; they may learn to conform to the rules imposed by members of their own group, when they might reject any standards which staff members might try to promote.

Patients suffering from alcoholism or from drug addiction may also be more able to function in a group of people who, they think, can understand them. They feel that, generally, doctors and nurses and the community as a whole are unsympathetic.

Special units for the treatment of specific personality disorders acquire a separate deviant culture pattern shared eventually by patients and staff. The kind of life which is led in such a community may acquire for the patients a worthwhileness which they may be unwilling to give up. Return to the wider community may be all the more difficult if patients have accepted the hospital culture as desirable and satisfying.

There are certain elements in the use of social therapy which are universally applicable. The environment in which the patient lives can be used to give him the support he needs for security and the freedom he needs for development. The way in which the patient spends his time can provide problems which must be solved.

The patient has experience of belonging to a group; he learns to co-operate with people and finds people who can help him to develop new modes of behaviour. He meets staff members whose behaviour is different from the authoritarian approach he has met before. The staff participate fully in the corporate life of the community, but they represent the normal non-deviant world. They help to form a bridge for the patient to cross when he is ready to leave hospital.

Further reading

Clark, D.H. (1981) *Social Therapy in Psychiatry*, 2nd edn. Edinburgh: Churchill Livingstone.

Kennard, D. (1983) *An Introduction to Therapeutic Communities*. London: Routledge & Kegan Paul.

Towell, D. (1975) *Understanding Psychiatric Nursing*. London: Rcn.

Appendix
Notes on The Mental Health Act 1983 and The Mental Health (Scotland) Act 1984

In the course of the last 100 years, legislation has been in existence to protect people who, by virtue of their mental disorder, are deemed to be vulnerable to abuse from members of the public and from unscrupulous members of staff of the institutions in which they are being cared for.

At the end of the nineteenth century, the Lunacy Acts and the Mental Deficiency Acts were primarily designed to prevent compulsory detention in an 'asylum' of anyone who was not a danger to others or to him/herself as well as suffering from a mental disorder. Apart from the many sections of these Acts which regulated admission to institutions, discharge from and care while in an institution, the Acts made provision for 'The Board of Control', a watchdog body with the duty to exercise protective functions on behalf of the mentally disordered.

The way the Lunacy Acts operated made it difficult, however, for people to obtain care and treatment unless they were in danger or a danger to others. In the 1930s, new legislation, the Mental Treatment Acts, made it possible to admit mentally disordered people, now referred to as 'patients', to institutions, renamed 'hospitals', on a voluntary basis. The protection against abuse which the Acts afforded applied also to voluntary patients.

To become a voluntary patient it was necessary to sign an application and patients had to give notice in writing of their intention to discharge themselves.

It was necessary to ensure that patients really understood what they were doing, and a medical officer had to ascertain that the patient was indeed 'volitional'. Many patients, though perfectly willing to be in hospital, were deemed not to be suitable for voluntary status because they were not regarded as volitional. Demented patients, confused patients, severely depressed patients or schizophrenic patients who were very

317

withdrawn, and severely mentally handicapped people had to be admitted under 'certificate' for this reason.

In the 1950s a Royal Commission recommended changes in legislation and in 1959 in England and Wales, 1960 in Scotland and 1961 in Northern Ireland, new legislation—'The Mental Health Acts'—came into operation. The main principles on which the Acts were based were:

1   That patients suffering from mental disorder should as far as possible be treated, in or outside hospital, on the same basis as patients suffering from any other disorder. They should be able to enter any hospital capable of offering treatment. They should enter hospital or leave hospital with no more formality or restrictions than any other patients.

2   That, outside hospital, provisions should be made for treatment and care comparable to those offered to people suffering from other disorders.

3   That hospitals which offered psychiatric treatment should be free to refuse admission if they felt unable to help the patient or for any other reason, just as other hospitals are.

4   That the provisions made for the fairly small number of patients who must be detained against their will should entail only a minimal amount of legal restriction.

5   In England and Wales, that special provisions for protection were no longer necessary.

In order to achieve these objectives, all previous legislation relating both to Mental Illness and what was formally known as Mental Deficiency was repealed. One Act replaced all former legislation and it covered disorders not formerly dealt with.

The term 'Mental Disorder' was used to cover all disorders dealt with under the Act. The definition in the Act of 'Mental Disorder' was: 'Mental illness, arrested or incomplete development, psychopathic disorder and any other disorder or disability of mind.' In Scotland the term 'Psychopathic Disorder' was not used.

There were four subdivisions of Mental Disorder recognized for the purposes of the compulsory provisions of the Act of 1959:

1   Mental illness
2   Severe subnormality
3   Subnormality
4   Psychopathic disorder

The Scottish Act did not define the categories. The term 'Mental Disorder' meant Mental Illness and Mental Defect. The latter term remained in use.

Admission without compulsion. Patients in all four of these categories could be admitted to any hospital without compulsion or application. It was not necessary that the patient should be capable of expressing a wish to be admitted. As long as he was not actively unwilling to enter hospital his admission could be informal.

Compulsory admission. In England and Wales and in Northern Ireland, for those patients who had to be admitted against their will, only the signatures of two specifically designated doctors were necessary. In Scotland, only emergency admissions were possible on the authority of medical officers. Within seven days an application to the Sheriff had to be made to obtain his authority for further compulsory detention.

In England and Wales and in Northern Ireland, no watchdog organization was appointed. When the Board of Control was dissolved in Scotland, the Mental Welfare Commission was appointed with the general brief of exercising protective functions. It had less power, however, than its predecessor, the Board of Control.

By the end of the 1970s it had become clear that the legislation of the 1960s had provided insufficient safeguards for patients. Following a review, a new Mental Health Act was passed in 1983 and a new Mental Health (Scotland) Act in 1984.

THE MENTAL HEALTH ACT 1983

Application of the Act

The Act concerns 'the reception, care and treatment of mentally disordered patients, the management of their property and other related matters'. The definition of Mental Disorder is a mental illness, arrested or incomplete development of mind, psychopathic disorder or any other disorder or disability of mind. For most purposes of the Act it is not enough for a patient to be suffering from one of the four specific categories of mental disorder set out in the Act:

1 Mental illness

2   Mental impairment
3   Severe mental impairment
4   Psychopathic disorder

It is important to note that no person shall be treated as suffering from mental disorder by reason of promiscuity or other immoral conduct, sexual deviancy, or dependence on alcohol or drugs.

The Scottish Act does not define the categories. The words Mental Subnormality and Mental Deficiency cease to have effect.

Admission without compulsion

Informal admission should be the normal mode of admission to hospital whenever a patient is willing to be admitted and be treated without the use of compulsory powers. It is not necessary that the patient should be capable of expressing a wish to be admitted. As long as he is not actively unwilling to enter hospital the admission can be informal. The majority of patients enter hospital as informal admissions.

Compulsory admission: England and Wales

Some patients suffering from mental disorder may have to be compulsorily admitted to and detained in hospital or received into guardianship. There are a number of different powers under which a patient may be compulsorily detained in hospital:

The emergency admission

An application may be made by an approved social worker or by the nearest relative of the patient in exceptional circumstances. The applicant must state that it is of urgent necessity that the patient should be admitted and detained for assessment, and that compliance with the normal procedures would involve undesirable delay. Only one medical recommendation is required, but the practitioner concerned must have seen the patient within the previous 24 hours. The application is effective for 72 hours.

Admission for assessment

Admission to and detention in hospital for assessment may be authorized where a patient is (a) suffering from mental disorder of a nature of degree which warrants the detention of the patient in hospital for assessment (or for assessment followed by medical treatment) for at least a limited period and (b) he ought to be so detained in the interests of his health or safety, or with a view to the protection of others. Detention is for up to 28 days. An application for admission must be made by either the patient's nearest relative or an approved social worker. An application for admission must be accompanied by written recommendations from two medical practitioners, one of whom must be approved as having special experience in the diagnosis and treatment of mental disorder.

Admission for treatment

The grounds for admission for treatment are first that the patient is suffering from one or more of the four forms of mental disorder as previously described. Secondly, the mental disorder must be of a nature or degree which makes it appropriate for the patient to receive medical treatment in hospital. Thirdly, for a patient suffering from psychopathic disorder or mental impairment there is an additional condition that medical treatment is likely to alleviate or prevent a deterioration in the patient's condition. Treatment need not be expected to cure the patient's disorder: medical treatment should enable the patient to cope more satisfactorily with his disorder or it should stop his condition from becoming worse. Fourthly, it must be necessary for the health or safety of the patient or for the protection of others that he should receive this treatment and it cannot be provided unless he is detained. Application for admission for treatment must be made by either an approved social worker or the patient's nearest relative. The person who is to be regarded as nearest relative is defined in the Act. This must be accompanied by written recommendations from two medical practitioners, one of whom must be approved as having special experience in diagnosis and treatment of mental disorder. Detention for treatment is for a maximum period of six months unless the order is renewed.

Patients already in hospital

A patient may be compulsorily detained for up to 72 hours if the doctor in charge of his treatment reports that an application for admission ought to be made. If the doctor is not obtainable, a first level nurse trained in nursing people suffering from mental illness or mental handicap may detain an informal patient on behalf of the managers for a period of up to six hours while a doctor is found. It must appear to the nurse that (a) the patient is suffering from mental disorder to such a degree that it is necessary for his health or safety, or for the protection of others, for him to be immediately restrained from leaving hospital and (b) it is not practicable to secure the immediate attendance of a doctor for the purpose of furnishing a report. The nurse must record these facts in writing.

Safeguards for patients and staff

Patients who feel they are wrongfully detained may apply to a *Mental Health Review Tribunal* to have their case considered. The tribunal has the power to discharge a patient from hospital. Patients admitted for assessment may apply within the first 14 days of detention. Patients admitted for treatment may apply within the first six months of detention, and again within six months if the detention order is renewed. In addition, a *Mental Health Act Commission* will ensure that hospitals have adopted and are following proper procedures for using the powers of detention. The Commission will also assist in giving staff guidance on good practice, which will be included in a Code of Practice. The Mental Health Act Commission is a new body. It has evolved a structure in which it will operate in independent groups from several regional offices.

Patients' information

The hospital managers must provide certain information to detained patients and their nearest relatives. This is to ensure that the detained patient understands the nature of his detention and his right to apply to a Mental Health Review Tribunal. They must also inform the person with whom the patient had last been living.

Consent to treatment

Compulsory detention does not mean that the patient may be

automatically compelled to accept treatment. There are safe-guards to ensure that either a second opinion or consent to treatment or both are obtained in the case of certain forms of treatment.

Treatment requiring consent and a second opinion
This section of the Act applies to the following forms of treatment where outcome is irreversible.
1 Psychosurgery—any surgical operation for destroying brain tissues or the function of the brain
2 Surgical implantation of hormones. The Mental Health Act Commission must be notified to consider the validity of the patient's consent. They will jointly issue a certificate but, before doing so, the medical member will consult with a nurse and one other professional who have been concerned with the patient's treatment.

Treatment requiring consent or a second opinion
This section of the Act applies to the following forms of treatment.
1 The administration of medicine if three months or more have elapsed since medicine was first administered during that period of detention
2 Electroconvulsive therapy

If the patient does not consent to a treatment, the Mental Health Act Commission must be consulted for a second opinion. In addition the medical member will consult with a nurse and one other professional and the responsible medical officer before giving a second opinion.

Urgent treatment
Special conditions are set out for treating patients in an emergency but they exclude those treatments mentioned above. Such treatments will be necessary to save the patient's life, to prevent serious deterioration of his condition, to alleviate serious suffering by the patient or to prevent the patient from behaving violently or being a danger to himself or to others. In cases where treatment is not immediately necessary or it is proposed to continue treatment after the initial urgent adminis-tration, it will be necessary to contact the Mental Health Act Commission.

Withdrawing consent

If a patient withdraws his consent to any treatment, the treatment must not be given or must cease to be given immediately.

Powers of the Courts and the Home Secretary

In certain circumstances patients may be admitted to and detained in hospital on the order of a Court, or may be transferred to hospital from penal institutions on the direction of the Home Secretary. The courts also have the powers: to remand to hospital for a medical report; to remand to hospital for treatment; and to obtain interim hospital orders.

Patients' property may be protected by the 'Court of Protection'.

APPLICATION OF THE MENTAL HEALTH (SCOTLAND) ACT 1984

Unlike the Mental Health Act Commission in England and Wales, *The Mental Welfare Commission* in Scotland is not new. Under the 1984 Act it has increased duties and increased power. It is concerned with exercising 'protective function in respect of mentally disordered persons who may be incapable of adequately protecting their persons or their interests', whether they are compulsorily detained or not, and wherever they are, whether in hospital or in the community. (The Mental Health Act Commission in England and Wales is concerned only with detained patients.)

In Scotland there is no Mental Health Review Tribunal. Detained patients may appeal for discharge either to the Sheriff or to the Mental Welfare Commission, which has the power to order the discharge of a patient against medical advice.

The Mental Welfare Commission has the duty to bring to the attention of the managers any matter which they consider appropriate to secure the welfare of any patient by:

1 Preventing ill treatment
2 Remedying any deficiency in care or treatment
3 Preventing or redressing loss or damage to his property

Curator bonis

The Mental Welfare Commission has the power to petition for the appointment of a *curator bonis* to administer a patient's property and affairs.

The duties of the Mental Welfare Commission to visit, interview and examine patients who are compulsorily detained and to visit patients on leave of absence, and the power to hold enquiries and require persons to give evidence, are laid down in the Act.

Compulsory detention of patients

Provisions for Emergency Admission are similar to those in England and Wales. The term 'short-term detention' is used for detention up to 28 days and 'long-term detention' for a period of detention beyond that. Short- and long-term detention must be authorized by the Sheriff.

Nurses have the power to detain a patient for only two hours.

The Mental Welfare Commission is informed at specified intervals of the movements in and out of hospital, of renewal of authority to detain a patient and of matters concerning guardianship.

Safeguards concerning consent to treatment are similar to those which apply in England and Wales.

Patients may be detained in hospital on the order of a court, under the Criminal Procedure (Scotland) Act 1975. The Secretary of State is empowered to make an order restricting discharge.

Glossary

We are indebted to the late Editor of the Royal Medico-Psychological Association's Handbook for Psychiatric Nurses *for permission to use extracts from the glossary in the Handbook.*

This glossary is intended to supplement the main text by providing an explanation, as well as a definition, of certain important terms. Some common terms are not included because they are adequately explained in the text.

Acting Out. Attempts by some patients undergoing individual long-term psychotherapy to reduce their emotional discomfort by releasing their feelings in disturbed behaviour. The latter is unconsciously determined and reflects previous unresolved conflicts and attitudes towards important figures during childhood. Such behaviour is consequently often aggressive and antisocial, but it is unsatisfactory to apply the term, as is sometimes done, to all disturbed behaviour shown by patients with neurotic or personality disorders.

The aim of treatment is often to help the patient to talk about his difficulties (to verbalize) instead of acting out.

Affect. Emotion, feeling or mood. Disturbances of affect of various kinds may occur in psychiatric disorders (for example, lability of mood, cyclothymia, flattening, incongruity [inappropriateness] of affect).

Affective Disorders. Psychiatric disorders in which the chief feature is a relatively prolonged affective change of abnormal degree, i.e. depression or mania.

Ambivalence. The existence, at the same time, of contradictory emotional feelings towards an object, commonly of love and hate for another person. Some ambivalence is a normal phenomenon in interpersonal relationships, but when it occurs to a marked degree it may lead to internal conflict and symptoms of psychological disturbance.

Amnesia. A loss or absence of memory which may cover a

variable period of time in the recent or remote past, and may be complete or partial (patchy).

Disturbance of memory is most commonly found in association with intellectual impairment as a symptom of dementia resulting from organic brain disease or degeneration. In such cases memory for recent events is lost first, but the impairment may later extend progressively back into the past and even into childhood. In the so-called dysmnesic (Korsakoff's) syndrome, however, it is the complete inability to remember current events and the fact that the patient may invent stories to fill in the gap (confabulation) that is the most striking feature, and there may be little or no evidence of any other intellectual deficit.

The first stage in the process of remembering is registration of the material to be subsequently recalled, and it is evident that this may be disturbed in states of impaired concentration. This may occur in functional psychotic disorders so that memory may be patchy for events during the acute stage of the illness, e.g. in severe depression. In the same way, a partial amnesia may be left after states of clouded consciousness and there is obviously a complete amnesia covering any period of unconsciousness.

The amnesia following head injury may, however, cover a period that exceeds the duration of unconsciousness. The loss of memory for events prior to the injury is spoken of as retrograde or pre-traumatic amnesia. The anterograde or post-traumatic amnesia extends from time of injury until continuous awareness by the patient. There may be some patchy memories towards the end of this period owing to the stage of clouded consciousness through which the patient passes before full consciousness is regained.

Amnesia may also occur as a hysterical phenomenon, sometimes associated with a fugue state. In such cases it often covers a long period, perhaps of many years, and there may be a discrepancy between the patient's ability to perform learned activities, or the knowledge he displays, and the extent of his amnesia.

Aphasia. The loss of the ability to express meaning by the use of speech or writing, or to understand spoken or written language, the former being described as motor and the latter as sensory aphasia. A lesser degree of impairment is known as dysphasia. Different types of aphasia arise from injury, disease or degeneration of various brain centres.

Aphonia. Loss of voice. May occur as a hysterical conversion symptom.

Ataxia. Loss or impairment of muscular co-ordination, resulting in an inability to perform accurate voluntary movement. In the upper limbs this is manifest as a clumsiness in handling and manipulating objects, and in the lower limbs as an unsteady or staggering gait. Ataxia may arise from injury, disease or degeneration of the brain or spinal cord, from toxic conditions or may be hysterical in origin.

Backward or Reverse Chaining. A behavioural technique used to teach tasks which can be broken down into their component parts. For example, when the patient is being taught or re-taught handwashing, drying the hands is taught first, followed by rinsing soap from the hands, and so on, backwards towards the beginning of the procedure, instead of starting, for example, with the insertion of the plug into the wash basin. The person who is taught by this method has the satisfaction of completing the task on each occasion (the therapist must of course socially reinforce, i.e. praise, the patient every time he manages to complete the task). This satisfaction is used to motivate the patient's learning of the earlier stages of the handwashing procedure.

Compulsion. A term restricted by some psychiatrists to an obsessional act, but used by others for all obsessional symptoms, i.e. compulsive words, phrases, ideas, thoughts, images and fears, as well as impulses. Compulsive actions are recognized by the patient to be morbid and irrational, and he struggles against them. Resistance is, however, usually associated with mounting anxiety which is relieved once the action is performed.

Conditioning. The process, described by Pavlov, by which a new stimulus, known as the 'conditioned' stimulus, comes to produce a response which is normally the result of another stimulus, the 'unconditioned' stimulus. Thus, Pavlov found

that, with a dog, the repeated association of food (the unconditioned stimulus) with the sound of a bell, eventually led to the
response of salivation elicited by the bell alone (the conditioned
stimulus).

In a similar way, the response of fear, which normally occurs
in situations of danger, may become conditioned to various
stimuli which are not in themselves usually fear provoking,
through some association with such a situation. Thus a pilot
may acquire a phobia for flying following an air crash, or a child
may become terrified of all dogs after being attacked by one.

It is uncertain to what extent such conditioning may contribute to the causes of phobic and some other psychiatric
disorders, but techniques for deconditioning (removal of conditioning) are being used with some success in the treatment of
selected cases of phobic anxiety. Conversely, the process of
conditioning an unpleasant response, such as vomiting, to the
hitherto pleasant stimulus of alcohol is used in the 'aversion'
treatment of alcoholism.

Conflict. In general psychiatric usage, the clash between
opposing wishes or desires which may give rise to emotional
tension and anxiety. According to the psychoanalytic theory of
psychological development, conflict in childhood may lead to
repression of one of the wishes together with the associated
painful memories.

Delusion. A false belief which, in the face of contrary evidence,
is held with conviction and is unmodifiable by appeals to reason
or logic that would be acceptable to persons of the same
religious or cultural background.

A delusion signifies a break with reality which justifies its
description as a psychotic symptom, and some psychiatrists
would further hold that any condition in which it is found
should be considered a psychosis. Beyond this, however, the
mere presence of a delusion is not diagnostic of any particular
psychiatric disorder, though some types of delusion may be
characteristic of certain conditions.

Delusions may be classified by (a) mode of origin, (b)
content, and (c) degree of systematization.

(a) By mode of origin, a distinction can be made between
'primary' and 'secondary' delusions. Primary, or autochtho-
nous, delusions appear suddenly, fully developed and without

warning, and are associated with schizophrenia. By contrast, secondary, or interpretative, delusions may occur in most psychotic disorders, and arise as a response of the patient to other symptoms of the illness. Thus, for example, delusions of guilt and unworthiness may arise in the setting of the depressive mood in involutional melancholia, or delusions of persecution in schizophrenia when auditory hallucinations are attributed to a hostile person or organization.

(b) In terms of their content, several types of delusion are recognized. Delusions of grandeur may occur in mania and schizophrenia. As the name implies, these are false beliefs concerning the patient's status and power. Paranoid is the term used to describe all delusions of being affected in some harmful or persecutory way. These may occur not only in schizophrenia and the paranoid states, but also in affective disorders, organic syndromes, and alcoholic and drug psychoses. In depressive illness, however, the patient will commonly accept such persecution as his just due, in keeping with his feeling of guilt and self-reproach. Delusions of reference are common in schizophrenia, but may also occur in affective illness and sometimes as a reaction in abnormally sensitive personalities. The patient believes that people, things and events refer to him in a special way. Thus people, even complete strangers in the street, look at him and he knows they are talking about him, or items on the radio and in the newspaper are really referring to him. Delusions of influence are often secondary to the disturbances of thought, perception and volition, which occur in schizophrenia. The patient complains that his thoughts, feelings and actions are influenced and controlled by some outside agency via radio waves, hypnotism or telepathy. These are also sometimes referred to as passivity feelings. Delusions of self-reproach, guilt and unworthiness are found in depressive illness and are in keeping with the prevailing mood of the patient. He reproaches himself for past failures and misdeeds which are often of a trivial nature. In involutional melancholia such delusions may become quite extravagant so that, for example, disasters and catastrophes in the world are held to be the result of the patient's sins. Hypochondriacal delusions are common in depressions of later life. A frequent complaint is of blockage of the bowels, and other beliefs include the presence of venereal disease and cancer. Somatic delusions may arise from unusual bodily sensations in schizophrenia. They are frequently bizarre, the patient believing, for example, that his appearance has completely changed and that he is turning into a woman. Nihilistic delusions may occur in psychotic depression. The patient believes that he is destroyed in part or totally, so that, for example, his inside has rotted away, or he is already dead and in hell.

(c) The degree of logical relationship between delusions may vary. At one extreme, patients to whom the diagnosis 'paranoia' is sometimes given may gradually develop, step by step, a system of delusions that is constructed in a logical manner and based on a single original false belief. Such delusions are said to be systematized. At the other extreme, delusions in delirium are commonly short lived, changeable and unconnected with each other, i.e. unsystematized. Between these two extremes any degree of connection can occur between co-existent delusions.

Depersonalization. A state in which the individual experiences a change in himself as a loss of his own identity or reality. It is characteristically very difficult to describe directly; the patient may use terms like odd, strange or peculiar, or expressions such as 'like an automaton' and 'as if in a dream' or may speak of feeling 'unreal'. Sometimes included under the term depersonalization is the comparable state of derealization in which it is the outer world that appears changed or unreal, rather than the individual himself. Again, this may be described in various ways, e.g. 'everything seems flat', 'as if the world is on the other side of a pane of glass'. Both states may be found in association, or either may occur alone.

Mild, transient depersonalization is a not uncommon occurrence in normal individuals, usually when fatigued. In a more severe form it can be a feature of most psychiatric disorders, and may simply represent the patient's way of interpreting changes in himself brought about by the illness.

It should be noted that in depersonalization the individual or the world is not described as actually changed, but 'as if' it is. A belief in an actual change may occur at times, but then denotes a delusional development.

Disorientation. Disturbance of the individual's appreciation of his position in time or space, or of his own identity, found in states of impaired consciousness, and revealed in his answers to questions concerning his identity, as to where he thinks he is, or what he believes to be the time, day of the week, or date.

Empathy. In psychiatric usage, the degree to which the observer is able to enter into the thoughts and feelings of the patient and establish good contact.

Endogenous and **Exogenous.** Endogenous—originating from within. Exogenous—originating from outside. May be used in psychiatry to distinguish between those cases of depressive illness which cannot easily be explained as a response to the patient's external circumstances and which are therefore assumed to be due to an innate predisposition to such illness (endogenous), and those which appear to be entirely related to the patient's situation (exogenous or reactive).

Euphoria. A feeling of well-being of pathological degree which may occur in some organic mental syndromes.

Extrapyramidal System. This is a clinical rather than an anatomical term. Broadly, it can be said to comprise all parts of the central nervous system concerned with the regulation of motor function, with the exception—as the name implies—of the pyramidal tracts, i.e. motor tracts connecting the cortex and the spinal cord. Disturbance of the extrapyramidal areas of the brain (such as may be caused by the administration of neuroleptics), especially of the corpus striatum, is manifest in the dyskinesias, e.g. unwanted superfluous movements, or reduced spontaneous motor activity.

Fugue. A state of altered awareness during which an individual suddenly forgets part or the whole of his life, leaves his home and wanders away. He often travels some distance until, just as suddenly, he becomes aware again of his identity. The place where he finds himself may be strange to him, but not infrequently it is somewhere that was of emotional importance at some earlier period in his life. He is likely to have, for a time at least, a complete amnesia for the period of the wandering or fugue itself.

The fugue is commonly a hysterical phenomenon, serving as a means of escape from some unpleasant situation or return to a place which was associated with a happier period in the patient's life which he (unconsciously) wishes to relive. Fugues may also occur occasionally in depressive illness, schizophrenia and epilepsy.

Hallucination. A false sensory perception which arises on its own, in the absence of a corresponding objective stimulus. Any form of sensation may be involved, so that in simple terms a hallucination can mean seeing, hearing, smelling, tasting or feeling something that is not present.

A hallucination should be distinguished from an illusion, another disorder of perception, i.e. mistaking something that is seen or heard for something else.

Hallucinations may be experienced by some normal individuals between the sleeping and waking state, i.e. just before going off to sleep or before fully awakening, and these are termed hypnagogic. In general, however, hallucinations are only found in mental disorder and are regarded as a psychotic symptom. Particular types of hallucination may be characteristic of some psychiatric disorders, or rarely found in others.

Visual hallucinations (i.e. of sight) usually occur in states of altered consciousness and should always suggest the possibility of an organic condition. In delirium and acute confusional states, visual hallucinations are more common than auditory, and characteristically take the form of people, animals or scenes which are well defined, detailed and frequently terrifying. Hallucinations in an epileptic aura are often visual and may be of a simple undifferentiated kind such as balls of fire, or more complex with scenes of elaborate detail. In epileptic twilight states, visual hallucinations are characteristically vivid, with complex scenes that are frequently coloured and moving. Visual hallucinations are rare in schizophrenia but may occur in the acute early stages of the illness. Visual hallucinations do not usually occur in depressive illnesses, but have been reported in acute manic states; the content is in keeping with the patient's prevailing mood of elation. Visual hallucinations very occasionally occur as a hysterical manifestation and the images which appear have a psychological significance to the patient, e.g. a dead parent or a religious figure.

Auditory hallucinations (i.e. of hearing) occur most frequently in schizophrenia but are also found less commonly in certain other psychiatric conditions, particularly in states of impaired consciousness. In delirium they tend to be of a simple undifferentiated kind such as buzzing or ringing, but threatening voices may occur in the subacute delirious states. One of the predominant symptoms in alcoholic hallucinosis is auditory hallucination, which initially is unformed, but gradually becomes differentiated into voices. Auditory hallucinations in an epileptic aura are usually unformed, but epileptic patients suffering from dreamy states or chronic paranoid hallucinatory states commonly hear voices that are accusatory and abusive. Auditory hallucinations may occur in severe depressive disorders and the content is then in keeping with the depressed mood. The patient may hear voices saying that he is an evil person, lives a sinful life and is due for punishment. In schizophrenia, auditory hallucinations are a common but not invariable feature. They may occur early or late in the illness, on only one occasion or repeatedly. The voices may be recognizable or not, distinct or indistinct, abusive or encouraging. They may describe all that the patient does, repeat aloud his thoughts, threaten or give him commands. They may appear to come from outside the body but are often located within the head and sometimes even other parts of the body such as the chest or abdomen.

Olfactory hallucinations (i.e. of smell) may occur in schizophrenia, a patient claiming, for example, that he can smell gas with which enemies are poisoning him. It is also characteristic for the seizures of temporal lobe epilepsy to commence with an olfactory hallucination.

Gustatory hallucinations (i.e. of taste) occur in the same conditions as those of smell. Thus a patient suffering from schizophrenia may complain of a change in the taste of food which indicates to him that he is being poisoned, and gustatory hallucinations may also occur as the aura of temporal lobe epilepsy.

Tactile hallucinations (i.e. of touch) may be found in states of altered consciousness and schizophrenia. They occur very characteristically in cocaine psychosis, which is a subacute delirious state due to prolonged exposure to the drug and probably arises from its effect on peripheral nerves. Patients complain that there are small animals, such as lice, on the skin and may even see them as visual hallucinations. Tactile hallucinations are not uncommon in schizophrenia and may lead to secondary delusional interpretation by the patient, e.g. that rays are being played upon him. They may be localized to the genital region and may then give rise to delusions of sexual interference.

Illusion. A false perception due to distortion of a real sensory perception. An illusion should be distinguished from a hallucination, which is a primary perception in the absence of objective stimulus. For example, if a patient mistakenly interprets a pattern on the wallpaper as grinning faces or eyes watching him, this is an illusion. If, on the other hand, he sees the figure of a man sitting in an empty chair, it is a hallucination.

Illusions may involve any of the senses, are more common at night, and generally occur in states of altered consciousness. It is not always possible, however, to be certain from a patient's account whether an abnormal perceptual experience is an illusion or a hallucination. This is particularly true in schizophrenia and some affective disorders when, for example, patients describe hostile remarks as having been made by people nearby, or see strange things in their room at night.

Insight. A term having more than one meaning in psychiatric usage, but most commonly applied to the recognition by a patient that he is ill. Insight in this sense may be complete, partial or absent, and may change during the course of an illness. Thus a patient who at the beginning of his illness holds delusions may later, with improvement in his condition, develop insight and realize that they were false beliefs arising out of illness. The presence or absence of insight is sometimes used as a criterion for distinguishing between neurotic and psychotic illness respectively, but the difference is seldom clear cut. The term is also used in a broader sense to mean the understanding by an individual of the underlying reasons for his feelings, attitudes and behaviour, the achieving of such insight being one of the aims of long-term individual psychotherapy.

Neologisms. New words coined by the patient. Occurs classically in schizophrenia.

Phobia. An excessive or irrational fear of a particular object or situation. Phobias for a very wide range of objects and situations can occur, but those which are found most commonly are sometimes given specific descriptive names, e.g. fear of enclosed places—claustrophobia, of open spaces—agoraphobia. Phobias may occur on their own or in association with other symptoms as part of an anxiety state. In such phobias, anxiety is aroused only by the particular object or situation.

However, the term phobia is also sometimes applied to fears with a compulsive quality which are found in obsessional disorder, e.g. those of contamination. Here, the fear is present in the mind most or all of the time, and has the characteristic features of an obsession, i.e. a subjective sense of compulsion and of internal resistance to it.

Psychodynamic. The understanding and interpretation of psychiatric symptoms or abnormal behaviour in terms of unconscious mental mechanisms, e.g. anxiety as the result of repressed aggression, or obsessional symptoms as a defence against forbidden wishes.

Psychopathology. Term used in various ways but generally applied to the study of psychiatric symptoms and disorders in terms of the psychological processes involved.

Restitution. This behavioural technique may be used to correct (redress) maladaptive behaviour. For example, a long-stay patient with incontinence may be socially unacceptable to the group. In the application of this method, the nurse encourages the patient, by physical prompting if necessary, to wash himself, mop up the urine from the floor, and launder his soiled underclothes each time incontinence occurs.

Sibling. One of two or more offspring of the same mother and father. Thus the brothers and sisters of an individual are spoken of as his 'siblings' or 'sibs' for short. If one of his parents has had children by a previous marriage, then they are his 'half-sibs' because he shares with them a common parent. If either his father or his mother remarries someone who already has children by a previous marriage, then these, who are not blood relatives, are described as his 'step-sibs', because they are the offspring of his step-parent.

Sympathomimetic. A substance, e.g. a drug, which mimics the adrenergic effect (i.e. of the adrenaline-releasing nerve fibres at the synapse) of the sympathetic nervous system.

Synaptic Cleft. The gap between neurones. Usually a chemical neurotransmitter (e.g. noradrenaline, dopamine) is released from the end of an axon (presynaptic) and diffuses across the cleft to bind with receptors on the cell membrane (postsynaptic) of the receiving neurone.

Syndrome. A group of symptoms and/or signs that are recognized as frequently occurring together and to which it is therefore convenient to give a label for descriptive purposes.

Teratogenic. Liable to produce developmental abnormalities in the fetus.

Index

Abreaction, drug-assisted, 262
Abstem (citrated calcium
    carbimide), 204–5
Acting out, 326
Action on Alcohol Abuse (AAA),
    198
Admission, newly admitted
    patients, 60–63, 144
Adolescent, disturbed, 125–34
    nurse as identification model,
      127, 128
    nursing care, 127–9
    parasuicide, 126
Affect, 28, 326
Affective disorders, 23
Aggression, 171–3, 267; see also
    Violent patients
Agoraphobia, 336
    treatment, 277
Agranulocytosis, 83, 223
Akathisia, 222
AL-ANON, 207
AL-ATEEN, 207
Alcoholics Anonymous, 206
Alcoholism, 197–8, 199, 282, 315
    aversion therapy, 281
    bout drinkers, 199
    drying-out, 205
    hallucinosis, 334
    treatment, 204–7
      family involvement, 207
    withdrawal state (delirium
      tremens), 200–1
Alpha House, 204
Alzheimer's disease, 12
    Society, 50
Ambivalence, 326
Amenorrhoea, 83
Amitriptyline (Tryptizol), 226

Amnesia, 18, 326
Anafranil (clomipramine), 226–7
Anorexia nervosa, 34–5, 101, 132
    behaviour therapy, 133
    mortality, 133
    nursing care, 132–4
    suicide, 133
Anorexic Aid, 134
Anoxia, cerebral, 13
Antabuse (disulfiram), 204–5
Antidepressant drugs, 134,
    226–34
    drug interactions, 234
    long-term administration, 230
    monoamine oxidase inhibitors,
      227–9
      unwanted effects, 228–9
    'second generation', 227
    tricyclic, 226–7
      unwanted effects, 229–30
Antiparkinsonian agents, 221
Anxiety states, 15–17
Aphasia, 327–8
Aphonia, 261, 328
Artane (benzhexol), 221
Assessment, 70, 71, 72, 73, 74, 77
Asthma, 34
Ataxia, 328
Atherosclerosis, cerebral, 13
Attention seeking, 92, 101, 297
Attitudes to psychiatric disorders
    historical, 38–40
    modern, 40–2
Autism, 117
    nursing care, 125
Aversion therapy, 281–2

Backward (reverse) chaining,
    153, 328

Barbiturates, 103
Bathing, 88
Behaviour therapy, 22, 260, 264,
273–83
anorexia nervosa, 133
aversion therapy, 281–2
backward (reverse) chaining,
153, 328
behavioural assessment, 274
exposure, 277
flooding, 277
operant conditioning, 275–81
'response prevention', 277
restitution, 92, 336
self-instructional training, 277
social skills training, 278–9
systematic desensitization, 275,
276–8
thought-stopping, 277
token economy, 279–81
treatment programmes, 93, 282
Benzhexol (Artane), 221
Benzodiazepines, 103, 224–5,
226
unwanted effects, 225
withdrawal fit, 225
Beta-blocking agents, 225
unwanted effects, 225–6
Bipolar illness (manic–depressive
psychosis), 23–5
Bolvidon (mianserin), 227
Bout drinkers, 199
Brain failure, chronic, 12
Brain substance laceration, 13
Bulimia nervosa, 36
Butyrophenones, 220

Camcolit (lithium carbonate), 231
Cannabis, 202
Carbamazepine, unwanted
effects, 195
Care plan writing, 86–6
Catharsis, 261
Cerebral abscess, 13
Cerebral tumour, 13

Cerebrovascular disease,
dementia due to, 13
Children, disturbed, 115–25
diagnostic difficulties, 116–18
family, 118–19
nurse's role, 122–5
treatment, 119–22
Children, mentally retarded, 116
Chlordiazepoxide (Librium), 224
Chlorpromazine (Largactil), 134,
219
Citrated calcium carbimide
(Abstem), 204–5
Class reality orientation, 154
Classical conditioning, 274
Classification of psychiatric
disorders, 10–37
Claustrophobia, 336
Clobazam (Frisium), 225
Clomipramine (Anafranil), 226–7
Clopenthixol decanoate
(Clopixol), 221
Clothes, 89–90
Cloxipol (clopenthixol
decanoate), 221
Cocaine psychosis, 334
Communication, 299, 306, 314
non-verbal, 92, 153, 160, 212
nurse–patient interactions, 293
patient–group, 306
psychotherapy, 259
skills, 213
talking, 294–303
techniques of, 299
Community care, 42–3
Community psychiatric nursing
care, 46–51
acutely disturbed patient, 47–8
family therapy, 48–9
long-term, 49
social, 50–1
Compulsion, 328
Conditioned response (Pavlov),
274, 328
Conditioning, 328–9
Confabulation, 327

Confidentiality, 63, 71, 267
Conflict, 15, 93, 126, 258, 269, 288, 329
Confusional state, acute (toxic), 11
Control, emotional, 301
Conversion hysteria, 17
Conversion reactions, 17
  treatment, 19
Conversion symptoms, 17, 18, 261
Coronary occlusion, 34
Counter-conditioning, 276
Court of Protection, 324
Creutzfeldt–Jakob's disease, 12
Criminal Procedure (Scotland) Act 1975, 325

Dangerous objects, 163–6
Day care facilities, 204
Day hospital, 47, 50
Delirious states, 11
Delirium tremens, 201
Deluded patients, 174–5
Delusions, 23, 26, 28, 30, 99, 329–31
  grandeur, 23, 330
  guilt and unworthiness, 330
  influence, 330
  nihilistic, 331
  paranoid, 330
  poverty, 23
  reference, 330
  sexual interference, 335
  somatic, 330–1
  systematized/unsystematized, 331
Dementia, 12, 14, 150–5
  cerebrovascular disease induced, 13
  multi-infarct, 13
  nursing care, 151–5
  post-trauma, 13
  senile, 12
Depersonalization, 331

Depixol (flupenthixol decanoate), 220
Depression, 22–3, 25–8, 126, 134, 158–70, 212, 267, 297
  atypical, 22
  elderly patient, 155
  endogenous (psychotic, unipolar), 25–8
  exogenous, 22
  food refusal, 98–100
  neurotic, 22
  nursing precautions, 163–6
  physical care, 160–1
  reactive, 22
  suicide, see Suicide
  symptoms, 159–60
Depressive pseudodementia, 155–6
Depressive reactions to stress, 22–3
Diazepam (Valium), 224, 225
  intravenous, 262
Difficult patients, 90–1
  food refusal, 98–102
Disabled Persons (Employment) Act 1944, 113
Disorientation, 331
Displaced anger, 174
Dissociation reactions, 18–19
Disulfiram (Antabuse), 204–5
Disturbed patients, 23, 28, 171–81; see also Violent patients
Drug administration, 216–18
Drug-assisted abreaction, 262
Drug dependence (addiction), 198–206, 315
  clinics, 201
  suicide, 205–6
  treatment and nursing care, 203–7
  withdrawal state, 200
  withdrawal symptoms, 200–1
Drug prescription, 217
Drug therapy, 214–34

Drug tolerance, 199
Drug trials, 214–16
Dyskinesias, 332
Dysmnesic (Korsakoff's)
        syndrome, 327
Dysphasia, 328
Dystonic reaction, acute, 221

Elderly patient, 135–57
    accidents, 138
    acute organic psychiatric
            disorders, 147–50
    alcoholism, 197
    chronic organic psychiatric
            disorders, 150–55
    depression, 155
    entertainment, 142–3
    long-stay, 146–7
    newly admitted, 144–6
    occupations for, 140–1
    physical health, 143–4
    physical requirements, 138–40
    reactions, 136–8
    subacute organic psychiatric
            disorder, 150
Electroconvulsive therapy (ECT),
        235–46
    after-treatment, 244–5
    behaviour after treatment, 245
    bilateral, 237–8
    care during treatment, 243
    electrode placement, 237–8
    indications, 235–6
    number/frequency of
            treatment, 237
    out-patient, 245–6
    physical contraindications, 236
    preparation
        physical, 239
        psychological, 239–41
    pre-treatment care, 241–2
    therapeutic effect, 237
    unilateral, 238
Electroencephalograph(y), 103,
        104, 192–3
Elimination, 90

Emotional
    bias, 79
    contact, 79
    detachment, 79
    difficulties, 302
    involvement, 291
    maturity, 126
    outbursts, 267
Empathy, 28, 71, 72, 131, 174,
        212, 213, 301, 332
Employment Rehabilitation Unit,
        113
Endogenous, 332
Epilepsy
    absence attacks, 183
    diagnostic investigations,
            192–3
        electroencephalography,
                192–3
    major (grand mal), 182
    minor (petit mal), 183
    temporal lobe, 185, 334
Epileptic patients, 182–96
    behavioural disorders, 185–6
    children, 186–7
    confusional state, post-fit,
            183–4
    drug intoxication, 185
    drug risks, 194–5
    emotional states, 184–5
    in hospital, 188
    nursing care, 188–9
    observation of fits, 189–92
    precautions against injury, 194
    prevention of fits, 193–4
    in society, 187–8
Euphoria, 332
Everyday living, basic activities,
        87–93
Excitable patients, 173–4
Exogenous, 332
Extensor plantar response, 192
Extrapyramidal system, 220, 332

Fainting, 34
Family therapy, 48, 271–2

Father–child relationship, 286
Fentazin (perphenazine), 219
Fetal alcohol syndrome, 197
Fluanxol (flupenthixol), 220
Flupenthixol (Fluanxol), 220
Flupenthixol decanoate
    (Depixol), 220
Fluphenazine decanoate
    (Modecate), 219
Food, 94–102
    child and, 95–6
        refusal, 96
    in home, 94–5
    nurse and, 97–8
    patient and, 96
    society and, 94
Fortanan (haloperidol), 220
Friends, patient's need of,
    289–90
Frisium (clobazam), 225
Fugue, 332–3

Glue sniffing, see Solvent abuse
Group, patient and, 304–6
Group homes, 43
Group hostels, 43
Group therapy, 268–71
Group working, 251–2

Hairdressing, 89
Halcion (triazolam), 224
Haldol (haloperidol), 220
Hallucinations, 26, 28, 333–4
    auditory, 23, 28, 30, 334
    gustatory, 334
    olfactory, 334
    visual, 11, 23, 333
    tactile, 334–5
Haloperidol (Haldol, Fortanan),
    220
Haloperidol decanoate, 220
History, psychiatric, 8, 70–1
Huntington's chorea, 12
Hygiene
    oral, 149, 195
    personal, 5, 87–93, 160

Hypertension, 34
Hyperthyroidism, 17, 34
Hypnosis, 261
Hypnotic drugs, 103, 107–8
Hypomania, 25
Hysteria, see Conversion
    reactions

Illusion, 335
Imipramine (Tofranil), 226
Incontinent patients, 91–2, 149,
    153, 336
Inderal (propranolol), 225
Industrial therapy organization
    movement, 43
Industrial training, 112–14
Information obtained
    from other people, 84–5
    by talking to patient, 83–4
Insight, 258, 270, 273, 301, 302,
    314, 335
Insomnia, 103–5
    relaxation techniques, 104
Institutional living, 109–10
Institutional neurosis, 109–10
Institutionalism, 109
Institutionalization, 109
Intellectual impairment, organic,
    12
Involutional depression, 27–8
Involutional melancholia, 26–7,
    330
Involvement, 290
    emotional, 291

Kemadrin (procyclidine), 221
Korsakoff's (dysmnesic)
    syndrome, 327

Largactil (chlorpromazine), 134,
    219
Leisure, see Recreation
Librium (chlordiazepoxide), 224

Lifeline Project, 204
Lithium, 230–4
  drug interactions, 233–4
  intoxication, 233
  patient preparation, 231
  preparations, 231
  serum level monitoring, 231–2
  unwanted effects, 232–3
Long-stay patient, 109–14, 251
  industrial training, 112–14
  money, 111–12
  visitors, 110–11
Ludiomil (maprotilene), 227
Lunacy Act 1890, 39
Lysergic acid diethylamide
        (LSD), 202

Mania, 173–4
  ECT for, 235
  food refusal, 100
  unipolar, 26
Manic–depressive patients
        (bipolar illness), 23–5
Maprotilene (Ludiomil), 227
Maudsley Hospital, 40
Melleril (thioridazine), 222
Menstruation, 90
Mental disorder, legal
        definitions, 318–19
Mental health, WHO definition,
        3
Mental Health Act 1959, 40–1
Mental Health Act 1983, 319–24
  admission without compulsion,
        320
  compulsory admission, 320–2
    admission for assessment,
        321
    admission for treatment, 321
    emergency admission, 320
    patients already in hospital,
        322
    patients' information, 322
    safeguards for patients and
        staff, 322

Mental Health Act (1983) (cont.)
  consent to treatment, 322–4
  urgent treatment, 323
  powers of Courts and Home
        Secretary, 324
Mental Health Act Commission,
        322
Mental Health Review Tribunal,
        41, 322
Mental Health (Scotland) Act
        1960, 41
Mental Health (Scotland) Act
        1984, 41, 324–5
  compulsory detention, 325
  curator bonis, 325
Mental Treatment Act 1930, 40
Mental Welfare Commission, 41,
        324, 325
Merital (nomifensine), 227
Mianserin (Bolvidon, Norval),
        227
Migraine, 34
MIND (National Association for
        Mental Health), 41
Misuse of Drugs Act 1971, 201
Misuse of Drugs Regulations
        1973, 201
Modecate (fluphenazine
        decanoate), 219
Mogadon (nitrazepam), 224, 225
Molipaxin (trazodone), 227
Money, patient's, 111–12
Mother–child relationships, 286
Mothering role of nurse, 287–9
Multidisciplinary team, 71, 74
Multi-infarct dementia, 13

Nardil (phenelzine), 228
National Health Service Nursing
        Home, 146
National Society for Epilepsy,
        187
Neologisms, 30, 335
Neurolepsis, 218

Neuroleptics, *see* Tranquillizers, major
Neuroses, functional, 14–23, 297, 315
  food refusal, 101
Newly admitted patient, 60–3, 144
Night sedation, 107–8
Nightmares, 105
Nitrazepam (Mogadon), 224, 225
Nomifensine (Merital), 227
Normal behaviour patterns, 78
  cultural difficulties, 78
Normality, 3–4
  activities, 6–7
    leisure, 7
    sexual adjustment, 7
    social contacts, 7
    work, 6
  adult, 5
Norval (mianserin), 227
Nurse–patient interactions, 292–303
Nurse–patient relationships, 284–291
Nursing process, 70–86

Observation, 77–83
  bias, 79–80
  constant, 167–9
  objectivity, 79
  observer effect, 71, 79
  opportunities, 81–2
  participant, 79
  physical symptoms, 82–3
  recording/reporting, 80
  selectivity, 79–80
  unusual events, 82
Obsessional patients, 93, 277
Obsessive–compulsive disorders, 19–22
  treatment, 277
Occupational retraining, 252
Occupational therapist, 74, 314
Occupational therapy, 251, 256

Opposite sex, nurse of, 296
Orap (pimozide), 219
Organic psychiatric disorders
  acute, 11
    elderly patients, 147–50
  chronic, 12–14
    elderly patients, *see* Dementia
  subacute, elderly patients, 150
Organic reactions (psychoses, states), 11
  chronic, 12
Oxprenolol hydrochloride (Trasicor), 225

Paranoia, 331
Parasuicide (attempted suicide), 126
Parent–child relationship, 286
Passivity feelings, 30
Patient status, 287
Penfluridol (Semap), 219
Peptic ulcer, 34
Perception, disturbance of, 23, 28
Perphenazine (Fentazin), 219
Personality disorders, 33–4, 78, 315
Phasal (lithium carbonate), 231
Phenelzine (Nardil), 228
Phenobarbitone, unwanted effects, 195
Phenothiazines, 219
  body weight increase, 223
  depot preparations, 219
Phenytoin, unwanted effects, 195
Phobia, 275, 336
Phoenix House, 204
Pick's disease, 12
Pimozide (Orap), 219
Pinel, Philippe, 38
Planning care, 75–7
Poisoning fears, 100
Poisons, care of, 166
Post-epileptic automatism, 182
Priadel (lithium carbonate), 231

Primary nursing, 148 (footnote)
Problem drug taker, 199
Prochlorperazine (Stemetil), 223
Procyclidine (Kemadrine), 221
Property, patients', protection of, 324
Propranolol (Inderal), 225
Pseudodementia (depressive pseudodementia), 155–6
Pseudoparkinsonism, 221–2
Psychiatric hospital
  desirable size, 58
  facilities, 58–9
Psychoanalysis, 260–1
Psychodynamic, 336
Psychologist, 93
  educational, 115
Psychopathic disorder, 315
Psychopathic personality, 33–4
Psychopathology, 78, 336
Psychoses
  acute organic, 11
  functional, 23–32
  symptomatic (exogenous), 11
Psychosomatic disorders, 34
Psychotherapy, 70, 116, 258–72
  behavioural, see Behaviour therapy
  children, 116
  family therapy, 48, 271–2
  group therapy, 268–71
  hypnosis, 261
  individual long-term, 259
    nurse's function, 266–8
  nurse's role, 263–8
  psychoanalysis, 260–1
  purpose, 258–60
  role therapy, 265–6
  supportive, 259–60
    nurse's role, 263–4

Rationalization, 16
Reality orientation, 153–4
Reciprocal inhibition, 276
Recreation and leisure, 252–7
  holidays, 253

Recreation and leisure (cont.)
  social activities, 253–7
Rehabilitation programmes, 110, 111–14
Relationships, 7, 46, 64, 82, 98, 127, 129, 137, 171, 206, 258, 262, 263, 264, 265, 266, 267
  interpersonal, 205, 251
  nurse–patient, 284–91
  patient–child, 286
  personal, 255
  private, 305
  therapeutic, 126, 176
Relaxation techniques for insomnia, 104
Reporting, 80
Respiratory tract mucous membrane congestion, 34
Restitution, 92, 336
Reverse (backward) chaining, 153, 328
Role, nurse's
  expressive, 212
  extended, 282
  instrumental, 212
  therapeutic, 211, 265–6
Routine, 66–9
  flexible/inflexible, 66–7
  patient adherence, 68–9
  patient initiative, 68–9
  patient involvement, 67–8

Schizophrenia, 28–32, 47, 78, 89, 91, 212, 297, 315
  catatonic, 30–1
  causation, 28, 29
  hebephrenic, 29–30
  paranoid, 31
  simple, 29
  Type I/Type II syndromes, 31–2
Self
  assurance, 171
  awareness, 7, 128, 172
  care, 88

Self (*cont.*)
  confidence, 69, 119, 124, 145
  destructive, 128
  esteem, 111, 153, 154, 180, 249
  reproach, 168, 330
  respect, 43, 145, 206, 315
  therapeutic use of, 212
Semap (penfluridol), 219
Senile dementia, 12
Sexual adjustment, 6, 7
  development, 7
  perversion, 281, 282
  problems, 205
  relationships, 7
Shaving, 88
Sheltered atmosphere, 43
  employment, 43, 113
Sibling, 336–7
  relationship, 286
Skill(s)
  communication, 213
  complex, 6
    coping, 213
  interpersonal, 211
  observational, 59
  social, 44, 264, 278, 279
  technical, 212
Sleep, 103–8
  electroencephalogram in,
    103–4
  factors affecting, 105–7
  paradoxical, 107
Social
  activities, 253–7
  awareness, 305
  care, 50
  causes of illness, 41
  class, 72
  climate, 64
  contacts, 7, 64
  factors, 43, 155
  influences, 7
  interaction, 256
  isolation, 155
  maladjustment, 42
  problems, 38

Social (*cont.*)
  skills, 44, 264, 278, 279
  therapy, 304–16
  workers, 314
Sociopath, 33
Solvent abuse (glue sniffing),
    129–31
  nurse's role, 131
Solvent Abuse (Scotland) Act
    1983, 130
Sotacor (sotalol hydrochloride),
    225
Sotalol hydrochloride (Sotacor),
    225
Staff attitudes, 59–60
Staff meetings, 306–7
Stemetil (prochlorperazine), 223
Subdural haematoma, 13
Suicide, 26, 27, 28, 88, 161–9,
    267
  anorexia nervosa, 133
  attempts, 168
  dangerous objects, 163–6
  drug dependence, 205–6
  elderly patient, 155
  observation of patient, 166–9
  poisons, precautions with, 166
  precautions against, 163–9
  by starvation, 99
  see also Parasuicide
Sympathomimetic, 229, 337
Symptomatology of psychiatric
    disorder, 78
Synaptic cleft, 226, 337
Syndrome, 337
Systems approach, 73

Talking
  by patient, 299–302
  to patient, 294–5
  with colleagues, 303
Tardive dyskinesia, 221, 222
Teratogenic, 232, 337
Therapeutic atmosphere, 180
Therapeutic community, 33, 264,
    312–16

Therapeutic environment, 55–65
Therapeutic intervention, 71, 76
Thiamine (vitamin B₁)
    deficiency, 13
Thioridazine (Melleril), 222
Thioxanthenes, 220
Thought
    blocking, 28, 29–30
    broadcasting, 30
    disturbance, 23
    processes, 28
Tofranil (imipramine), 226
Token economy, 92, 279–81
Tranquillizers, 218–26
    major, 218–23
        acute dystonic reaction, 221
        akathisia, 222
        extrapyramidal effects,
            220–2
        haematological effects, 223
        hypotensive effects, 222
        metabolic effects, 222–3
        miscellaneous effects, 223
        pseudoparkinsonism, 221–2
        tardive dyskinesia, 222
    minor, 224–6
        unwanted effects, 225
Transference, 263, 291
Trasicor (oxprenolol
    hydrochloride), 225
Trazodone (Molipaxin), 227
Triazolam (Halcion), 224
Tryptizol (amitriptyline), 226
Tuke, William, 38
Tyramine, 228

Ulcerative colitis, 34
Uniform, nurse's, 292–3
Urticaria, 34

Vaginal discharge, 83
Valium (diazepam), 224, 225
    intravenous, 262
Viloxazine (Vivalan), 227
Violence, outbreaks of, 175–6
Violent patients, 171–81
    isolation, 179
    manual restraint, 179–80
    treatment, 176–7, 178
    weapons used by, 177–8
Visiting, 82
Vitamin B₁ (thiamine) deficiency,
    13
Vitamin B complex, 205
Vitamin C, 205
Vivalan (viloxazine), 227
Voluntary organizations, 204

Ward
    locked, 59–60
    meetings, 307–12
    morale, 63–4
    size, 58–9
    structure/arrangement, 56–7
    therapeutic activities in, 76
Ward sister, 296–7
Withdrawal, 28, 29, 32, 109, 125,
    159
    into fantasy, 117, 118
    state, 200
    symptoms, 200–1
Work, 247–52
    aid to treatment, 249–50
    group, 251–2
    mentally ill patient, 248–9
    society and, 247–8
    time factor, 250–1